The Ethics of Reproductive Technology

The Ethics of
Reproductive Technology

EDITED BY

Kenneth D. Alpern

DePaul University

New York   Oxford
OXFORD UNIVERSITY PRESS
1992

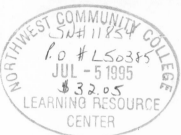

Oxford University Press

Oxford   New York   Toronto
Delhi   Bombay   Calcutta   Madras   Karachi
Kuala Lumpur   Singapore   Hong Kong   Tokyo
Nairobi   Dar es Salaam   Cape Town
Melbourne   Auckland

and associated companies in
Berlin   Ibadan

Copyright © 1992 by Oxford University Press, Inc.

Published by Oxford University Press, Inc.
200 Madison Avenue, New York, NY 10016

Oxford is a registered trademark of Oxford University Press

Library of Congress Cataloging-in-Publication Data
The Ethics of reproductive technology / edited by Kenneth D. Alpern.
p. cm.   Includes bibliographical references.
ISBN 0-19-507435-1
1. Human reproductive technology—Moral and ethical aspects.
I. Alpern, Kenneth D.
RG133.5.E85   1992
176—dc20   92-8252

1 3 5 7 9 8 6 4 2

Printed in the United States of America
on acid-free paper

To my father
and the memory of my mother

Preface

This anthology examines normative and conceptual issues raised by recent technological and social innovations in human reproduction such as in vitro fertilization, embryo transfer, and parenting through contract (surrogate motherhood). The aim of the anthology is to identify and work toward solutions to normative problems of morality, public policy (including law), and personal prudence. The approach of the anthology is decidedly philosophical in that it focuses on fundamental conceptual relations that underlie popular debates about the goods and bads of innovations in human reproduction. Thus, though these debates are represented and specific reproductive techniques are discussed, the anthology is organized around analysis of key concepts and does not attempt to comment on each specific technique and its peculiar problems.

The anthology begins with a general introduction that explains the intent of the anthology and the nature of the problems addressed. Separate introductions to each of the eight parts describe the issues that are the focus of the part and summarize the articles and their relationships to each other. Suggestions for further reading are given in the introductions and in a list at the end of the book. A glossary of medical, scientific, and legal terms is also included.

A brief outline of the anthology is as follows. The first set of articles provides background material necessary for informed examination of the normative issues. These articles describe the biology of natural reproduction, the causes and psychology of infertility, and the procedures involved in the reproduction-aiding techniques.

The analytical portion of the anthology opens with a series of articles debating the ethics of parenting through contract and in vitro fertilization. These articles raise a wide range of normative issues and introduce the most important and widely discussed issues, positions, analyses, and arguments.

The next set of articles begins deeper conceptual analysis, addressing the most fundamental conceptual issues: the desire to have children and the significance of genetic, gestational, and social relations with children. These articles explore such questions as: What sense is there to the idea that a child is a continuation of the parents? What is the importance of relationships of genes and of the process of gestation to the value of having children? More broadly, what precisely is valued and valuable in having children, and to what extent is the desire for children to be understood in the context of desires for such things as loving relationships, community, power, status, and gender realization? How much should such desires be indulged, and how does having children through reproductive technology serve appropriate desires? Only when we attain some clarity on these issues will we be able to address confidently questions of the prudent, moral, and socially responsible use of innovations in reproduction.

Conceptual analysis is carried further by the next set of articles, which examines the significance of carrying out reproduction within commercial and technological frameworks of meaning and value. These readings address such questions as: Does it matter how babies are made, as long as a child is the result? Does it matter whether the child is created or transferred for monetary considerations or that reproductive activities can become marketable services?

The anthology then turns to several general normative issues that arise in connection with innovations in reproduction. One part considers the significance of reproductive technology for women. To what extent does it offer opportunities for greater choice and new freedom, and to what extent does it express and contribute to the oppression of women? Another part considers the proper legal status of reproductive technology. Is use of reproductive technology protected by the Constitution, perhaps as part of a right to privacy or as a right deriving from rights recognized in connection with sterilization, contraception, and abortion? On what grounds and in what ways should the government act to ban, restrict, regulate, facilitate, or support and promote specific practices? The final set of analytical readings asks how health care professionals and institutions should see their roles in the use of reproductive technology. Are they duty bound to provide whatever services are legal? How are practitioners to determine and balance their competing obligations to patients, society, their professions, the institutions in which they practice, and their own moral values? What is the role of professional codes of ethics and hospital policies in guiding and regulating practice?

The anthology closes with a set of articles presenting a number of prominent case studies, including the famous Baby M case and other actual disputes over children and embryos. These cases illustrate the sorts of conflicts that can arise in the use of reproductive technology and offer concrete situations in which to apply and test the insights gained from the readings that precede them.

The anthology is appropriate for lower- and upper-level undergraduate students, as well as for students in graduate and professional programs and for anyone interested in ethical or public policy concerns in philosophy, religion, political science, sociology, medicine, women's and gender studies, the sciences, or technology studies. The articles, often paired in debate, are by prominent practitioners and commentators, including Lori Andrews, Gena Corea, R. G. Edwards, Leon Kass, and John Robertson. Classic writings from Aristotle and Simone de Beauvoir are also brought to bear. These writers represent a wide range of theoretical perspectives—liberal, conservative, and radical—and disciplinary backgrounds, including philosophy, religion, law, medicine, the sciences, and health care administration.

Acknowledgments

I would like to thank Doris Zallen for interesting me in the topic and Bat-Ami Bar on, Patrick Callahan, Anil Gupta, Stephen Houlgate, Mark Levine, Anita Malebranche, Joseph Pitt, and especially Ronald McLaren and Waiva Worthley for helping me to see this project through to its completion. All of these individuals have made helpful suggestions and given me the support of their friendship. More formal support has been provided by a competitive research leave from DePaul University and by Kenyon College during my tenure there as an Affiliated Scholar.

Evanston   K.D.A.
December 1991

Contents

VIII   Case Studies   315

Contributors

Kenneth D. Alpern is Associate Professor of Philosophy, DePaul University.

The American Fertility Society is a professional organization dedicated to studying and promoting reproductive health. The members of the Ethics Committee, 1984–85, were Lori B. Andrews, J.D., Celso-Ramon Garcia, M.D., Clifford Grobstein, Ph.D., Gary D. Hodgen, Ph.D., Howard W. Jones, Jr., M.D., Richard J. McCormick, S.J., Richard Marrs, M.D., C. Alvin Paulsen, M.D., John Robertson, J.D., Edward E. Wallach, M.D., and LeRoy Walters, Ph.D.

Lori B. Andrews is an attorney and project director in medical law at the American Bar Foundation.

Aristotle was a Greek philosopher of the fourth century B.C. A student of Plato's, Aristotle is one of the most important thinkers in Western culture, having written classic works in virtually every branch of philosophy, and in biology and other sciences as well.

Simone de Beauvoir was an existentialist philosopher, literary figure, and leading French feminist.

Gena Corea is a feminist writer specializing in issues of obstetrics and gynecology.

R. G. Edwards is Professor of Human Reproduction, Cambridge University, and Scientific Director, Bourn Hallam Clinics.

Samuel Gorovitz is Professor of Philosophy and Dean of the College of Arts and Sciences, Syracuse University.

Roberto Iraola is a lawyer practicing in Washington, D.C.

Carolyn M. Kaplan has been instructor in chemistry and in biology, Williams College.

Lawrence J. Kaplan is Professor of Chemistry, Williams College.

Leon Kass, M.D., is Addie Clark Harding Professor, The College and Committee on Social Thought, The University of Chicago.

Noel P. Keane is a lawyer and founder of the Infertility Center of New York.

Herbert T. Krimmel is Professor of Law, Southwestern University School of Law, Los Angeles.

Miriam D. Mazor is Clinical Instructor in Psychiatry, Harvard Medical School, Senior Associate in Psychiatry, Beth Israel Hospital, Boston, and a psychiatrist in private practice, Brookline, Massachusetts.

Ann Neale holds a doctorate in philosophy and is Vice-President for Advocacy in Corporate Ethics, Franciscan Health Systems, Aston, Pennsylvania.

Oliver O'Donovan is Regius Professor of Moral and Pastoral Theology in the University of Oxford and Canon of Christ Church.

Margaret Jane Radin is Professor of Law, Stanford Law School.

John A. Robertson is Thomas Watt Gregory Professor of Law, the University of Texas at Austin.

George P. Smith III is Professor of Law, the Catholic University of America.

Rosemarie Tong is Thatcher Professor in Philosophy and Medical Humanities, Davidson College.

The Vatican Congregation on the Doctrine of the Faith oversees the official teachings of the Roman Catholic Church to ensure doctrinal correctness.

Mary Anne Warren is Associate Professor of Philosophy, San Francisco State University.

Leonard J. Weber holds a doctorate in religious studies and is Director of The Ethics Institute, the University of Detroit Mercy.

The Ethics of Reproductive Technology

Introduction

Louise Brown, the first child conceived through in vitro fertilization, was born in July 1978. Since that time, innovations in human reproduction have been the subject of regular media attention and constant public controversy. Louise Brown herself was touted as a "test-tube baby," invoking images of mad scientists conjuring up human beings from chemicals in the laboratory. This was not the case,[1] but the term exemplifies the sorts of misconceptions, hopes, and fantasies that can be created by the intersection of technology, communications media, and basic human values.

A little less than eight years later, Mary Beth Whitehead gave birth to a baby girl in an arrangement for parenting through contract (so-called surrogate motherhood). She had agreed, for the sum of $10,000 beyond her expenses, to be artificially inseminated with the sperm of William Stern, to carry the resulting pregnancy to term, and, upon giving birth, to surrender the child to Mr. Stern and his wife. For more than two years the story, known as the "Baby M" case, was front page news across the country as Mary Beth Whitehead sought to keep the child, first absconding with her out of the state and then fighting the Sterns in a protracted legal battle for custody. During the public controversy that accompanied the Baby M case, conflicting calls were made variously to enforce the contract, to outlaw the practice entirely, to recognize a woman's right to a child she bears regardless of contract, and to ban the payment of money; analogies were drawn with adoption, divorce, artificial insemination, and prostitution; claims were made of the oppression of women, economic exploitation, and the sanctity of contract. At the end of the legal battles, the courts awarded custody to Mr. Stern and regular visitation rights to Mary Beth Whitehead, who remained the child's legal mother.

Other cases continue to be in the news: frozen embryos "orphaned" by the death of their "parents"; refusals to accept a child born in a parenting through contract arrangement; and battles for control of sperm, eggs, embryos, and children. Beyond the fascination and frenzy stirred up by media exploitation of these events are serious questions about what is good for us as individuals, in our relations with others, and in our social institutions. How should we go about developing, using, and controlling the technologies?

The problems of recognizing and balancing competing interests and rights are great enough. But at a deeper level, we are puzzled about how even to conceptualize the problems. Our difficulty in finding appropriate terms in which to discuss the issues indicates that our normal ways of thinking about such matters, the very categories we use in our thinking—parenthood, procreation, being the child of, property, person, etc.—are being challenged. Technological achievements and novel social arrangements have created possibilities of which we have never even conceived, let alone determined the value.

The aim of this anthology is to work toward the resolution of these problems, first by identifying issues, surveying positions, and setting out arguments and then by digging more deeply into the foundations of the concepts and values appealed to in these first approaches. The anthology does not seek to comment on each specific reproduction-aiding technique and service (RT) and the problems peculiar to it.[2] Rather, my hope is that by seeking clearer understanding of fundamental concepts and their relations, we will be better able to see our way through the intricacies of whatever techniques are developed in this rapidly changing field. In this introduction, I characterize the *kinds* of issues to be addressed. Later in the anthology, at the beginning of each part, further introductory material briefly summarizes and draws connections between the various readings.

Types of Normative Issues

At their heart, the RTs change the activities and processes by which children come into existence, and they intimately involve individuals beyond the traditional mother and father in those activities and processes (e.g., donors of eggs, sperm, or embryos; technicians who collect eggs, facilitate fertilization, sort embryos, and reintroduce them into a woman's body; lawyers who stipulate medical procedures and legal arrangements). As a result of these changes, the RTs potentially affect the relationships of the people involved in reproduction and the nature and significance of the activities and processes of reproduction themselves. Even more deeply, the RTs may change the very frameworks through which we understand things and form our values and so may ultimately change our conception of ourselves. At issue in controversies over the RTs are exactly what changes the RTs do or might bring about, whether these changes are good or bad, and what should be done about them. Thus, the RTs raise normative issues—issues concerning values and better and worse actions. More precisely, three sorts of normative issues can be distinguished: those of prudence, of morality, and of policy.

Prudence

Concerns of prudence, as philosophers use the term, are concerns about whether a certain course of action serves the interests (happiness, well-being, good) of the party undertaking the action. For example, in connection with the RTs, concerns of prudence include, among other things, weighing the potential benefits and harms that face a woman who chooses to bear a child in an arrangement for parenting through contract, or considering whether in vitro fertilization (IVF) is a wise choice for a person if it involves spending thousands of dollars and enduring repeated hormone treatments and operations with at best a 15–20% chance of success.

Answers to such questions may be up to the individuals involved in that persons have their own values and should be free to make their own decisions and judge their own satisfactions. But we also recognize that what may appear to be best for us, or what we feel like doing, may not be in our best interest. We can be misinformed, impulsive, self-deceived, or simply mistaken. For these reasons, when faced with difficult decisions, we are wise to seek the advice of others and to recognize that their insights may be valid for us.

Morality

Morality concerns, roughly, whether persons show proper regard for the interests of all parties affected by their actions and for any relevant rights, principles, or values.[3] The nature and content of these moral considerations are much debated issues in ethical theory, but a few comments can be made here to guide practical consideration of the moral issues in reproductive technology.

Whereas prudence concerns the interests only of the person who is performing the act, morality involves according proper place to the interests of other people as well. Exactly what the morally proper balance is between one's own and others' interests is a controversial question in moral theory, but neither complete self-sacrifice nor exclusive self-regard is generally demanded or found acceptable.

Moral rights are variously conceived, but in the two leading modern traditions of moral philosophy—utilitarianism and Kantian deontology—moral rights have been held to be, respectively, either (1) particularly vital interests which, if not secured, would be catastrophic for a person's well-being or (2) demands made by basic respect for persons as such. Moral rights (so too moral principles and, in some instances, moral values) are usually held to outweigh concerns of mere interest; for example, a right to privacy, as some claim for procreative activities, would normally be held to override concerns about how nonvital elements of persons' well-being might be affected by recognizing that right.

Moral principles and moral values may ultimately be based on and reducible to moral rights, but it is useful to distinguish them since they usually take a different form. Moral principles state or imply a rule of action, such as "the sanctity of contract" or, more broadly, "keeping one's promises." Principles determine fairly specifically what one should do. Moral values, such as "the family" or "the unity of body and spirit in procreation," indicate something that should be given weight in moral deliberations and preserved in action, though they may leave wider latitude as to how that is to be accomplished. Appeals to moral rights, principles, and values are constantly being made in the debates over the RTs, but it is essential to keep in mind that these appeals are subject to critical examination: it may be questioned whether the right, principle, or value applies as claimed; whether in fact it applies to the case in question; or even whether such a right, principle, or value exists at all.[4] The resolution of such issues must ultimately take one beyond "applied" ethics to philosophical ethical theory.[5]

Policy

A third sort of normative issue concerns the responsibilities and policies of social institutions. Falling under this heading are questions about whether a certain practice should be made illegal and whether the government has legitimate power to do so. More broadly, questions of policy extend beyond government action to include practices of other social institutions, such as hospitals and the professional organizations of health care providers and lawyers.[6] And even within government action, it is important to note that the functions of government and the legal system include not only allowing or outlawing practices, but also regulating, protecting, facilitating, and supporting practices and adjudicating disputes occurring within them. Thus, for example, among possible government policies toward parenting through contract are not only banning it outright by criminal sanction, but regulating the practice by license or through state-run agencies (as in the case of adoption); a hands-off policy except when called in to adjudicate disputes, (as with business contracts); actively promoting it (as in the case of organ donorship); or banning only parts of the practice (e.g., banning third-party brokering or payments, as is the policy in Britain).[7]

A Note on Religion

The normative significance of religion is not entirely agreed upon. Some people feel that religion is the foundation of morality, providing its content and ultimate justification. Philosophers from Plato to the present, some of them devoutly religious, have rejected this view. But even so, religion can be involved in normative decisions at least as a personal commitment, and so can provide insight, guidance, and meaning to those who have such commitments. Just how far respect for religious commitments can be demanded of others, however, is another controversial issue of ethical and political theory that is beyond the scope of this introduction. In any case, it should be borne in mind that a religious commitment does not automatically have a claim in policy, or indeed in the moral deliberations of nonbelievers.

Conceptual Issues

In addressing the normative issues of prudence, morality, and policy, we are called upon to identify and adjudicate among various interests, rights, principles, and values. This is rarely an easy task, even when we have clear conceptions of the persons, relations, and processes involved. But with the RTs we often do not have such clear conceptions. The concepts and frameworks of understanding upon which we commonly depend were developed without a view to the possibilities raised by the RTs. As a result, the inferences we are accustomed to make (e.g., between something's being of a certain kind and its having a certain moral status) become problematic.[8] For example, we normally accord to parents certain rights and responsibilities regarding their children; we generally think that procreative activities are intimate and that their privacy should be protected. But we are less assured about these inferences when the RTs throw into question who counts as a parent (the sperm donor or the husband of the woman who born the child? the woman who carried and gave birth to the child or the woman who bears a genetic relation to it?) or what sorts of things procreative acts are (what sorts of technological intervention destroy the intimacy between a man and a woman; should this matter?). The possibilities raised by the RTs often just do not fit perfectly, or perhaps at all, into our traditional categories. Still, we generally would like to find some way to accommodate these previously unrecognized possibilities within our established categories and ways of thinking. For our frameworks of understanding—the ways in which we find meaning and significance in things and arrive at our feelings, desires, and judgments—have been formed in terms of these categories. Thus, some of the most difficult problems raised by the RTs concern how to extend, modify, or replace our concepts and categories so that we may find a place for the RTs in our frameworks of understanding. Of course, the possibility also exists that we may have to abandon our traditional ways of thinking. In any event, the following paragraphs survey a number of ways in which the RTs challenge these ways of thinking and point out several alternatives for trying to meet the challenges.

1. The RTs present us with cases in which the criteria for the application of our traditional concepts are satisfied imperfectly, as when they are satisfied incompletely, only analogically, or with significant discrepancies. In such cases, we must decide whether or not to extend our traditional concepts to include the new possibilities. For example, in artificial insemination with donor sperm (AID), a married woman may have a child by a man who is not her husband. By this criterion, should we deem the woman's actions adulterous and the child illegitimate? Who should be considered the child's father? There is no definite procedure by which to decide, though presumably we should try to analyze more closely exactly what it is about our traditional notions of adultery and legitimacy that matters to us and try to judge just how significant are the divergences of the new case. What has in fact happened, at least in the law, is that a husband who consents to his wife's use of AID is deemed to be the legal father of any resulting children, and the children are deemed his legitimate offspring. In no case is AID held to constitute adultery. With these concepts in place, parental rights and responsibilities before the law follow according to the normal implications of the concepts of paternity, legitimacy, and adultery. Decisions of this sort are more complex and difficult outside formal systems such as the law, where concepts and their implications are not defined by authorities acknowledged as serving that function.

Expressions such as "surrogate mother" or "donor" (of sperm, eggs, or embryos) illustrate how apparently convenient terminology may affect the meaning and implications of traditional concepts without our realizing it. The term "surrogate mother" is by now notorious. The label insinuates that the woman who bears and is genetically related to the child has less claim to the status of mother (with its traditional rights and interests) than does the woman who takes custody of the child. And even though the term "donor" is widely accepted, at least in the case of sperm donors in AID, we should recognize that this usage does involve an extension of our concept of donorship, and we should be aware of the implications before according that status to providing sperm.

2. In what may be a special case of the first sort of conceptual challenge, the RTs appear to split apart concepts that we have traditionally treated as unified. For example, motherhood has historically been a fairly unproblematic notion: a mother is a woman who bears and raises a child. With greater scientific sophistication, we have incorporated the further idea that mothers share genes with their children.[9] The RTs, however, make it possible that different women stand in the genetic, gestational, and social relations comprised by our traditional, unified concept of motherhood. Given this possibility, we have to decide how to regard the three now separate relations and how the interests, rights, and responsibilities of the single woman who satisfied all the criteria of motherhood should be reallotted among the several women who now satisfy only one.[10] Our lack of confidence about how to proceed in this case is signaled, I think, by our retaining the term "mother" in labeling each separate element of the traditional concept: "genetic mother," "gestational mother," and "social mother."

This same sort of splitting occurs with other concepts important to reproduction—indeed, with the process of procreation itself. For we find that elements of the unified, continuous bodily processes of procreation can be carried out in different ways and by different individuals.

3. We may try to preserve our traditional concepts in the face of these conceptual problems, but at a certain point the application of a traditional concept to a new possibility may become too attenuated, unilluminating, or confused, especially when several conflicting analogues may be claimed, as is the case with parenting through contract mentioned above. In such cases, we might abandon our traditional concepts and categories and seek to develop a new way to conceive of the problematic case within our larger world view. Indeed, we might opt for this alternative from the start if a possibility is sufficiently unusual and distinctive, such as using human clones or synthesizing humans entirely from chemicals in the laboratory. Creating new concepts and categories is a familiar practice in formal systems, such as the law or organized sports, where the meanings and relations of new concepts can be largely stipulated, such as "corporation" or "designated hitter." The manner in which new concepts can be created in less formalized spheres of activity may not be as clear, but it would seem that many of the new concepts in formalized activities developed from concepts in less formalized social relations. (Thus more formalized concepts such as custody, guardianship, and adoption developed out of concepts of possession, control, and power.) In any

case, inventing a new concept, whether by explicit definition or through evolving social practice, is another possible conceptual move in coming to terms with the RTs.[11]

4. Conceptual problems may also arise when one sort of framework of meaning and significance is extended into the domain of another, as when economic, technological, or legal frameworks encroach on the domain of personal relationships.[12] For example, it is charged that in parenting through contract, babies and reproductive relations are priced, bought, sold, and in general subjected to forces of supply and demand, and that these practices degrade persons to commodities (objects of commerce) and intimate personal relationships to forms of economic exchanges. Similarly, it is claimed that when reproduction is conceived in terms of technological concerns of control, design, power, and manufacture, the consequence is that embryos are reduced to materials, private personal intimacies are transformed into rational public ventures, and in general procreation is degraded to production and persons to things. Such conceptual shifts change not only the terms of evaluation of reproduction, but also the nature of the entities (persons), relations, and activities involved.

To make such charges is not to substantiate them. Indeed, it could be argued in rebuttal that the interpenetration of frameworks is not necessarily objectionable.[13] In order to make the case, the idea of frameworks of meaning and significance must be more fully spelled out and the character of their illicit extensions explained. Whatever its resolution, though, this sort of conceptual issue is at the heart of many of the normative disputes occasioned by the RTs.

5. Finally, and most radically, it may be proposed that our traditional ways of thinking are just not adequate for the new possibilities. What we require is not the extension or piecemeal supplementation of traditional concepts, but a revolution in our world view, what has been called a "paradigm shift."[14] In such revolutions, basic categories, methods, modes of explanation—all conceptual relations—are completely transformed or, even more radically, abandoned and replaced. The most familiar examples of conceptual revolutions come from the physical sciences—for instance, the Copernican, Newtonian, and Einsteinian revolutions. Closer to our concerns, the works of Darwin and Freud are widely held to have radically transformed our conceptions of human beings and their relations.

The nature and conditions of conceptual revolutions are much debated, but one of the conditions for radical transformation in our ways of thinking is continuing failure to resolve problems through the basic categories we have been using. Perhaps the RTs are creating such a condition. To the extent that it is revolutionary, the result of a radical reworking of our ways of understanding personal relations and reproductive activities cannot be described until it is actually carried out. Such a monumental task has not been done specifically with respect to reproductive activities.[15] Still, it may turn out that nothing short of a conceptual revolution is necessary to resolve the difficulties raised by the RTs.

The possibilities surveyed here—extension, splitting, and replacement of concepts, framework encroachment, and revolution in world view—do not exhaust the conceptual challenges raised by the RTs. But these characteristic examples serve to illustrate how normative questions may rest on more fundamental issues concerning the proper way to conceive of the entities, relations, and processes in terms of which those questions are formulated.

The Articles

The articles in this anthology are organized into eight parts. Part I provides factual background information about the nature of natural and of aided human reproduction and about the psychology of infertility. Part II introduces a wide range of normative issues raised by the RTs and presents representative positions, arguments, and analyses. The next five parts examine more closely specific normative issues and several of the fundamental conceptual issues underlying normative disputes. Part III examines the various meanings and values that can be accorded to the initial desire to have children and to the various activities and events involved in natural reproduction. Part IV addresses the significance of carrying out reproduction in the context of commercial and technological frameworks of meaning and value. Parts V, VI, and VII consider specific normative issues: respectively, the significance of the reproductive technologies for women, the proper constitutional and legal status of the RTs, and the problems for the health care professions in accommodating professional responsibility and personal values. Part VIII comprises a number of case studies. Each part is preceded by a more detailed description of the content and relationships of the articles, which also contains suggestions for further reading.

This anthology attempts to work toward solutions to the normative problems of prudence, morality, and policy arising out of the RTs, and in particular to identify and better understand the conceptual structures underlying these normative problems. The case studies are an appropriate way to conclude. They remind us of the human beings whose happiness and well-being are at issue in the theoretical debates. The theoretical debates must be informed by recognition that human feeling and human lives are at stake in these philosophical and legal arguments. But it is equally important to recognize that without this deeper theoretical understanding, human happiness and human values cannot be securely and successfully served.

Notes

1. In vitro fertilization does not replace all the processes of natural reproduction. Rather, it involves collecting eggs and sperm, combining them in a glass dish, growing any resulting fertilized eggs to the two- to eight-cell stage, and introducing them into a woman's uterus. A more detailed description is given in the article by Lawrence Kaplan and Carolyn Kaplan included in this anthology.

2. The RTs include a wide range of procedures and social arrangements. Some involve sophisticated technology: in vitro fertilization, embryo transfer, cryopreservation, or gamete intrafallopian transfer. Some are quite simple and are not particularly new: artificial insemination has been widely practiced for over 40 years and can be accomplished at home. Some variants of parenting through contract are just social arrangements, involving no technology at all; indeed, something quite like parenting through contract appears in the Bible (Genesis 16:1–6). Some worries about the RTs concern the use of more general medical techniques in carrying them out, such as amniocentesis, laparoscopy, lavage, and embryonic biopsy.

3. The idea of moral responsibilities can be accommodated within this formulation as particular patterns of the demands made by interests, rights, principles, and values.

4. For example, would the existence of something called a "right to privacy" mean that procreation through the RTs must be allowed? Does the mere fact that there is such a thing as a right to property determine whether clinics or couples or one rather than another member of a couple should have control over frozen embryos? Should the principle of the sanctity of contract apply even when it stipulates conditions in which a woman in a contract for parenting must have an abortion? Should any special moral value be accorded to sex being engaged in only in marriage and only when open to having children?

5. For a brief overview of moral theories, see James Rachels, *The Elements of Moral Philosophy* (New York: Random House, 1986), or Tom L. Beauchamp, *Philosophical Ethics: An Introduction to Moral Philosophy* (New York: McGraw-Hill, 1982).

6. The obligations and responsibilities of professional organizations and roles are complex matters, especially as professions are often accorded special status by government. See Alan H. Goldman, *The Moral Foundations of Professional Ethics* (Totowa, NJ: Rowman and Littlefield, 1980).

7. On the variety of functions of government, see Robert S. Summers, "The Technique Element in Law," *California Law Journal* 59 (1971), pp. 733–746.

8. I do not mean to imply that conceptual problems of the meaning and nature of concepts and categories are independent of questions of values.

9. My account, of course, is simplified, and I am speaking as if we have had a single, shared understanding of motherhood and its implications. These simplifications, however, should not affect the points I am trying to make.

10. As should be clear, this sort of problem does not originate with the RTs. Social circumstances have long created splits between genetic and gestational roles, on the one hand, and the role of rearing children, on the other. The split created by the RTs here is just more sensational and unanticipated.

11. An example of this sort of strategy in connection with the RTs is Leon Kass's approach to the status of embryos. Kass, in the article in this anthology, seems to be trying to craft a new category for human embryos distinct from both the categories of person and of thing. The possibility of the need for new categories is also raised in the final case study in the anthology in which one question is whether destroyed embryos and frozen embryos should be considered under property law or under custody law.

12. Terms commonly used in making charges of improper extension include "objectification," "commodification," "commercialization," and "turning people into things."

13. For example, Elisabeth M. Landes and Richard Posner, in "The Economics of the Baby Shortage" [*Journal of Legal Studies* 7 (1978), pp. 323–348], appear to be

advocating a market in babies to relieve the perceived shortage of adoptable babies; Alison M. Jaggar and William L. McBride, in " 'Reproduction' as Male Ideology" [*Hypatia*, WSIF 3 (1985), pp. 185–196], argue that reproduction *should* be seen as a form of production.

14. The term "paradigm shift" has been made popular by Thomas Kuhn's classic, *The Structure of Scientific Revolutions* (Chicago: University of Chicago Press, 1962).

15. Though a number of feminist writers are working in this direction. See, for example, Mary Daly, *Gyn/ecology* (Boston: Beacon Press, 1978), and Carol Gilligan, *In a Different Voice* (Cambridge, MA: Harvard University Press, 1982).

I

BIOLOGICAL, TECHNOLOGICAL, AND PSYCHOLOGICAL BACKGROUND

The articles in this section provide background information necessary for informed examination of the normative issues raised by reproductive technology. In the first article, Lawrence Kaplan and Carolyn Kaplan describe the biology of natural reproduction, the causes of infertility, and the most significant RTs and services. In the second article, psychiatrist Miriam Mazor relates the psychological experiences common to individuals and couples who encounter problems with fertility in their attempts to have children.

Natural Reproduction and Reproduction-Aiding Technologies

Lawrence J. Kaplan and Carolyn M. Kaplan

[M]any people think that we should control scientific progress and prohibit its application to new human problems. But if we do that, we are choosing to have all the misery and suffering that we could prevent by further scientific progress. *We have no choice but to make choices. We had better understand and be ready for them.*[1]

The development and availability of various reproduction-aiding technologies requires careful evaluation from many perspectives. While it would be unreasonable to expect every lawyer, philosopher, and individual faced with the hard decisions raised by these technologies to become an expert in reproductive biology, they should have a basic understanding of the principles and fundamental science upon which these technologies are based. With this understanding they can better appreciate the technical, social, legal, ethical, and moral issues raised by these technologies, as well as the advantages and risks associated with the techniques. In order to help accomplish these goals, this essay presents a brief overview of the basic scientific and technological facts of natural reproduction and the reproduction-aiding technologies.

Sexual Reproduction

We begin our discussion with the biology and physiology of natural reproduction, that is, the conception of a child by a man and a woman through unaided and unsupplemented sexual intercourse and the subsequent biological processes.

Humans reproduce sexually, that is, through the union of two cells (gametes): the egg (ovum; plural, ova)[2] from the female and the sperm from the male. These gametes carry the genetic code of the male and the female. In reproduction the egg and sperm combine to form a single cell from which a new individual develops. The genetic makeup of this new cell is a combination of the genes from the egg and the sperm.

15

The Male Reproductive System

The functions of the male reproductive system[3] are to produce, store, and deliver sperm into the female's reproductive tract. The small sperm cell, about 0.06 mm in length, looks and moves like a tadpole, with a head and a long, wriggling tail. The head carries the vital genetic information in the nucleus of the cell, while the tail serves to propel the sperm in the reproductive tract of the female.

The primary structures of the male reproductive system are as follows:

Testes: two glandular organs in the scrotal sac that produce sperm and the
male hormone testosterone
Penis: the external sex organ, with the urethral canal traversing its length
Tubes: the epididymis, vas deferens, and ejaculatory ducts that conduct
sperm from the testes to the penis
Glands: several glands along the ejaculatory duct contributing secretions
that constitute seminal fluid

Sperm is continuously produced in the mature male, and is stored in the epididymis and the first portion of the vas deferens. The stored sperm cells are haploid; that is, they contain only 23 chromosomes, half the original genetic information of the male. When a haploid sperm cell is combined with a haploid egg cell from the female, a diploid embryo results, each cell of which contains 46 chromosomes in 23 pairs. For the discussion of sex preselection below, it is important to note that the male sperm cell determines the sex of any offspring: whereas the sex chromosomes of females are always X chromosomes (female-determining), the sex chromosomes of males may be either X or Y chromosomes (male-determining). The sex of a child, then, is determined by whether the sperm that fertilizes the egg from which it develops happens to carry an X chromosome or a Y chromosome.

The production of sperm is controlled by a complex and delicate system of hormones: testosterone, follicle-stimulating hormone (FSH), and luteinizing hormone (LH). These hormones maintain a relatively constant number of sperm through negative feedback. When there is a dearth of sperm cells in the testes, hormones send a signal that increases production. Once sperm are replenished, production is shut down. Sperm cells take about 60–72 days to mature and are best produced at a temperature of around 95°F, slightly below normal body temperature—hence the location of the testes outside the body mass in the scrotal sac. Unejaculated sperm are reabsorbed into the body.

At ejaculation, muscular contractions propel sperm through the ejaculatory ducts, where fluids from the various glands are secreted to form semen. The seminal vesicles secrete a viscous alkaline fluid containing fructose (which supplies energy) and prostaglandins (which increase sperm motility and induce uterine contractions that help propel the sperm). The prostate gland contributes a milky fluid that protects the sperm from the acidic environment of the vagina, and a mucus-like lubricating substance is also added. The resulting semen (sperm and seminal fluids) is expelled through the urethra of the penis and into the woman's vagina. From there, the sperm move toward the egg, located higher in the female's reproductive tract, by whipping their tails and through involuntary muscular contractions of the uterus and fallopian tubes. During this period, the essential process of capacitation takes place, in which the sperm become capable of penetrating and fertilizing the egg. Only about 100 to 1000 sperm of the 50 to 250 million in a normal ejaculate reach the egg, taking about 15 minutes. Normally, only one sperm is able to unite with the egg and complete the process of fertilization.

The Female Reproductive System

The primary structures of the female reproductive system are as follows:[4]

> *Ovaries:* two walnut-sized organs located on either side of the lower abdomen in which eggs (ova) develop
> *Fallopian tubes or oviducts:* thin tubes leading from each of the ovaries to the uterus, through which eggs travel and in which they are fertilized
> *Uterus:* the womb, where the fertilized egg implants and develops in pregnancy
> *Cervix:* passage from the uterus to the vagina
> *Vagina:* a canal extending from the cervix to the outside of the body

The primary processes in the female reproductive system are as follows:

- Production of mature eggs
- Transportation of eggs from the ovaries to the uterus, during which time fertilization may occur
- Preparation of the uterus to receive the fertilized egg
- Development of the embryo[5] in the uterus
- Parturition (giving birth)

The female reproductive system involves two distinct but intertwined systems under strict hormonal control. One system is the ovarian system, which is responsible for the production of eggs. The other is the uterine system, which prepares the lining of the uterus for implantation of a fertilized egg. These systems are regulated and synchronized by cyclical increases and decreases in the concentration of several hormones: estrogen, progesterone, gonadotropin-releasing hormone (GnRH), FSH, and LH.

Ovarian System

The ovaries contain cells (primordial sex cells) that, during a woman's reproductive life, mature into eggs. A woman's full complement of primordial sex cells (eggs in an incompletely developed form) is present from before birth, numbers about 7 million at the fifth month of fetal development, and declines to about 400,000 at birth. About 400–500 will mature during her active reproductive life.

In order to be capable of union with sperm, primordial sex cells must undergo further cell division and maturation. This ovarian process, along with the process of uterine development, takes place in a cycle of about 28 days throughout a woman's reproductive life (roughly from the early teens to the mid-forties).

Usually one egg will mature during each cycle, though more than one may develop, creating the possibility of fraternal twins, triplets, and so on. The cycle begins when FSH and LH secreted by the pituitary gland stimulate one or more primordial sex cells to resume development and the follicle surrounding the cells to enlarge. At about the middle of the 28-day cycle, ovulation takes place: FSH secretion decreases, the LH level rapidly rises (in what is often called the "LH surge"), and the enlarged follicle ruptures, releasing the maturing egg into the fallopian tube. Once in the fallopian tube, the egg is propelled down the tube toward the uterus.

Uterine System

After rupturing, the follicle in the ovary is transformed into a new structure called a corpus luteum. The corpus luteum secretes large amounts of estrogen and progesterone, which act on the wall of the uterus to prepare it for implantation and nourishment of the embryo. If fertilization does not occur, the enriched lining of the uterus will disintegrate and pass out of the body, along with the remains of the unfertilized egg, at menstruation.

Fertilization

Normally fertilization, if it is to occur, takes place in a fallopian tube and generally occurs within 10–15 hours of ovulation. In fertilization, a sperm penetrates the egg's jelly-like coat, the coat changes to prevent additional sperm from entering, and the egg undergoes one further cell division, allowing for the last stage of fertilization, the union of genetic materials of the egg and sperm. The result, if all goes well, is a single cell containing in its nucleus the full human complement of 23 pairs of chromosomes, half contributed by the sperm and half by the egg.

Implantation and Pregnancy

The fertilized egg is at first called a zygote. During the four or five days it takes to reach the uterus, the zygote undergoes several cell divisions. When it reaches the uterus, the mass of about 16 cells rearranges itself into a hollow ball of cells called a blastocyst. The cells in the blastocyst continue to divide until the outer layer of cells makes contact with the uterine lining and attaches to it in the process called implantation. Some of the cells of the blastocyst develop into the placenta and fetal membrane, and some develop into the fetus itself.

Following implantation, additional connections are made between the mother and the embryo to ensure that sufficient nutrients are available for development. As the embryo grows, membranous structures known as chorionic villi project into the uterine wall and provide firm attachment. The region of attachment is known as the placenta—the primary nutritive, respiratory, and excretory system for the embryo. A second membrane, the amnion, surrounds the embryo and provides the local environment in which the embryo grows. This extensive tissue system provides for the maintenance of the embryo during its continued division, differentiation, and development throughout pregnancy.

A number of important stages or events in the development of the embryo should be noted:

- At the two- and four-cell stage each cell is totipotential; that is, separated cells retain the potential to form separate embryos, which could result in the birth of identical twins.
- By about day 14 or 15 a heap of cells, called the "primitive streak," develops in the embryo. Two primitive streaks may develop; this is the last point at which identical twins can occur.
- Brain activity: primitive brain waves have been claimed to occur as early as the 40th day, though it is not clear how these electrical impulses relate to what we know as consciousness.[6]
- Viability: the point at which the fetus can survive outside the womb. This point depends on the state of neonatal technology and presently occurs at around 24 weeks.
- Parturition: birth, usually around 40 weeks after conception.

Fertility and Sterility

As we have seen, reproduction relies upon a number of anatomical and hormonal systems. So it is not surprising that reproduction is not always successful. It has been estimated, for example, that even when sperm do reach the egg in natural reproduction, for every 100 eggs only 84 are fertilized, 69 implant, 42 survive the first week of pregnancy, and 31 survive to birth. For many individuals even this proportion does not hold. The figure of 15% is widely cited as the incidence of infertility among couples in the United States of childbearing age under the standard definition of infertility as the inability to produce offspring after one year of regular sexual relations.[7] Infertility also has been generally held to be on the rise. Both the 15% figure and the rising incidence of infertility have been disputed, but even on lower estimates 2.4 million couples were infertile in 1982, and a total of $1 billion was spent in 1987 by couples seeking professional help for infertility.[8]

Many of the conditions and living patterns of modern society have been cited as causing infertility. Environmental pollutants and day-to-day stress are commonly thought to be partially at fault. The relatively new pattern of short and varied sexual encounters, resulting disease, the unforeseen side effects of extensive use of birth control methods, and greater awareness in certain sectors of the population have probably contributed to the increasing number of infertile individuals seeking help. Perhaps most significant, couples today are choosing to start families later in life, even though the incidence of infertility increases with age, dramatically so for women after the age of 30.

Physiologically, two leading causes of fertility disorder are hormonal malfunctions and anatomical abnormalities, congenital or acquired, such as occluded fallopian tubes or an enlarged blood vessel in a testis. In about 10% of couples who seek treatment, no physical or metabolic cause can be found. Psychological factors are now less credenced as a cause of infertility. In about 5% of all cases, infertility is cured spontaneously (i.e., without treatment).

Current therapy for infertility generally approaches it as a problem for the couple, rather than as the fault of the man or woman. In order to discuss in more detail the conditions that may lead to infertility, however, it is necessary to return to the reproductive functions of each partner.

Male Infertility

For natural fertilization to occur, the ejaculate must be potent and present in the female genital tract so that the sperm and egg can join. Each typical ejaculate contains from 50 to 250 million sperm in a semen volume of 1.0 to 3.5 ml. Generally speaking, if the sperm count is consistently below 20 million sperm per milliliter, fertility is likely to be impaired. Not just sperm count and concentration are important for fertility; so too are the volume and quality of the seminal fluid and the morphology (size, shape, structure) and motility of the sperm. Low semen volume, for example, may impair the ability of sperm to be carried to the woman's cervix or may inadequately protect sperm against the acidity of the vagina. An unusually high volume of semen may result in an insufficient concentration of sperm.

Even if both the volume of seminal fluid and the sperm count are normal, the morphology or motility of sperm may be impaired. In order to reach the egg, sperm must be able to propel themselves by rapidly whipping their tails back and forth. If more than half the sperm in an ejaculate are slow or have trouble moving in a straight line, fertility may be impaired. Although all men produce some abnormally formed sperm (e.g., sperm with deformed heads or curled or kinked tails), if the rate of deformity is consistently above 40%, infertility is likely. Sperm production may also be impaired by hormonal problems and by malfunction of the testes, due to disease, physical injury, or genetic defect, or by excessive heat.

Although any of these problems can lead to infertility, many can be readily diagnosed and treated. Since optimal sperm production occurs below normal body temperature, the remedy may be as simple as switching from brief-style underwear to boxer shorts. Occasionally, minor surgery may be successful in opening various blocked ducts and tracts. Finally, hormonal therapy may be used to induce higher levels of sperm production. Yet, though many techniques exist to enhance or restore fertility, some problems cannot be overcome using traditional methods. These formerly insoluble problems may be resolved by one of the technologies reviewed below.[9]

Female Infertility

Female fertility problems can arise at any of the steps in the reproductive process: interaction of sperm and cervical mucus, ovulation, tubal transport, implantation of the embryo, or pregnancy maintenance. Hormonal as well as anatomical problems may lead to dysfunction in any or all of these processes.

When sperm are introduced into the woman's genital tract, they must first pass through the cervix and its mucus. Throughout most of the menstrual cycle the mucus is thick, designed to protect the uterus from infection. During ovulation, rising estrogen levels cause the mucus to become thin and stretchy. At this time, the cervical mucus actually protects sperm from the woman's white blood cells and from the extreme acidity of the reproductive tract itself. The mucus also provides nutrients for sperm and filters out abnormal sperm. If the mucus fails to thin, sperm will have difficulty passing through the cervix and reaching the egg.

As discussed above, ovulation is controlled by hormones. Inadequate levels of any one of the five hormones involved in ovulation can prevent it from occurring. Absence of ovulation due to radical change of diet, extreme dieting, intensive exercise, or stress may be treated by altering these practices. Hormonal supplements, at an average cost of $6,000 to $12,000, are a remedy for about half the women who fail to ovulate.

The most serious cause of absence of ovulation is premature ovarian failure. This condition may be the result of damaged ovaries. In some cases, however, the egg supply is exhausted early in the woman's reproductive life. Premature ovarian failure cannot be treated medically at this time.

Tubal transport problems are among the leading causes of infertility in women. Since the fallopian tubes connect the ovaries to the uterus, if they are blocked, the egg cannot be fertilized or pass to the uterus. Normally, the walls of the tubes contract rhythmically in order to create a constant flow that propels the egg down toward the uterus. If the walls are damaged or blocked by scars or adhesions, they may fail to contract or to move the egg effectively. The walls may be damaged by infection (such as by sexually transmitted diseases or rupture of the appendix), irritation, or pelvic inflammatory disease (which may result from use of an intrauterine device or prior medical treatment). In some cases, blocked tubes may be opened surgically using a laparoscope and a laser or surgical knife, though surgery also increases the chances of ectopic pregnancy (a pregnancy developing in a fallopian tube instead of in the uterus).

Normally, when the blastocyst reaches the uterus, the endometrium (uterine lining) is thick and lush, ready to accept the clump of cells. The necessary build-up of the uterine wall depends upon progesterone secreted by the corpus luteum. If production of progesterone is delayed or is insufficient in amount, the uterine wall will not be ready and implantation cannot occur, a condition called "luteal phase defect." Treatment for this condition involves a regimen of hormone therapy, with about a 50-50 chance of success.

Repeated miscarriages (spontaneous abortions) are a particularly distressing type of infertility because, while conception and implantation occur, the body rejects the developing embryo. The problem may be due to environmental factors that are relatively easy to adjust, such as smoking, excessive alcohol consumption, and exposure to certain chemicals. But the most common cause of spontaneous abortion (40–60%) is the body's rejection of embryos with chromosomal defects. This is a natural safeguard that prevents the development of defective embryos. At present, a physician cannot treat random chromosomal defects. If the problem is recurring, it is likely that one parent is contributing irregular genetic information. Anatomical abnormalities of the uterus may also cause spontaneous abortion. In these cases, the only present option for a couple desiring a child genetically related to at least one of them is the donation of sperm or eggs using one of the reproduction-aiding technologies described below.[10]

Reproduction-Aiding Technologies

We have seen that reproduction is an intricate and delicate series of interactions between the woman, the man, her eggs, his sperm, and the fertilized egg and the woman's body. Still, the process does work for the large majority of people. But we have also seen that for millions of couples, natural reproduction does not work and often therapies fail to result in the desired child. In an effort to aid those couples with severe problems, alternatives to natural reproduction have been developed. The reproduction-aiding techniques discussed below fall into two categories: those in which the roles of genetic, gestational, and social parents remain as they are in natural reproduction; and those in which the provider of sperm, egg, or gestational functions is other than one of the social parents. In the first category, we will discuss in vitro fertilization and artificial insemination using the husband's sperm. In the second category, we will include in vitro fertilization coupled with egg donation, artificial insemination using donor sperm, embryo transfer, and surrogate motherhood. These techniques, used in various combinations, form the basis of reproductive technology.[11]

Home Diagnostic Techniques

Before entering into a discussion of high-tech approaches to conception, we will consider several of the less complicated and less expensive alternatives. These techniques seek to predict the day of ovulation so that intercourse may be planned for maximal probability of fertilization.

Keeping a basal temperature chart is one simple technique that has been in use for many years. The basic idea is that ovulation is thought to occur one or two days before a slight (0.4° F) rise in basal (that is, "at rest") body temperature. Thus, to use the technique, the woman each morning, before getting out of bed or engaging in any activity, takes her temperature with a normal household thermometer. By charting her temperature over a period of several months, the woman may be able to predict when she is about to ovulate and adjust intercourse accordingly. Though simple and inexpensive, this technique is fairly crude, given variations in the timing of menstrual cycles and factors such as illness, amount of sleep, and diet, all of which cause variation in basal temperature. Apart from keeping temperature charts, some women are able without aids to detect small changes in their bodies that indicate when ovulation will occur.

In the past few years, kits for the home determination of ovulation have become available over the counter. These relatively simple and inexpensive kits respond to the LH in urine that remains from the LH surge occurring 12 to 36 hours before ovulation. One need only collect an uncontaminated urine sample, insert a test stick, and observe any color change on the stick. In addition to the biochemical test kits, a somewhat more sophisticated technique employs small electrodes to detect changes in body chemistry. The woman places the electrodes in her mouth each morning, beginning about a week to 10 days before ovulation is expected. Readings are taken, looking for a peak that usually occurs six days before ovulation. The timing of intercourse is adjusted accordingly.

All these techniques of predicting ovulation are relatively safe, simple, and increasingly reliable. They do not offer help for all problems of infertility, but they do promise significant help for many. These techniques and devices represent sophisticated scientific knowledge and technological developments that allow people to control their reproductive lives without the direct intervention of others.

Artificial Insemination and Cryopreservation of Semen

Artificial insemination (AI)[12] is the most widely used reproduction-aiding technology today. In essence, it is a relatively simple procedure: semen is collected (usually by masturbation) and mechanically introduced into the vagina near the cervix. The first report of human AI with the husband's sperm (AIH) dates from 1790. AI with donor sperm (AID, where sperm is from a man other than the woman's husband) was first recorded in 1884.

From the biological point of view, it is irrelevant whether the sperm used in AI is from the husband or from a donor. In general, the husband's sperm is used if it does not have impaired ability to fertilize the egg and no genetic disorders are suspected. AI can aid a male with a low sperm count, as several ejaculates can be collected and concentrated before being introduced into the woman's vagina. AIH has the advantages of being safe, simple, and (compared to other reproduction-aiding techniques) inexpensive. Further, both husband and wife are biologically related to the child. Because it is so attractive, home kits for AI, similar to those used in testing for pregnancy, may soon be available over the counter.

The approved procedure for donor insemination is carried out by a physician, who obtains sperm from a licensed sperm bank and carries out the insemination with the consent of the woman and her partner. Sperm banks acquire sperm from males—quite often medical students—who are paid in the range of $25 per ejaculate. Sperm donors are almost always anonymous and legally have no duties or rights to any resulting children when the proper consent forms are filed. Sperm samples *are* sufficiently characterized, however, to allow recipients or their doctors the opportunity to select for desired traits such as race and general physical resemblance to the woman's husband or partner.[13] Even today, surprisingly few records are kept of donors and recipients,[14] and such records as are maintained are accessible only under very restrictive conditions.

AID is valuable where the male produces no sperm, has a sperm count too low for effective pooling, has an rH factor or antibody incompatibility with his partner, or has a severe hereditary disorder. AID is also being used increasingly by women who seek to conceive children without having sexual relations with a man. Many physicians, however, are reluctant to perform AID for unmarried women.

Chances for success with AID are very good, with estimates running as high as 30,000 births per year in the United States. This represents about a 60% success rate within three to six ovulatory cycles. The cost of AI varies but ranges between $400 and $600 per cycle.

AI with stored or pooled samples relies heavily upon a scientific technique known as cryopreservation, that is, preservation by freezing.[15] The freezing of biological samples containing cells has always been problematic due to the formation of ice during freezing and degeneration of the samples during thawing. Recently, new techniques involving liquid nitrogen have been successful: semen in a small vial is suspended over liquid nitrogen and cooled first to −76°F and then to −196°F, at which temperature it can be stored indefinitely. The survival rate for sperm frozen and thawed is approximately 67%. Although over 5,000 infants have been born from frozen sperm, the long-term genetic and biological consequences are unknown.

Cryopreservation of sperm has made sperm banks widespread and allows for the transfer of sperm over large distances and stretches of time. It also makes it possible for a man to store sperm in anticipation of a dangerous work environment, chemotherapy, or other conditions threatening his continued fertility.

In Vitro Fertilization

In vitro fertilization (IVF)[16] is the procedure whereby the so-called test-tube babies are conceived. Actually, "in vitro" simply means in glass, and IVF is the union of sperm and egg outside the body—usually in a glass petri dish.

Though it may sound simple, it is a complex and delicate procedure. Years of research and many failures preceded the first successful IVF birth, that of Louise Joy Brown in 1978, under the care of Robert G. Edwards and Patrick Steptoe.

Because fertilization takes place outside the woman's body, care must be taken to ensure that the biological materials survive in the foreign environment. Furthermore, coordinating and partially duplicating the complex functions of the many hormones controlling normal ovulation, fertilization, and implantation require great knowledge and technological ability. The key to successful IVF is timing: eggs must be retrieved when they are mature, but just before the follicle would naturally burst; the woman must be hormonally prepared to accept a developing embryo; sperm must be collected and mixed with the eggs; and the embryo must be grown and implanted.

Eggs can be retrieved after predicting the time of natural ovulation. More usually, the retrieval of eggs is facilitated by regulating and enhancing the maturation of the follicle and subsequent ovulation by hormonal treatment: hormonal drugs are used to stimulate follicles to mature at a desired time and in greater numbers than would occur naturally.

The most common way to retrieve eggs is through laparoscopy. In this procedure, the woman is placed under general anesthesia and an incision is made in her abdomen near the navel. A laparoscope—a long, thin fiberoptic tube that allows viewing inside the body—is inserted into and guided through the abdominal cavity to the ovary. Through a second incision, a long, hollow double aspirating needle is inserted to puncture the follicle and to suck out fluid and maturing eggs. The procedure takes about 30 minutes. Laparoscopy is now being replaced by the use of a needle directed by ultrasound, inserted through the vagina, through which eggs can be aspirated. Only local anesthesia is needed for this new, nonsurgical procedure.

As soon as it is retrieved, the fluid from the follicle is examined to determine if any eggs are present and to sort out and discard any damaged or malformed eggs. This step is necessary because a mature follicle often fails to yield a mature egg. If one or more eggs are recovered, they are immediately washed and placed in petri dishes in a nutrient solution; then they are placed in an incubator for four to eight hours to begin cell division.[17]

Although most of the physician's attention is focused on the recovery and incubation of eggs, sperm also must be obtained and treated in preparation for IVF. Once obtained, the sperm are separated from the seminal fluid, washed, and concentrated by centrifugation. Washing simulates conditions the sperm would encounter in their passage through the woman's reproductive tract, and bathing the sperm removes various components and aids capacitation. The concentrated sperm are then placed in a culture medium and incubated for an hour. The most active sperm swim to the upper layer of the medium and are used for fertilization.

Actual fertilization takes place in a petri dish. The eggs are removed from the incubator, and each is placed in a separate dish in a small droplet of medium. A few drops of highly concentrated sperm are pipetted onto each egg. The mixture is replaced in the incubator and, if all goes well, fertilization occurs within 24 hours.

Development of the embryo outside the uterus is critically important to IVF. If the embryo is introduced into the uterus either too early or too late, implantation will not occur. While the embryo is incubating, the woman is given a progesterone injection to prepare her uterus for implantation. Two days after fertilization, the conceptus has developed to about two to eight cells. At this stage, it is ready to be placed in the uterus. The woman lies face down, with her knees drawn up to her chest, in a position that is thought to cause minimal disturbance to the embryo. The embryo is introduced into the uterus through a long catheter inserted through the vagina and cervix. Then the woman assumes a prone position and remains still for four hours in order to increase the likelihood of implantation.

For reasons not yet fully understood, implantation seems to work best if several embryos are placed in the uterus; four appear to be the optimal number. When multiple embryos are introduced, usually only one implants and develops; the others are discharged from the woman's body. Occasionally, more than one embryo implants, and multiple births result.

Overall, success rates for IVF are not very high, though the American Fertility Society has deemed IVF an established (no longer an experimental) technique when properly practiced. Even the best clinics claim no more than a 15–20% success rate, and many have had no successes. The cost per attempt is usually about $10,000, and the total cost of treatment is several times that amount, with no assurance of success. Apart from monetary costs, IVF can be an ordeal both psychologically and physically. Still, IVF has grown rapidly in popularity. Approximately 200 clinics operate in the United States, and around 15,000 IVF babies have been born worldwide (nearly 3,500 in the United States in 1989). For many couples, IVF is the last chance, at the end of a long and trying struggle, to have a child who is biologically their own.

Gamete Intrafallopian Transfer and Transvaginal Oocyte Retrieval

Variations on IVF have been developed with the hope of improving the rate of success and reducing trauma to the potential mother. In gamete intrafallopian transfer (GIFT), for example, eggs are retrieved as in normal IVF, but the equipment is not removed. The eggs are mixed with concentrated sperm, and then the egg–sperm mixture is placed back into the fallopian tube. The advantages of GIFT over IVF include the fact that sperm and egg fuse and develop in their natural environment, the fact that the procedure takes only one day, and the reduction of costs for potential parents.

Another variation on IVF is called transvaginal oocyte retrieval. In this procedure, the eggs are obtained from the ovaries by inserting a needle through the vaginal wall rather than through the abdominal wall. Though this procedure is more difficult for the physician, who must guide the needle to the ovary without puncturing other vital organs, it is much easier for the patient because only a local anesthetic is used and no surgery is required.

Egg Donation, Embryo Transfer, and Embryo Freezing

A number of reproduction-aiding procedures may be used in conjunction with IVF.[18] One is egg donation, which is simply the retrieval of eggs from one woman and their implantation into another. Egg donation might be practical for a woman whose ovaries are damaged but whose uterus is capable of normal functioning. Still, egg donation requires extensive hormonal regulation. For without the ability to freeze eggs or embryos readily, *two* women's cycles must be synchronized so that the donor ovulates at the time the recipient is ready to receive the egg. An attraction of this technology is that a woman, even though not the genetic parent of the child, can be both the gestational and the social parent.

Embryo transfer, in essence, is the transfer of a developing fertilized egg before implantation from one woman to another. The second woman gestates the embryo and ultimately gives birth. In the most common variant of this still fairly rare technique, the first woman is artificially inseminated with sperm from the recipient's husband. The embryo is removed from the donor by the technique of lavage, that is, by flushing the uterus with a solution introduced and recovered through a catheter.

Embryo transfer assists the same women as does egg donation. It may also be of use to women with normal ovaries but a dysfunctional uterus: husband and wife can initiate fertilization naturally or by AIH, and the resulting embryo can be transferred to the uterus of a surrogate gestator. Though embryo transfer is much easier than IVF in that it can be done in the physician's office without anesthesia or surgery, the cycles of the two women still must be synchronized, and lavage increases the chances of uterine infection.

Another emerging technique, embryo freezing, offers a number of technological advantages. This technique is commonly used in breeding cattle. The first successful human birth from a frozen embryo was in 1983. The baby was born to an Australian patient who had miscarried during an attempt at IVF but who successfully bore a child from an embryo frozen at her request as a precaution during the initial attempt. Development of the ability to freeze and then thaw embryos at a later date frees IVF and embryo transfer from certain time constraints: embryo transfer no longer requires synchronization of two women's cycles, and a woman can store embryos for multiple attempts at implantation, without further need to collect eggs, or as insurance against damage to her eggs or reproductive organs. Embryo freezing also offers the option of storing excess fertilized embryos rather than destroying them.

Surrogate Motherhood

In its most popular form, surrogate motherhood[19] requires little scientific knowledge or technological ability: a woman is artificially inseminated with the sperm of a man who is not her husband, but she agrees from the outset to give up any resulting child to the man and, typically, his wife. Indeed, surrogacy of this sort need not even involve AI: the surrogate and the man can just have sexual intercourse—though this variation also raises the question of adultery. In either of the above cases, the child will be the genetic and gestational offspring of the surrogate and the contracting male. Though surrogacy does not require much technology, surrogate motherhood is usually discussed together with the more scientifically and technologically revolutionary techniques because it has flourished at the same time, is an option for many of the same individuals, and may be coupled with the sophisticated techniques previously discussed. For example, using egg or embryo transfer, a surrogate could agree to gestate a child who was not genetically related to her. Thus, a couple in which the woman had functioning ovaries but no uterus could have a child that was genetically derived from both of them. In a more radical scenario, a third woman could be enlisted to supply the egg—indeed another male could be enlisted to supply the sperm—thus involving separate individuals in the roles of genetic father, genetic mother, gestational mother, rearing mother, and rearing father.

By far the most common form of surrogate motherhood, however, involves AI of a surrogate by the husband of a couple to whom the surrogate has contracted to give up the child at birth. Typically, the contract is arranged by a broker, usually an attorney, who advertises for women willing to be surrogates, matches couples and surrogates, screens surrogates for physical and psychological fitness, and oversees the process. Fees for brokers are in the range of $5,000 to $10,000. Payment to the surrogate is typically about $10,000 beyond medical and other expenses related to the pregnancy. Couples who seek a child through surrogate motherhood can thus count on spending a minimum of $30,000. A few cases have been noted of surrogacy without contract or fee, such as a woman's sister (and, in one case, a woman's mother!) agreeing to carry a child for her. Estimates are that approximately 2,000 children were born from traditional surrogacy arrangements in the period 1988–1990 and about 80 from arrangements for gestational surrogacy. Though most surrogacy arrangements have gone smoothly, spectacular disagreements such as the Baby M case have arisen, and the legality of commercial surrogacy is currently under intensive scrutiny by courts and legislatures.

Sex Preselection

The reproduction-aiding technologies described so far aim at the birth of a child. Many other startling and far-reaching techniques are being developed for goals that are ancillary to the production of a child. One such goal is the prediction and selection of the traits of one's child. Particular energy is being spent in the attempt to preselect the child's sex.[20] Though claims have outstripped actual success, the ability to select one's child's sex has been growing.

Sex preselection is in fact quite an old endeavor, and a great deal of folklore tells how to ensure the birth of a boy or (less frequently) a girl. For example, it has been held that the birth of a girl would be more likely if the mother ate sweet foods and a boy more likely if she ate sour foods, or, alternatively, if boots were worn to bed or if the male hung his pants on the right side of the bed.

Most recent scientific attempts at sex preselection have sought to determine the child's sex by selecting for or giving advantage to the type of sperm that would fertilize the egg (sperm carrying an X chromosome for females, a Y chromosome for males). While controversy exists, several differences between sperm carrying X chromosomes and those carrying Y chromosomes have been proposed: the former are larger, more dense, slower-moving, and inhibited by alkaline environments, whereas the latter die sooner, are more numerous in each ejaculation, and are slowed by acidic environments.

One procedure developed in light of these proposed differences involves the separation of sperm in a glass column containing a protein called serum albumin. Semen is layered on top, and the more motile sperm containing Y chromosomes are supposed to swim more efficiently through the dense layers of albumin. These sperm are then collected at the bottom of the column and used in AI in attempts to produce male babies. Other methods of sex preselection are based on separating sperm containing X and Y chromosomes in a centrifugal field (taking advantage of differences in density) or an electrical field (taking advantage of differences in electrical charge). In addition to these clinical methods, a number of procedures that can be used at home have been proposed. Timing intercourse to take advantage of changes in the pH of the woman's reproductive tract is widely used, based on the belief that sperm carrying an X chromosome are more likely to survive the acidic environment that exists just prior to ovulation, while sperm carrying a Y chromosome are favored in the alkaline environment at the time of ovulation. Use of a douche, jelly, or foam to alter the pH of the woman's reproductive tract has also been tried. Future developments in this field may include a pill for the male, which would alter the ratio of sperm carrying X and Y chromosomes produced, and a pill for the female, which would alter the physiological conditions in her reproductive system to favor survival of one or the other type of sperm. Though many claims have been made for the techniques of sex preselection, so far none has achieved widely accepted success, but it is almost certain that the option of sex preselection is close at hand.

Conclusion

Human reproduction involves complex and delicately regulated systems. As we have seen, many inventive and exciting techniques are being developed to aid or, more often, to replicate various functions of these sytems. These techniques are powerful tools and promise many benefits. However, they also raise serious legal and moral questions. Indeed, finding answers to these questions of value may be a greater challenge than that of developing the technologies themselves.

Notes

1. H. D. Swanson, *Human Reproduction: Biology and Social Change* (New York: Oxford University Press, 1974), p. 15.

2. The generation of fully mature ova (the process is called "oogenesis") involves several cell divisions with special names for each of the several resulting cells. For simplicity, the term "egg" will be used in following the cell that becomes the mature ovum through all its stages of development.

3. On the male reproductive system, see L. Browder, *Developmental Biology* (Philadelphia: Saunders, 1980), pp. 146–172; J. G. Creager, *Human Anatomy and Physiology* (Belmont, CA: Wadsworth, 1983), pp. 730–735; and D. D. Ritchie and R. Carola, *Biology,* 2nd ed. (Reading, MA: Addison-Wesley, 1983), pp. 270–272.

4. On the female reproductive system, see G. Karp and N. H. Berrill, *Development,* 2nd. ed. (New York: McGraw-Hill, 1981), pp. 116–138; Browder, *Developmental Biology,* pp. 173–231; and P. Grant, *Biology of Developing Systems* (New York: Holt Rinehart & Winston, 1978), pp. 265–282.

5. Unless it is clear from the context, the term "embryo" here and in what follows is used to refer to all stages of development after fertilization.

6. See, for example, Hannibal Hamlin, "Life or Death by E.E.G.," *JAMA* 190 (12 October 1964), p. 113.

7. Infertility is not necessarily permanent or untreatable, in contrast to sterility, which is irreversible by therapeutic intervention, as in the case of a woman who lacks ovaries or a man who lacks testes. Among infertile patients, primary infertility (infertility occurring in those who have never conceived) and secondary infertility (infertility occurring in those who have previously conceived) are also distinguished. On infertility and sterility generally, see D. Epel, "The Program of Fertilization," *Scientific American* 237 (1977), pp. 128–138 and "Fertilization," *Endeavour* (New Series), 4 (1980), pp. 26–31; Creager *Human Anatomy and Physiology,* pp. 758–762; and V. Davajan and D. R. Mishell, "Evaluation of the Infertile Couple," in V. Davajan and D. R. Mishell, eds., *Infertility, Contraception and Reproductive Endocrinology,* 2nd ed. (Oradell, NJ: Medical Economics Books, 1986).

8. U.S. Congress, Office of Technology Assessment. *Reproductive Hazards in the Workplace,* OTA-BA-266. (Washington, DC: U.S. Govt. Printing Office, December, 1985). This report claims that the rate of infertility dropped from 11.2% in 1965 to 8.4% in 1982, and that some sort of infertility treatment is sought by 51% of couples with primary infertility and by 22% of couples with secondary infertility.

9. On male infertility, see M. Perloe and L. G. Christie, "Male Fertility," in M. Perloe and L.G. Christie, eds., *Miracle Babies and Other Happy Endings for Couples with Fertility Problems* (New York: Rawson Associates, 1986), pp. 45–88, and R. H. Glass and R. J. Ericsson, "The Male Factor in Infertility," in Robert H. Glass, ed., *Getting Pregnant in the 1980's* (Berkeley: University of California Press, 1982), pp. 37–55.

10. On female infertility, see M. Perloe and L. G. Christie, "Female Fertility," in *Miracle Babies,* pp. 89–156, and R. H. Glass and R. J. Ericsson, "The Male Factor in Infertility," in *Getting Pregnant in the 1980's,* pp. 1–36.

11. On reproductive-aiding technologies in general, see R. H. Blank, "Making Babies: The State of the Art," *The Futurist* 19 (1985), pp. 11–17.

12. L. B. Andrews, *New Conceptions,* Ch. 7, (New York: St. Martin's Press, 1984), pp. 159–196.

13. More notorious examples of selection include the so-called Nobel Sperm Bank that advertises sperm from intellectually superior males.

14. Nearly half of the physicians in a recent study by the Office of Technology Assessment do not keep records that allow matching of a donor and a recipient after the fact, as reported in Judith Gaines, "A Scandal of Artificial Insemination," *New York Times, Good Health Magazine,* Oct. 7, 1990, p. 29.

15. J. J. Nagle, *Heredity and Human Affairs,* 3d. ed. (St Louis: Times Mirror/ Mosby, 1984), pp. 143–144.

16. C. Grobstein, "External Human Fertilization," *Scientific America* 240 (1979), pp. 57–67; P. C. Steptoe and R. G. Edwards, "Laparoscopic Recovery of Preovulatory Human Oocytes After Priming of Ovaries with Gonadotropins," *Lancet* 1 (1970), pp. 683–689; R. G. Edwards, P. C. Steptoe, and J. M. Purdy, "Fertilization and Cleavage *in vitro* of Preovulation Human Oocytes, *Nature* 229 (1971), pp. 132–133; M. Gold, "The Baby Makers," *Science 85* 6 (April 1985), pp. 26–38.

17. Experiments with freezing eggs at this stage to allow greater flexibility have not been as successful as freezing them after eggs have been fertilized and have divided to about the eight-cell stage. See the discussion of embryo freezing below.

18. Andrews, *New Conceptions,* Ch. 11, pp. 243–266; J. A. Treichel, "Embryo Transfers Achieved in Humans," *Science News* 124 (1983), p. 69; A. E. Beer and R. E. Billingham, "The Embryo as a Transplant," *Scientific American* 230 (1974), pp. 36–46.

19. Andrews, *New Conceptions,* Ch. 8, pp. 197–241.

20. R. H. Glass and R. J. Ericsson, "Sex Preselection," in *Getting Pregnant in the 1980's,* pp. 113–128, and R. H. Blank, *Redefining Human Life: Reproductive Technologies and Social Policy* (Boulder, CO: Westview Press, 1984), pp. 68–70.

Emotional Reactions to Infertility

Miriam D. Mazor

For a long time, the subject of infertility has been rather neglected in the psychiatric literature or has been treated in a manner that has lagged far behind our medical understanding of the problem. The focus of this paper will be on reactions to infertility as a developmental crisis in adult life. . . .

Most of the discussion that follows is based on my clinical work,[1] from 1975 to 1979, with slightly over 100 couples and a few single women, concerned about their infertility. . . . In general, the sample was skewed toward middle-class business and professional people between the ages of 28 and 40 who were involved in rather long-term, stable relationships.

Initially, most patients were surprised, even shocked, to learn that they were unable to conceive once the decision to have a baby was made. The decision was often arrived at after years of careful use of birth-control, years of study, training, or career building. Most were distressed and indignant about the loss of control of their life plans implicit in the situation, and many of them handled their feelings of helplessness by becoming experts in areas of particular concern to them. On the whole, these patients were better informed than the average medical school graduate about the physiology of reproduction, significance of various tests (e.g., gonadotropin levels), side effects of treatment modalities, and so on. By and large, this style of defending against helplessness proved to be useful to the patients and allowed them to work collaboratively with the infertility specialist who was treating them, although an occasional doctor felt threatened by what he or she felt was a questioning of his/her competence and expertise, and an occasional patient was more interested in competitive argument with the doctor than in acquiring information and understanding the process of the infertility investigation.

Most patients seem to go through three phases in dealing with the infertility crisis;[2] these stages may vary in length and often overlap. The first phase revolves around the narcissistic injury. Acknowledgment of an infertility problem, whether it is after six months, one year, or several years of attempting to achieve a pregnancy, is a tremendous blow. Patients are preoccupied with the

From Miriam D. Mazor and Harriet F. Simons, eds. *Infertility: Medical, Emotional and Social Considerations*. New York: Human Sciences Press, Inc., 1984, pp. 23–35. Abridged. Used by permission.

medical workup and with their own bodies. Prior to this time, many of them have had minimal contact with doctors and have considered themselves as basically healthy people. The infertility study is often a long-term project requiring a high degree of patient participation and cooperation. Other aspects of their lives, such as career plans and social relationships, are often subordinated to the critically timed tests and procedures. Patients must expose their bodies for examination and manipulation; they must reveal intimate details of their sexual lives, and often their private wishes and fears surrounding their desire for a child.

Infertility patients often feel damaged, defective, and "bad." This sense of "badness" may not remain confined to reproductive function alone but may encompass sexual function and desirability, physical attractiveness, performance, and productivity in other spheres as well. Something as basic as core gender identity may be consciously called into question. Several female patients have described feeling like "neuters," not belonging to any group classifiable as male or female; male patients referred to intercourse as "shooting blanks."[3] Concerns about sexual identity and sexual function are almost universal among infertility patients, no matter which partner has the medical problem. In both men and women there is usually a significant diminution of sexual desire, with ejaculatory disturbances of a temporary nature reported by over half of the men.[4] The depression of both partners consequent to their unsuccessful efforts to achieve a pregnancy, the necessity for sexual relations on demand at specified times in the woman's cycle, and the concern about whether this time will be successful contribute heavily to the problems in sexual function commonly seen in infertile couples.[5] Sex is no longer a spontaneous, pleasurable activity; it is an assignment, a mission with a definable goal, i.e., pregnancy. Although some authors[6] report an increased incidence of promiscuity and extramarital affairs in an effort to "prove" one's masculinity or femininity, in my experience infertile couples complain largely of loss of libido and depression. Many try to be extra good to atone for whatever sins, real or imagined, they may feel caused their infertility.[7] They may carry a heavy load of guilt, sometimes focused on a past event (e.g., an abortion), which may or may not be related to the current problem. Often the guilt is experienced in a diffuse way—guilt about Oedipal wishes, guilt about masturbation, guilt about sexual fantasies of any kind.

There is usually a tremendous escalation of anxiety as the couple awaits the onset of the next menstrual period. The woman becomes preoccupied with changes in her body, searching for signs of pregnancy. All of the tension cannot be attributed to the physiologic changes toward the end of the cycle, as many husbands also report great anxiety at this time. Some drugs used to stimulate ovulation, e.g., Clomid, may prolong the second half of the cycle and increase the hope of pregnancy. As the menses begin, many women are plunged into a stage of despair—"the cataclysm," as one patient called it; the recurrent barren cycles become exhausting.

Relations between the partners become strained and tense. The infertile spouse may fear actual or emotional abandonment by the other; some will continally test and provoke the partner with comments like "If you had married someone else you'd have a family by now." The fertile partner may feel an obligation to maintain a front of unswerving loyalty, to disavow any disappointment or anger. In situations where a combined problem exists, there may be a great deal of tension around the issue of who is "really to blame" for the problem. And, since the bulk of the tests and diagnostic procedures involve the woman, there may be resentment on her part at having to shoulder most of the responsibility for the workup. The daily basal body temperature charting may serve as a constant reminder that *her* body is not producing a baby, regardless of where the medical problems lie. Some husbands choose to become involved in the temperature charting as a means of affirming their support and involvement.

Oedipal wishes and fears are rekindled with a new intensity—e.g., the wish to present the parent of the opposite sex with the treasured gift of a baby. Some patients have elaborate fantasies about how their infertility is in some way the product of parental revenge; they feel betrayed and "cheated" by the parents who promised them the power to make babies when they grew up.

Rivalry with siblings is reactivated, especially when the siblings have proven their fertility. The jealousy often extends to the entire fertile population. Many patients seriously restrict their lives and cut off old friendships in order to avoid confrontation with pregnant women or families with young babies. The isolation only serves to increase their sense of defectiveness. A peculiar kind of jealousy may emerge in groups of infertile patients. Women who have had a series of miscarriages are viewed as "more fortunate" by those who have never conceived; those who ovulate regularly are seen as "more normal" by those who do not; patients argue about whether it is "better" or "worse" to have a male infertility problem (which is usually less treatable, although the option of donor insemination exists), whether it is "better" or "worse" to have a diagnosis of absolute infertility or to go on thinking that there is a lingering chance for a pregnancy. Themes of deprivation and relative degrees of suffering are common in such groups: rarely will they tolerate a member with a secondary infertility problem (one who has borne a living child), and they have difficulty in dealing with the issue of what to do about group members who become pregnant, with the initial impulse being to expel the offending member.

For many women the wish for the pregnant state, as distinct from parenthood, is endowed with many magical properties. Pregnancy is viewed romantically as the "blossoming" of a woman; labor and delivery are her chances for a starring role.

Many patients see their infertility as a pronouncement of "unfitness" for parenthood. They are disproportionately enraged by those who seem to take it for granted—e.g., people who abuse or neglect their children or those who favor abortion on demand. Some patients express more abstract fears about not being able to produce anything of value, accomplish anything of worth. During the tumult of the infertility workup it is, in fact, more difficult to concentrate on studies or career.

Therapy with patients going through this first phase involves recognizing and acknowledging the feelings evoked by the situation, offering support to help the narcissistic wounds heal, restoring a sense of self-esteem, and helping the patient regain some sense of control over his or her life by clarifying those areas in which elements of choice remain (e.g., choice of a doctor, the time-table for diagnostic and treatment procedures, etc.). It may be sufficient to help patients remember how they have coped with disappointments and frustrations in the past and to remind them to utilize those coping skills in their current situation.

Patients usually enter the second phase when they are ready to call a halt to the infertility investigation. It may be an agonizingly difficult decision, especially for those couples whose infertility remains unexplained or for those who have a small, lingering chance to achieve a pregnancy. During this phase the couple reexamines their own feelings about parenthood and goes through a period of grieving for the loss of their reproductive function, of mourning for the biologic children they could not have together. It is in some ways a more painful but less intense process. Although there are now fewer social pressures to have children, for most people parenthood remains an integral part of their development as adults. Frustration in attaining that goal requires a significant reorganization of one's identity in relation to the self and to others.

In her paper "Women and Mid-Life,"[8] Notman discusses how the phases of a woman's life, viewed by herself and others, are often defined by events related to her reproductive function. The awareness of her own mortality, her sense of differentiation from older and younger generations, her assessment of herself in relation to her social environment, are all closely interwoven with the experiences of childbirth, parenting, and the eventual launching of her children into the adult world. Even unmarried or voluntarily childless women may go through a period of depression and mourning somewhere in their thirties or forties, grieving for a part of themselves and for potential life plans that may never be realized.

Most of the literature on male development takes the reproductive role of the male for granted, secondary to the all-important area of work and career development.[9] However, some recent work has examined more thoroughly the meaning of fatherhood to men. Ross's[10] work on "Paternal Identity" is an excellent example. Much of his discussion is applicable to women as well as men, and can also serve as a useful framework in which to examine the difficulties facing the infertile person. In his discussion he defines identity as the individual's continuing sense of self, a very private experience of the self in relation to others.

There are several aspects of identity that are interrelated. During the first year of life the child forms a constant sense of self as distinct from others; in the second year he or she consolidates what Stoller[11] calls "core gender identity." i.e., a firm cognitive and emotional conviction that one is a male or a female and that other people can be similarly classified. Later on, a sense of sexual identity emerges, evolving throughout the life cycle and referring to the sense of the kind of man or woman a person is.

Generational identity refers to the individual's appreciation of where he or she belongs in the generational flow—his or her status as child, parent, grand-child, grandparent.

Parental identity refers to one's fantasies and actual achievements in the imagined or real role of a generator and nurturer of products, human and otherwise. In other words, biological parenthood does not automatically be-stow a sense of parental identity, nor is it impossible to achieve a parental identity in the absence of biological parenthood. In some ways the entire developmental process, from infancy onward, is a preparation for forthcom-ing parenthood, or at least for the capacity to assume a parental role. The decision to have children optimally represents a wish to experience love in a new way, to consolidate a positive identification with parents or parental figures who taught us what love is or should be. There may be self-centered aspects to the desire for children—e.g., fantasies of being reborn, of creating an extension or better version of oneself, of filling a lonely void. For women the wish for the pregnant state may be charged with narcissistic fantasies, with wishes to be valued and admired. To some extent everyone is also ambivalent about becoming a parent. The responsibility is awesome, requiring a major reorganization of one's life style and priorities, sacrifices of freedom and privacy. These fantasies and fears are universal, but the fertile population is afforded the opportunity to test them in reality. The infertile person must struggle harder with them.

Ross[12] discusses how the birth of a first child allows a man to look at his own father in a new light—as a man very much like himself. Until then he may have idealized him or devalued him, but in any case perceived him mainly in relation to this paternal function. Similarly the woman begins to view her mother as a woman like herself, with strengths and vulnerabilities. Becoming a parent allows the adult to view the world from the other side of the Us-Them split (with "Us" being the children until that point, "Them" being the parents). The infertile man or woman must work out his or her own ways of renegotiating the relationship with the actual parents of adult life and must put to rest the larger-than-life parents of childhood.

Concerns about generational identity are often expressed in a variety of ways. Many patients express their concern about forever remaining the child of their parents, never fully achieving adult status. Some talk about feeling "old," about being confronted prematurely with a sense of their own mortality (it must be borne in mind that the major non-reproducing populations are the very young and the very old). They worry about being the end of the genetic line. Some patients in my practice who are themselves the children of Holo-caust survivors feel this very acutely, as if they must somehow reproduce not only for themselves but for the sake of extended families annihilated during World War II. Others describe their fears of a lonely, grandchildless old age.

Therapy during this phase must focus on the sorting out of issues so that the infertility problem can be put into some perspective in the totality of the patient's life. The individual must reassess his or her own inner resources and make some decision about how best to realize his or her own creative, generative, and nurturant potentials in the absence of biological children. For each individual the resolution of the problem is a very personal matter. At this time, too, the couple must reassess their relationship with each other. Together they must come to terms with the loss of their reproductive function and mourn the loss of the biologic children they could not have together. The infertility experience has the potential to damage or disrupt the relationship; hostility may be generated if one spouse is more heavily invested than the other in having children. There are few social supports to assist the couple in the grieving process because the loss is so vague, invisible, and potential; in a sense they become more dependent on each other for a while. Some couples report that the experience actually brought them closer together, confirming the strength of the bond of love that held them together. In some ways they must complete at an earlier stage a task many couples postpone until after their children are grown.

The third phase involves making some decision about whether and how to pursue the difficult alternate routes to parenthood—adoption or, in cases of male infertility, artificial insemination by donor. Through this phase the therapist should be aware that there will be a great deal of reworking of old issues. The processes a couple must undergo in order to adopt or use donor insemination are full of their own stresses, discussion of which is beyond the scope of this chapter. The loss of the unborn biologic children is periodically re-mourned, as the world is full of reminders that other people go on having babies. The grief work is never "totally finished," and it is not at all uncommon for the old feelings about infertility to recur at other major transition points in people's lives—retirement, menopause, developments in the lives of adopted children, relatives, and close friends—but it is hoped that the infertile man or woman will have achieved enough satisfaction from life to be able to handle the old disappointment.

The third phase is somewhat different for those couples who do achieve a pregnancy. For them it feels like a "miracle," and they may find that the reality of pregnancy and parenting fails to live up to their long cherished illusions. Or they may feel that they have no right to ambivalent feelings, no right to complain or feel tired; they must be perfect parents and produce a perfect child in order to compensate for their feelings of inadequacy in the area of reproduction. I have been surprised at the number of patients who return to therapy after the birth of a child with concerns about what "normal" parents are supposed to feel. Interestingly, the incidence of clinical depression or other major psychiatric symptoms in the postpartum period seems to be lower among formerly infertile women than in the general population.[13]

For some couples, the third phase may involve the working out of a life style without children that is acceptable to both partners. This may be especially difficult for those couples who have for many years focused their lives around the single-minded goal of pregnancy. For them the infertility workup and treatment have become a substitute for a child, perhaps their only common interest or the only way in which they can demand or give each other emotional support. It may be difficult to wean such couples from their dependence on their infertility problem (one couple had been working at it for over thirteen years and had seen over ten infertility specialists; they entered psychotherapy seeking a referral for a "new infertility doctor").

For each individual and couple, the resolution of the problem is unique and is often contingent on prior experiences in coping with disappointment and loss. Patients must prepare themselves to use resources other than reproduction in order to consolidate a comfortable identity as a middle-aged and older adult whether or not parenthood is achieved.

Notes

This paper was presented at the 133rd Annual Meeting of the American Psychiatric Association, in San Francisco, on May 7, 1980, as part of a Symposium (#43) on Emotional Aspects of Problems in Reproduction.

1. M. Mazor, "The Problem of Infertility," in *The Woman Patient,* Vol. I, M. Notman and C. Nadelson, eds., New York: Plenum, 1978), pp. 137–160; "Barren Couples," *Psychology Today* 12 (May 1979), pp. 101, 103–104, 107–108,110; "Psychosexual Problems of the Infertile Couple," *Medical Aspects of Human Sexuality* 14 (1980).

2. Mazor, "Barren Couples."

3. B. E. Menning, *Infertility: A Guide for the Childless Couple* (Englewood Cliffs, New Jersey: Prentice-Hall, 1977).

4. Mazor, "Psychosexual Problems"; C. Debrovner and R. Shubin-Stein, "Sexual Problems Associated with Infertility," *Medical Aspects of Human Sexuality* 10 (Mar. 1976), pp. 161–162; and H. E. Walker, "Sexual Problems and Infertility," *Psychosomatics* 19 (1978), pp. 477–484.

5. Menning, *Infertility;* Mazor, "Psychosexual Problems"; Debrovner and Shubin-Stein, "Sexual Problems"; Walker, "Sexual Problems."

6. Walker, "Sexual Problems."

7. Debrovner and Shubin-Stein, "Sexual Problems."

8. M. Notman, "Women and Mid-life: A Different Perspective," *Psychiatric Opinion* 15 (15 September 1978), pp. 15–25.

9. D. Levinson, C. Darrow, et al., *The Seasons of a Man's Life* (New York: Knopf, 1978).

10. J. M. Ross, "Paternal Identity: Reflections on the Adult Crisis and Its Developmental Reverberations," in *On Sexuality: Psychoanalytic Observations,* T. Byram Karasu and C. W. Socarides, eds., (New York: International Universities Press, 1979).

11. R. Stoller, *Sex and Gender* (New York: Science House, 1968).

12. Ross, "Paternal Identity."

13. Menning, *Infertility.*

II

CONFLICTING PERSPECTIVES: ISSUES, POSITIONS, AND ARGUMENTS

The articles in this part survey many of the major normative issues raised by reproductive technology and serve as an overview of the positions, arguments, and analyses common to recent discussions. The articles by law professors Robertson and Krimmel debate the morality of parenting through contract. The remaining four articles, from Edwards, the Vatican, Kass, and Gorovitz, address normative issues centering on the practice of IVF.

Robertson

John Robertson defends the morality of parenting through contract, focusing primarily on the benefits and harms of the practice, especially the charge that harm will result from separating genetic, gestational, and social relationships with the child. Robertson also addresses worries about physical and psychological harm to the mother, commercialization of reproduction, and the possibility that children produced through the practice may be unwanted. Robertson's main argument in defense of parenting through contract is that certain other well-established practices—AID, divorce, adoption, and even natural reproduction—exhibit the same features that have caused concern about parenting through contract. In fact, Robertson suggests that in the final analysis, parenting through contract is little different from the widely accepted practice of independent (nonagency) adoption.

Krimmel

In response to Robertson, Herbert Krimmel argues that parenting through contract is morally objectionable because it treats children not as valuable in themselves but as commodities, that is, as things to be bought and sold and valued for their utility in satisfying other persons' desires. The core of parenting through contract, Krimmel asserts, is creation of a child "with the premeditated intention to transfer him at birth." In Krimmel's view, this feature not only distinguishes parenting through contract from adoption, it reverses the implication that Robertson sought to draw. For children born through contracts can be expected, like adopted children, to have a strong interest in the circumstances of their birth and transfer, and, Krimmel maintains, the commercial and contractual elements in their history can only diminish their security and sense of self-worth. Even though such children may have much to be thankful for, they can never escape the fact that they were created with the express intention of being given, or rather, sold, away.

In this line of argument, Krimmel has identified one of the central moral concerns raised by parenting through contract and by reproductive technology in general. As procreation is conceived and practiced to a greater extent within commercial and technological frameworks of meaning and value, our conceptions of children and procreation may be fundamentally changed for the worse. This theme is expanded upon most directly in articles from the Vatican, Kass, Warren, Keane, and Tong, the latter two of which also specifically address the proper legal status of parenting through contract. The underlying concepts of commercialization, commodification, and technological control are analyzed in the articles by Radin and O'Donovan. Also relevant to this issue are the articles in Part III, which examine the nature and significance of the "natural" relationship between parents and children.

Edwards

R. G. Edwards, famous, along with Patrick Steptoe, for having perfected the techniques that resulted in the first successful human birth by IVF, defends the morality of IVF research and clinical use of IVF. Edwards briefly reviews the research and testing that went into the early development of human IVF and enumerates the many benefits of IVF to infertile couples and the spin-off benefits of IVF for contraception, embryology, and other areas.

Among the main moral issues Edwards addresses are informed consent, the treatment of embryos, and, under the heading "the dehumanization of procreation," concerns about commercialization and technological control. Edwards quickly dismisses worries about informed consent[1] but addresses at greater length the other ethical concerns he has identified.

In this anthology, a number of different approaches are offered to the status of embryonic life[2] (see also the articles from the Vatican, Kass, and Gorovitz). Edwards argues that embryos should not be accorded full human rights at the moment of conception because the biological processes leading to life are continuous and do not justify picking an arbitrary point for life to begin. The point of conception is arbitrary because, in his view, the same potential for life exists in ova and sperm *before* fertilization, yet few people are particularly exercised about the mistreatment of unfertilized ova or sperm.

On worries about commercialization and technology, Edwards's position is simply that we have God-given creative powers of intellect and action, and we should use them. To the objection that children, marriage, and procreation are degraded when procreation is removed from the sphere of bodily love, he replies, similarly to Robertson, that family values have survived assaults from contraception, divorce, and other elements of modern life that separate love, sex, marriage, and family, and it is hard to see how family values are better protected by withholding treatment from infertile couples. If the persons' motives are love and commitment, then, Edwards concludes, why should the assistance of technology be denied to them?

Vatican Statement

This last set of issues addressed by Edwards is central to the excerpt from the Vatican's official statement on reproductive technology. In its statement, the Vatican attempts to articulate a principled basis from which to judge the morality of reproductive technology. The philosophy underlying these principles is that human life is not to be conceived merely in biological terms or merely in terms of what a person happens to desire, but in terms of the unity of the person, including body, soul, and the capacity for communion with other persons and with God. More specifically, the principles from which the Vatican's statement reasons are, briefly, as follows.

Respect for Life

The cell formed at fertilization has life. This life is not identical to either the mother or the father but is a new human individual. A human individual is a human person. So, embryos from the moment of fertilization on must be respected as innocent human beings. It is not that embryos merely have the potential to develop into human persons, but that they *are* human persons from the moment of fertilization. Thus, as innocent persons, they must be protected from harm and from violation of their integrity and must receive every chance to live.[3]

Union of Functions

Marriage involves the spiritual and bodily union of two people, which attains its true significance only when it is open to expression and completion in having children. To remove or replace any of these elements—marriage, sexual union, openness to and full participation in conception and birth—is to destroy the unity that confers ultimate value upon any of the elements. In particular, the unity of procreation is destroyed if any element of natural procreation is replaced by a reproductive technique or performed by a third party (donor, doctor, etc.). Furthermore, only in the unity of these elements is the child secure in his or her relationship to the parents and thereby able to realize his or her own identity and proper human development.

On these grounds, the Vatican statement holds that experimentation and research involving embryos are acceptable only if they are not invasive in any way or if they do not harm those particular embryos; additional embryos should not be produced. On these grounds, virtually all reproduction-aiding techniques, including AID, IVF, and parenting through contract, are judged morally illicit. Even AIH is suspect, though here the Church appears to be trying to walk a very thin line between its principles and an extremely widespread practice. Strictly, a technique can be morally acceptable according to the Vatican only if it does not replace but merely "facilitates the conjugal act or helps it reach its natural objectives."

Certain of these positions of the Catholic Church are familiar from its positions on abortion and contraception. Even so, the virtually complete condemnation of reproductive technology is an extreme position. Still, the theme of the importance of the unity of procreative activities and processes has been advocated from a number of different perspectives—secular, religious, and feminist—and is examined further in the articles by Kass, Alpern, O'Donovan, and Corea.

Kass

Leon Kass addresses the slippery slope argument, the status of embryos, the separation of sexuality and procreation, and the policy issue of federal funding for IVF. Kass's worry about the slippery slope is not that practices presently engaged in will predictably lead to even more objectionable practices, but that our acceptance of present practices already exemplifies attitudes that would justify those objectionable practices. His discussion of the status and treatment of embryos can be seen as illustrating this point. "To be human," he claims, "means not only to have human form and powers; it means to have a human context and to be humanly connected." Thus, when we focus, as Kass charges is typical in IVF, exclusively on the end product of obtaining a functioning biological human, regardless of the processes by which it comes to be, we fundamentally degrade what we are as humans. IVF does not inevitably lead to laboratories growing babies in test tubes, but the *attitudes* expressed in IVF already embody the same conception of humanness portrayed in Huxley's *Brave New World*. Embryos, though they are not complete persons, are still in a distinctive way human and should be regarded with a special sense of awe. Kass's position on embryonic life, however, is not the same as the Vatican's. He holds that early embryos, lacking actual human functions, are not yet fully human. Rather, it is in virtue of their *potential* to become full human beings by normal, self-initiated development that embryos must be accorded a certain degree of respect. In Kass's estimation, this respect entails a position similar to the Vatican's on research involving embryos, but it does allow the most common form of clinical IVF, even recognizing that embryos will be destroyed. For, Kass argues, this loss of embryos is analogous to the loss of embryos in natural reproduction. He then attempts to restrain the use of his principle— that what occurs spontaneously in natural reproduction may be mimicked by deliberate action—from extensions that are unacceptable to him.

On federal funding, Kass reviews arguments in favor of funding of IVF research: the similarity of IVF research to other funded programs, the benefits of IVF, the greater ability to regulate funded activities, and the promoting of U.S. leadership in the field. He concludes, however, that IVF research should not be funded, largely because of the greater importance and benefits to be gained from other uses of those funds, but also because federal money should not be allotted easily for activities about which a large portion of the population has ethical qualms.

Gorovitz

The article by philosopher Samuel Gorovitz was written in response to arguments such as those presented in the article from Kass and in the Vatican statement. Gorovitz's central observation on slippery slope arguments is that they can be, and in medicine characteristically have been, safely negotiated. Abortion, for example, has not led to infanticide. Gorovitz applies the same reasoning to feared effects of IVF on the family, marriage, and our conception of ourselves. Whether or not to worry depends on the empirical likelihood that sound judgment will prevail, and Gorovitz finds no particular reason to worry.

On the status of embryos, Gorovitz attempts to rebut arguments that grant early embryos either the status of human persons or a special status in virtue of their potential. On the first, he observes that embryos do not satisfy even the most minimal necessary condition of personhood: sentience. On the argument from potential, he remarks, as does Edwards, that the egg and sperm that unite to form a fertilized egg have the same potential to be a specific individual before their union as they do afterward. Further, Gorovitz continues, Kass's argument that since embryos are objects of awe they are worthy of a special sort of respect misfires, for many things are objects of awe (single strands of DNA, hydrogen atoms, cadavers) without meriting the treatment Kass advocates.[4]

The article by Gorovitz also contains a useful analysis of senses of the term "natural" (in connection with charges that IVF is unnatural and therefore unacceptable) and a defense of reproductive technology as a proper use of medicine even though it does not cure patients of their malady.

Notes

1. For a sharply critical appraisal of standards of informed consent in the development and use of IVF, see Gena Corea, *The Mother Machine* (New York: Harper & Row, 1985), Part Three, especially chapter 9.

2. For simplicity, the term "embryo" will be used to refer indifferently to all of the early stages of cell development from fertilization on.

3. A sense of the scope of this principle can be gained from its application to embryos that are not viable, i.e., devoid of scientifically confirmable prospects for development or long-term life. Since on this principle even a nonviable embryo *is* human life, a human person, the embryo cannot morally be subjected to adventitious experiments or be casually discarded.

4. The issue of the status of embryos is not the focus of further articles in this anthology. This issue has been at the center of controversies over abortion, and doing justice to these voluminous debates would overwhelm the other important issues raised by reproductive technology. A good anthology of analytical writings on abortion and the status of embryos is Joel Feinberg, ed., *The Problem of Abortion,* 2nd ed. (Belmont, Calif.: Wadsworth, 1984).

Surrogate Motherhood: Not So Novel After All

John A. Robertson

All reproduction is collaborative, for no man or woman reproduces alone. Yet the provision of sperm, egg, or uterus through artificial insemination, embryo transfer, and surrogate mothering makes reproduction collaborative in another way. A third person provides a genetic or gestational factor not present in ordinary paired reproduction. As these practices grow, we must confront the ethical issues raised and their implications for public policy.

Collaborative reproduction allows some persons who otherwise might remain childless to produce healthy children. However, its deliberate separation of genetic, gestational, and social parentage is troublesome. The offspring and participants may be harmed, and there is a risk of confusing family lineage and personal identity. In addition, the techniques intentionally manipulate a natural process that many persons want free of technical intervention. Yet many well-accepted practices, including adoption, artificial insemination by donor (AID), and blended families (families where children of different marriages are raised together) intentionally separate biologic and social parenting and have become an accepted thread in the social fabric. Should all collaborative techniques be similarly treated? When, if ever, are they ethical? Should the law prohibit, encourage, or regulate them, or should the practice be left to private actors? Surrogate motherhood—the controversial practice by which a woman agrees to bear a child conceived by artificial insemination and to relinquish it at birth to others for rearing—illustrates the legal and ethical issues arising in collaborative reproduction generally.

An Alternative to Agency Adoptions

Infertile couples who are seeking surrogates hire attorneys and sign contracts with women recruited through newspaper ads. The practice at present probably involves at most a few hundred persons. But repeated attention on *Sixty Minutes* and the *Phil Donahue Show* and in the popular press is likely to engender more demand, for thousands of infertile couples might find surro-

From *Hastings Center Report* 13 (1983), pp. 28–34. Reproduced by permission. © The Hastings Center.

gate mothers the answer to their reproductive needs. What began as an enterprise involving a few lawyers and doctors in Michigan, Kentucky, and California is now a national phenomenon. There are surrogate mother centers in
Maryland, Arizona, and several other states, and even a surrogate mother
newsletter.

Surrogate mother arrangements occur within a tradition of family law that
gives the gestational mother (and her spouse, if any) rearing rights and obligations. (However, the presumption that the husband is the father can be challenged, and a husband's obligations to his wife's child by AID will usually
require his consent.)[1] Although no state has legislation directly on the subject
of surrogate motherhood, independently arranged adoptions are lawful in
most states. It is no crime to agree to bear a child for another and then
relinquish it for adoption. However, paying the mother a fee for adoption
beyond medical expenses is a crime in some states and in others will prevent
the adoption from being approved.[2] Whether termination and transfer of
parenting rights will be legally recognized depends on the state. Some states,
like Hawaii and Florida, ask few questions and approve independent adoptions very quickly. Others, like Michigan and Kentucky, won't allow surrogate
mothers to terminate and assign rearing rights to another if a fee has been
paid or even allow a paternity determination in favor of the sperm donor. The
enforcibility of surrogate contracts has also not been tested, and it is safe to
assume that some jurisdictions will not enforce them. Legislation clarifying
many of these questions has been proposed in several states but has not yet
been enacted.*

Even this brief discussion highlights an important fact about surrogate
motherhood and other collaborative reproductive techniques. They operate
as an alternative to the nonmarket, agency system of allocating children for
adoption, which has contributed to long queues for distributing healthy
white babies. This form of independent adoption is controlled by the parties,
planned before conception, involves a genetic link with one parent, and
enables both the father and mother of the adopted child to be selected in
advance.

Understood in these terms, the term "surrogate mother," which means
substitute mother, is a misnomer. The natural mother, who contributes egg
and uterus, is not so much a substitute mother as a substitute spouse who
carries a child for a man whose wife is infertile. Indeed, it is the adoptive
mother who is the surrogate mother for the child, since she parents a child
borne by another. What, if anything, is wrong with this arrangement? Let us
look more closely at its benefits and harms before discussing public policy.

---

*Since the original publication of this essay, the New Jersey Supreme Court has invalidated
contracts for surrogacy in the famous Baby M case (see the case study in this anthology), and
several states have passed legislation limiting commercial transactions. Michigan, for example,
has made commercial brokering of surrogacy a criminal offense punishable by a $50,000 fine and
one year in prison—Editor.

All the Parties Can Benefit

Reproduction through surrogate mothering is a deviation from our cultural norms of reproduction, and to many persons it seems immoral or wrong. But surrogate mothering may be a good for the parties involved.

Surrogate contracts meet the desire of a husband and wife to rear a healthy child, and more particularly, a child with one partner's genes. The need could arise because the wife has an autosomal dominant or sex-linked genetic disorder, such as hemophilia. More likely, she is infertile and the couple feels a strong need to have children. For many infertile couples the inability to conceive is a major personal problem causing marital conflict and filling both partners with anguish and self-doubt. It may also involve multiple medical workups and possibly even surgery. If the husband and wife have sought to adopt a child, they may have been told either that they do not qualify or to join the queue of couples waiting several years for agency adoptions (the wait has grown longer due to birth control, abortion, and the greater willingness of unwed mothers to keep their children[3]). For couples exhausted and frustrated by these efforts, the surrogate arrangement seems a godsend. While the intense desire to have a child often appears selfish, we must not lose sight of the deep-seated psychosocial and biological roots of the desire to generate children.[4]

The arrangement may also benefit the surrogate. Usually women undergo pregnancy and childbirth because they want to rear children. But some women want to have the experience of bearing and birthing a child without the obligation to rear. Phillip Parker, a Michigan psychiatrist who has interviewed over 275 surrogate applicants, finds that the decision to be a surrogate springs from several motives.[5] Most women willing to be surrogates have already had children, and many are married. They choose the surrogate role primarily because the fee provides a better economic opportunity than alternative occupations, but also because they enjoy being pregnant and the respect and attention that it draws. The surrogate experience may also be a way to master, through reliving, guilt they feel from past pregnancies that ended in abortion or adoption. Some surrogates may also feel pleased, as organ donors do, that they have given the "gift of life" to another couple.[6]

The child born of a surrogate arrangement also benefits. Indeed, but for the surrogate contract, this child would not have been born at all. Unlike the ordinary agency or independent adoption, where a child is already conceived or brought to term, the conception of this child occurs solely as a result of the surrogate agreement. Thus even if the child does suffer identity problems, as adopted children often do because they are not able to know their mothers, this child has benefited, or at least has not been wronged, for without the surrogate arrangement, she would not have been born at all.[7]

But Problems Exist Too

Surrogate mothering is also troublesome. Many people think that it is wrong for a woman to conceive and bear a child that she does not intend to raise, particularly if she receives a fee for her services. There are potential costs to the surrogate and her family, the adoptive couple, the child, and even society at large from satisfying the generative needs of infertile couples in this way.

The couple must be willing to spend about $20,000–25,000, depending on lawyers' fees and the supply of and demand for surrogate mothers. (While this price tag makes the surrogate contract a consumption item for the middle classes, it is not unjust to poor couples, for it does not leave them worse off than they were.) The couple must also be prepared to experience, along with the adjustment and demands of becoming parents, the stress and anxiety of participating in a novel social relationship that many still consider immoral or deviant. What do they tell their friends or family? What do they tell the child? Will the child have contact with the mother? What is the couple's relationship with the surrogate and her family during the pregnancy and after? Without established patterns for handling these questions, the parties may experience confusion, frustration, and embarrassment.

A major source of uncertainty and stress is likely to be the surrogate herself. In most cases she will be a stranger and may never even meet the couple. The lack of a preexisting relation between the couple and surrogate and the possibility that they live far apart enhance the possibility of mistrust. Is the surrogate taking care of herself? Is she having sex with others during her fertile period? Will she contact the child afterward? What if she demands more money to relinquish the child? To allay these anxieties, the couple could try to establish a relationship of trust with the surrogate, yet such a relationship creates reciprocal rights and duties and might create demands for an undesired relationship after the birth. Even good lawyering that specifies every contingency in the contract is unlikely to allay uncertainty and anxiety about the surrogate's trustworthiness.

The surrogate may also find the experience less satisfying than she envisioned. Conceiving the child may require insemination efforts over several months at inconvenient locations. The pregnancy and birth may entail more pain, unpleasant side effects, and disruption than she expected. The couple may be more intrusive or more aloof than she wishes. As the pregnancy advances and the birth nears, the surrogate may find it increasingly difficult to remain detached by thinking of the child as "theirs" rather than "hers." Relinquishing the baby after birth may be considerably more disheartening and disappointing than she anticipated. Even if informed of this possibility in advance, she may be distressed for several weeks with feelings of loss, depression, and sleep disturbance.[8] She may feel angry at the couple for cutting off all contact with her once the baby is delivered and guilty at giving up her child. Finally, she will have to face the loss of all contact with "her" child. As the reality of her situation dawns, she may regret not having bargained harder for access to "her baby."

As with the couple, the surrogate's experience will vary with the expectations, needs, and personalities of the parties, the course of the pregnancy, and an advance understanding of the problems that can arise. The surrogate should have a lawyer to protect her interests. Often, however, the couple's lawyer will end up advising the surrogate. Although he has recruited the surrogate, he is paid by and represents the couple. By disclosing his conflicting interest, he satisfies legal ethics, but he may not serve the interests of the surrogate as well as independent counsel.

Harms to the Child

Unlike embryo transfer, gene therapy, and other manipulative techniques (some of which are collaborative), surrogate arrangements do not pose the risk of physical harm to the offspring. But there is the risk of psychosocial harm. Surrogate mothering, like adoption and artificial insemination by donor (AID), deliberately separates genetic and gestational from social parentage. The mother who begets, bears, and births does not parent. This separation can pose a problem for the child who discovers it. Like adopted and AID children, the child may be strongly motivated to learn the absent parent's identity and to establish a relationship, in this case with the mother and her family. Inability to make that connection, especially inability to learn who the mother is, may affect the child's self-esteem, create feelings of rootlessness, and leave the child thinking that he had been rejected due to some personal fault.[9] While this is a serious concern, the situation is tolerated when it arises with AID and adoptive children. Intentional conception for adoption—the essence of surrogate mothering—poses no different issue.

The child can also be harmed if the adoptive husband and wife are not fit parents. After all, a willingness to spend substantial money to fulfill a desire to rear children is no guarantee of good parenting. But then neither is reproduction by paired mates who wish intensely to have a child. The nonbiologic parent may resent or reject the child, but the same possibility exists with adoption, AID, or ordinary reproduction.

There is also the fear, articulated by such commentators as Leon Kass and Paul Ramsey,[10] that collaborative reproduction confuses the lineage of children and destroys the meaning of family as we know it. In surrogate mothering, as with ovum or womb donors, the genetic and gestational mother does not rear the child, though the biologic father does. What implications does this hold for the family and the child's lineage?

The separation of the child from the genetic or biologic parent in surrogate mothering is hardly unique. It arises with adoption, but surrogate arrangements are more closely akin to AID or blended families, where at least one parent has a blood tie to the child and the child will know at least one genetic parent. He may, as adopted children often do, have intense desires to learn his biologic mother's identity and seek contact with her and her family. Failure to connect with biologic roots may cause suffering. But the fact that adoption through surrogate mother contracts is planned before conception does not increase the chance of identity confusion, lowered self-esteem, or the blurring of lineage that occurs with adoption or AID.

The greatest chance of confusing family lines arises if the child and couple establish relations with the surrogate and the surrogate's family. If that unlikely event occurs, questions about the child's relations with the surrogate's spouse, parents, and other children can arise. But these issues are not unique. Indeed, they are increasingly common with the growth of blended families. Surrogate mothering in a few instances may lead to a new variation on blended families, but its threat to the family is trivial compared to the rapid changes in family structure now occurring for social, economic, and demographic reasons.

In many cases surrogate motherhood and other forms of collaborative reproduction may shore up, rather than undermine, the traditional family by enabling couples who would otherwise be childless to have children. The practice of employing others to assist in child rearing—including wet-nurses, neonatal ICU nurses, day-care workers, and babysitters—is widely accepted. We also tolerate assistance in the form of sperm sales and donation of egg and gestation (adoption). Surrogate mothering is another method of assisting people to undertake child rearing and thus serves the purposes of the marital union. It is hard to see how its planned nature obstructs that contribution.

Using Birth For Selfish Ends

A basic fear about the new reproductive technologists is that they manipulate a natural physiologic process involved in the creation of human life. When one considers the potential power that resides in our ability to manipulate the genes of embryos, the charges of playing God or arrogantly tampering with nature and the resulting dark Huxleyian vision of genetically engineered babies decanted from bottles are not surprising. While *Brave New World* is the standard text for this fear, the 1982 film *Blade Runner* also evokes it. Trycorp., a genetic engineering corporation, manufactures "replicants," who resemble human beings in most respects, including their ability to remember their childhoods, but who are programmed to die in four years. In portraying the replicants' struggle for a long life and full human status, the film raises a host of ethical issues relevant to gene manipulation, from the meaning of personhood to the duties we have in "fabricating" people to make them as whole and healthy as possible.

Such fears, however, are not a sufficient reason to stop splicing genes or relieving infertility through external fertilization.[11] In any event they have no application to surrogate mothering, which does not alter genes or even manipulate the embryo. The only technological aid is a syringe to inseminate and a thermometer to determine when ovulation occurs. Although embryo manipulation would occur if the surrogate received the fertilized egg of another woman, the qualms about surrogate mothering stem less from its potential for technical manipulation, and more from its attitude toward the body and mother-child relations. Mothers bear and give up children for adoption rather frequently when the conception is unplanned. But here the mother conceives the child for that purpose, deliberately using her body for a fee to serve the needs of others. It is the cold willingness to use her body as a baby-making machine and deny the mother-child gestational bond that bothers. (Ironically, the natural bond may turn out to be deeper and stronger than the surrogate imagined.)

Since the transfer of rearing duties from the natural gestational mother to others is widely accepted, the unwillingness of the surrogate mother to rear her child cannot in itself be wrong. As long as she transfers rearing responsibility to capable parents, she is not acting irresponsibly. Still, some persons assert that it is wrong to use the reproductive process for ends other than the good of the child.[12] But the mere presence of selfish motives does not render reproduction immoral, as long as it is carried out in a way that respects the child's interests. Otherwise most pregnancies and births would be immoral, for people have children to serve individual ends as well as the good of the child. In terms of instrumentalism, surrogate mothering cannot be distinguished from most other reproductive situations, whether AID, adoption, or simply planning a child to experience the pleasures of parenthood.

In this vein the problems that can arise when a defective child is born are cited as proof of the immorality of surrogate mothering. The fear is that neither the contracting couple nor the surrogate will want the defective child. In one recent case* (*New York Times,* January 28, 1983, p. 18) a dispute arose when none of the parties wanted to take a child born with microcephaly, a condition related to mental retardation. The contracting man claimed on the basis of blood typing that the baby was not his and thus he was not obligated under the contract to take it or to pay the surrogate's fee. It turned out that surrogate had borne her husband's child, for she had unwittingly become pregnant by him before being artificially inseminated by the contracting man. The surrogate and her husband eventually assumed responsibility for the child.

An excessively instrumental and callous approach to reproduction when a less than perfect baby is born is not unique to surrogate mothering. Similar reactions can occur whenever married couples have a defective child, as the Baby Doe controversy, which involved the passive euthanasia of a child with Down syndrome, indicates. All surrogate mothering is not wrong because in some instances a handicapped child will be rejected. Nor is it clear that this reaction is more likely in surrogate mothering than in conventional births, for it reflects common attitudes toward handicapped newborns as much as alienation in the surrogate arrangement.

*See the case study in this anthology entitled "Parenting through Contract When No One Wants the Child"—Editor.

As with most situations, "how" something is done is more important than the mere fact of doing it. The morality of surrogate mothering thus depends on how the duties and responsibilities of the role are carried out, rather than on the mere fact that a couple produces a child with the aid of a collaborator. Depending on the circumstances, a surrogate mother can be praised as a benefactor to a suffering couple (the money is hardly adequate compensation) or condemned as a callous user of offspring to further her selfish ends. The view that one takes of her actions will also influence the role one wants the law to play.

What Should the State's Role Be?

What stance should public policy and the law take toward surrogate mothering? As with all collaborative reproduction, a range of choices exists, from prohibition and regulation to active encouragement.

However, there may be constitutional limits to the state's power to restrict collaborative reproduction. The right not to procreate, through contraception and abortion, is now firmly established.[13] A likely implication of these cases, supported by rulings in other cases, is that married persons (and possibly single persons) have a right to bear, beget, birth, and parent children by natural coital means using such technological aids (microsurgery and in vitro fertilization, for example) as are medically available. It should follow that married persons also have a right to engage in noncoital, collaborative reproduction, at least where natural reproduction is not possible. The right of a couple to raise a child should not depend on their luck in the natural lottery if they can obtain the missing factor of reproduction from others.[14]

If a married couple's right to procreative autonomy includes the right to contract with consenting collaborators, then the state will have a heavy burden of justification for infringing that right. The risks to [the] surrogate, couple, and child do not seem sufficiently compelling to meet this burden, for they are no different from the harms of adoption and AID. Nor will it suffice to point to a communal feeling that such uses of the body are—aside from the consequences—immoral. Moral distaste alone does not justify interference with a fundamental right.

Although surrogate mothering is not now criminal, this discussion is not purely hypothetical. The ban in Michigan and several other states on paying fees for adoption beyond medical expenses has the same effect as an outright prohibition, for few surrogates will volunteer for altruistic reasons alone. A ban on fees is not necessary to protect the surrogate mother from coercion or exploitation, or to protect the child from abuse, the two objectives behind passage of those laws. Unlike the pregnant unmarried woman who "sells" her child, the surrogate has made a considered, knowing choice, often with the assistance of counsel, before becoming pregnant. She may, of course, choose to be a surrogate for financial reasons, but offering money to do unpleasant tasks is not in itself coercive.

Nor does the child's welfare support a ban on fees, for the risk is no greater than in natural paired reproduction that the parents will be unfit or abuse the child. The specter of slavery, which some opposed to surrogate mothering have raised, is unwarranted. It is quibbling to question whether the couple is "buying" a child or the mother's personal services. Quite clearly, the couple is buying the right to rear a child by paying the mother to beget and bear one for that very purpose. But the purchasers do not buy the right to treat the child or surrogate as a commodity or property. Child abuse and neglect laws still apply, with criminal and civil sanctions available for mistreatment.

The main concern with fees rests on moral and aesthetic grounds. An affront to moral sensibility arises over paying money for a traditionally non-commercial, intimate function. Even though blood and sperm are sold, and miners, professional athletes, and petrochemical workers sell some of their health and vitality, some persons think it wrong for women to bear children for money, in much the same way that paying money for sex or body organs is considered wrong. Every society excludes some exchanges from the market-place on moral grounds. But the state's power to block exchanges that inter-fere with the exercise of a fundamental right is limited. Since blocking this exchange stops infertile couples from reproducing and rearing the husband's child, a harm greater than moral distaste is necessary to justify it.

Although the state cannot block collaborative reproductive exchanges on moral grounds, it need not subsidize or encourage surrogate contracts. One could argue that allowing the parties to a surrogate contract to use the courts to terminate parental rights, certify paternity, and legalize adoption is a sub-sidy and therefore not required of the state. Similarly, a state's refusal to enforce surrogate contracts as a matter of public policy could be taken as a refusal to subsidize rather than as interference with the right to reproduce. But given the state's monopoly of those functions and the impact its denial will have on the ability of infertile couples to find reproductive collaborators, it is more plausible to view the refusal to certify and effectuate contracts as an infringement of the right to procreate. Denying an adoption because it was agreed upon in advance for a fee intereferes with the couple's procreative autonomy as much as any criminal penalty for paying a fee to or contracting with a collaborator. (The crucial distinction between infering with and not encouraging the exercise of a right has been overlooked by the Michigan and Kentucky courts that have held constitutional the refusal to allow adoptions or paternity determinations where a fee has been paid to the surrogate mother. This error makes these cases highly questionable precedents.[15])

A conclusion that surrogate contracts must be *enforced,* however, does not require that they be specifically carried out in all instances. As long as damage remedies remain, there is no constitutional right to specific performance. For example, a court need not enjoin the surrogate who changes her mind about abortion or relinquishing the child once it is born. A surrogate who wants to breach the contract by abortion should pay damages, but not be ordered to continue the pregnancy, because of the difficulty in enforcing or monitoring the order. (Whether damages are a practical alternative in such cases will depend on the surrogate's economic situation, or whether bonding or insurance to assure her contractual obligation is possible.) On the other hand, a court could reasonably order the surrogate after birth to relinquish the child. Whether such an order should issue will depend on whether the surrogate's interest in keeping the child is deemed greater than the couple's interest in rearing (assuming that both are fit parents). A commitment to freedom of contract and the rights of parties to arrange collaborative reproduction would favor the adoptive couple, while sympathy for the gestational bond between mother and child would favor the mother. If the mother prevailed, the couple should still have other remedies, including visitation rights for the father, restitution of the surrogate's fee and other expenses, and perhaps money damages as well.

The constitutional status of a married couple's procreative choice shields collaborative arrangements from interference on moral grounds alone, but not from all regulation. While the parties may assign the rearing rights according to contract, the state need not leave the entire transaction to the vagaries of the private sector. Regulation to minimize harm and assure knowing choices would be permissible, as long as the regulation is reasonably related to promoting these goals.

For example, the state could set minimum standards for surrogate brokers, set age and health qualifications for surrogates, and structure the transaction to assure voluntary, knowing choices. The state could also define and allocate responsibilities among the parties to protect the best interests of the offspring—for example, refusing to protect the surrogate's anonymity, requiring that the contracting couple assume responsibility for a defective child, or even transferring custody to another if threats to the child's welfare justify such a move.

Not What We Do—But How We Do It

The central issue with surrogate mothering, as with other collaborative reproduction, is not the deliberate separation of biologic and social parentage, but how the separation is effected and the resulting relationship with the third party. If the third party's involvement in the reproduction is discrete and limited, collaborative reproduction is easily tolerated. Thus few people question the anonymous sperm donor's lack of rights and duties toward the offspring, except in the case where the mother and donor have expressly agreed that he would have some access to the rearing of a child.[16] The donor's claim—and possibly the child's need to connect—is less strong in such cases. Egg donations, though involving more risk and burden for the donor, should be similarly treated, for they are also discrete and limited.

Collaborative reproduction involving gestational contributors poses more difficult problems, because the nine-month gestational period creates a unique and powerful bond for both donor and offspring that seems to justify a claim in its own right. Yet in adoption we allow those claims to be nullified by the gestational mother's choice. Surrogate motherhood presents the same issue. The difference is that it is planned before conception, but that hardly seems to matter once the child is born and the mother wishes to fulfill her commitment. The issue of whether the mother should be held to a promise on which others have relied is distinct from the question of whether mothers can relinquish children deliberately conceived for others outside the agency-controlled adoption process.

Surrogate mothering casts particular light on one other collaborative technique that may soon be widely available—the transfer of the externally (or internally) fertilized egg of one woman to another woman who gestates and births it.[17] The third party in this situation is a gestational surrogate for a genetic and rearing mother, who is unable or unwilling to bear and birth her child. At first glance the gestational mother's claim to the child seems less compelling than the claim of the surrogate mother because the child is not genetically hers. Yet concerns will arise, as with surrogate mothers, over the severing or denial of the gestational bond, the degree to which the contract should be honored, and the gestational mother's relationship (if any) with the child.

The moral issues surrounding surrogate mothering also cast light on the problems with manipulative techniques such as genetic alteration of the embryo and nonuterine gestation of the fertilized egg. Since those techniques will be used primarily for paired reproduction, the main concerns will be the safety of the offspring and the morality of genetic manipulation. However, when manipulation and collaborative reproduction are combined, the relationship of the offspring to the third-party contributor will come into question.

Surrogate mothering for a fee is neither the evil nor the panacea that many have thought. It is barely distinguishable from the many current practices that separate biologic and social parentage and that seek parenthood for personal satisfaction. The differences do not appear to be great enough to justify prohibition, active discouragement, or for that matter, encouragement. Like many human endeavors, in the final analysis, what matters is not *whether* but *how* it is done. In that respect public scrutiny, through regulation of the process of drawing up the contract rather than its specific terms, could help to assure that it is done well.

Notes

The author gratefully acknowledges the comments of Rebecca Dresser, Mark Frankel, Inga Markovits, Phillip Parker, Bruce Russell, John Sampson, and Ted Schneyer on earlier drafts.

1. People v. Sorenson, 68 Cal. 2d 280, 437 P.2d 495; Walter Wadlington, "Artificial Insemination: The Dangers of a Poorly Kept Secret," *Northwestern Law Review* 64 (1970), 777.

2. See, for example, Michigan Statutes Annotated, 27.3178 (555.54)(555.69) (1980).

3. Elisabeth Landes and Richard Posner, "The Economics of the Baby Shortage," *Journal of Legal Studies* 7 (1978), 323.

4. See Erik Erikson, *The Life Cycle Completed* (New York: Norton, 1980), pp. 122–124.

5. Phillip Parker, "Surrogate Mother's Motivations: Initial Findings," *American Journal of Psychiatry* 140:1 (January 1983), 117–118; Phillip Parker, "The Psychology of Surrogate Motherhood: A Preliminary Report of a Longitudinal Pilot Study" (unpublished). See also Dava Sobel, "Surrogate Mothers: Why Women Volunteer," *New York Times,* June 25, 1981, p. 18.

6. Mark Frankel, "Surrogate Motherhood: An Ethical Perspective," pp. 1–2. (Paper presented at Wayne State Symposium on Surrogate Motherhood, Nov. 20, 1982.)

7. See John Robertson, "In Vitro Conception and Harm to the Unborn," *Hastings Center Report* 8 (October 1978), 13–14; Michael Bayles, "Harm to the Unconceived," *Philosophy and Public Affairs* 5 (1976), 295.

8. A small, uncontrolled study found these effects to last some four to six weeks. Statement of Nancy Reame, R.N., at Wayne State University, Symposium on Surrogate Motherhood, Nov. 20, 1982.

9. Betty Jane Lifton, *Twice Born: Memoirs of an Adopted Daughter* (New York: Penguin, 1977); L. Dusky, "Brave New Babies," *Newsweek,* Dec. 6, 1982, p. 30.

10. Leon Kass, "Making Babies—the New Biology and the Old Morality," *The Public Interest* 26 (1972), 18; "Making Babies Revisited," *The Public Interest* 54 (1979), 32; Paul Ramsey, *Fabricated Man: The Ethics of Genetic Control* (New Haven: Yale University Press, 1970).

11. The President's Commission for the Study of Ethical Problems in Medicine and Biomedical and Behavioral Research, *Splicing Life: The Social and Ethical Issues of Genetic Engineering with Human Beings* (Washington, D.C., 1982), pp. 53–60.

12. Herbert Krimmel, Testimony before California Assembly Committee on Judiciary, Surrogate Parenting Contracts (November 14, 1982), pp. 89–96.

13. Griswold v. Connecticut, 381 U.S. 479 (1964); Eisenstadt v. Baird, 405 U.S. 438 (1972): Roe v. Wade, 410 U.S. 113 (1973); Planned Parenthood v. Danforth, 428 U.S. 52 (1976); Bellotti v. Baird, 443 U.S. 622 (1979); Carey v. Population Services International, 431 U.S. 678 (1977).

14. Although this article does not address the right of single persons to contract with others for reproductive purposes, it should be noted that the right of married persons to engage in collaborative reproduction does not entail a similar right for unmarried persons. For a more detailed exposition of the arguments for the reproductive rights of married and single persons, see John Robertson, "Procreative Liberty and the Control of Conception, Pregnancy and Childbirth," *Virginia Law Review* 69 (April 1983), 405, 418–420.

15. See Doe v. Kelley, 106 Mich. App. 164, 307 N.W.2d 438 (1981); Syrkowski v. Appleyard, 9 Family Law Rptr. 2348 (April 5, 1983); In re Baby Girl, 9 Family Law Reptr. 2348 (March 8, 1983).

16. See C.M. v. C.C., 152 N.J. 160, 377 A.2d 821 (man who provided sperm for artificial insemination held to have visitation rights because of express agreement with the mother).

17. See Richard D. Lyons, "2 Women Become Pregnant with Transferred Embryos," *New York Times,* July 22, 1983, p. A1, B7.

Surrogate Mother Arrangements from the Perspective of the Child

Herbert T. Krimmel

A dozen or so years from now, when the children already born from surrogate mother arrangements start to ask questions about the way in which they were brought into this world, what will we tell them? What can we expect their feelings to be?[1]

They will learn that they were different from other babies, that they were the product of what some call "collaborative reproduction."[2] They will discover that what this means in their cases is that their biological mothers decided to conceive them, not because their biological mothers wanted to raise, know, and love them, but for some other reasons. That, for these other reasons, their biological mothers entered into contracts to transfer custody of them to their biological fathers and their biological fathers' wives,[3] in order to fulfill a need that those couples had: the desire to experience the joys of having a baby.

If the emotional experiences of adopted children are a guide,[4] the children born under surrogate mother arrangements will want to know why their mothers gave them up. How will these children feel about the various reasons surrogate mothers[5] are giving today for why they enter into surrogate mother arrangements? And, if the experiences of adopted children are a guide, the children born under surrogate mother arrangements will want to know more than just the why of it. They will also want to know *how* it was possible for their biological mothers to have given them up. Will these children find complete solace for the fact that their mothers were able to part with them in the love of the parents who raised them?

And how will these children feel about the parents who raised them? What will they think about their parents' arranging for their existence with contracts, terms, conditions, and warranties? How will they feel that they had to meet specifications before their intended parents had to accept them?

How will these children feel about the language that surrogate mothers use to describe themselves and them?

From *Logos: Philosophic Issues in Christian Perspectives* 9 (1988), pp. 97–112. Notes abridged. Reprinted with permission.

The purpose of this article is to address the practice of surrogate parenting from the perspective of the children who will be born under these arrangements in order, I hope, to convince you that surrogate mother arrangements are both unethical and inimical to the interests of children and of society.

The Ethical Problem with
Surrogate Mother Arrangements

What is fundamentally unethical about surrogate mother arrangements is that they, of necessity, treat the creation of a person as the means to the gratification of the interests of others, rather than respect the child as an end in himself.[6] They treat a person (the child) as though he were a thing, a commodity.

Essential and indispensible to the operation of each and every surrogate mother arrangement is the shared and common intention of the parties to transfer the baby at birth from his biological mother to his adopting parents. But surrogate mother arrangements are more than just contracts about the custody of children vis-à-vis their biological parents. They are also contracts for the creation of children,[7] the irreducible core of which is that the surrogate mother must be willing to create a child with the premeditated intention to transfer him at birth. By the very nature of the transaction, the surrogate mother cannot desire to keep the child. Nor can she make a pretense to valuing the child in and for himself, since she would not otherwise be creating the child but for the monetary and other emotional consideration she receives under the surrogate mother contract.[8] Indeed, the very purpose and designs of the surrogate mother arrangement is to separate in the mind of the surrogate mother her decision to create the child from the decision to have and raise that child. Her desire to create the child must necessarily be the result of some motive other than the desire to be a parent. The child is conceived, not because he is wanted by his biological mother, but because he can be useful to her and others. He is conceived in order to be given away.

The Motivations of Surrogate Mothers

Why do the women who sign up to be surrogate mothers enter into surrogate mothers arrangements? According to the reasons thus far advanced by surrogate mothers themselves and those who have studied them:[9]

1. Most do it for the money. Ninety percent of surrogate mothers say they would not be surrogates if they were only reimbursed for their expenses.
2. Many do it in order to deal with some past emotional trauma. About one-third of the surrogate mothers in the Parker study say that an important reason for them is to work through guilt, or other negative

feelings, associated with a past abortion or with the giving up of a child for adoption.

3. Some of them do it, at least in part, because they enjoy being pregnant. These women cite as reasons both enjoyment of the physical sensations of being pregnant and of receiving the cultural deference and attention accorded pregnant women.
4. Many cite the so-called "altruistic" motive. They want to do something nice for someone else, often expressed as wanting to give an infertile couple "the gift of life."
5. The vast majority normally give some combination of the above as their motivation.

What is clearly absent from this list of reasons for procreating a child, and what *must* be absent for surrogate mother arrangements to work, is the motive of wanting the child. For, if the desire to have and raise the child were more important to surrogate mothers than the motives listed above, they could never enter into a surrogate mother arrangement.

However one may feel about the relative merits of the surrogate mothers' various motives, common to them all is the use of the child as a means to the surrogate mother's happiness. Each of the motives given above clearly indicates that the child is being *valued* by the surrogate mother primarily, if not exclusively, for his utility as a means to her economic or psychological well-being. The child is a source of income, therapy, self-esteem, or good feelings. That, is his raison d'etre. Implicitly, if not explicitly, the child has a price.

Even the so-called "altruistic" motive is not altruistic at all when viewed from the perspective of the child. Children should not be given away as elegant gifts to make others happy for the same reason one does not give one's spouse to a lonely friend. To do so is to treat them as things and not as persons. Moreover, it quite clearly communicates to the person being given away that he is of less importance to you than the happiness of the third party.

Regarding the Motives of Parents in Natural Procreation

But, it has been asked,[10] how are the motives of surrogate mothers really all that different from those of parents who use natural means of procreation? Professor Robertson argues that with natural parents "ends and means intertwine. Children are instruments for parental meaning and satisfaction, at the same time that they are loved for themselves."[11] He goes on to argue that "[p]ersons making this charge [that surrogate mother arrangements are ethically wrong because they use children as a means] usually overlook how traditional reproductive practices could also be condemned on this basis."[12] Professor Robertson's comparison is erroneous for two reasons: first, because one evil does not justify another; and second, because it overlooks a very important distinction.

For any parent to treat his child, however conceived or acquired, solely as a means,[13] seems to me to be a pretty good theoretical definition of child abuse. We readily perceive and condemn this type of behavior in the case of overly ambitious parents, for example, those more interested in having a famous child actress, Olympian, pianist, and so on, than they are in their child's welfare. Surrogate mother arrangements, however, are not justified because parents using natural means of procreation *could* commit equal evils.[14] They are condemned because they cannot, by their very nature, rise to an ethical treatment of children that is possible for natural parents. Which, leads to the second fallacy in Professor Robertson's comparison.

Interestingly enough, though, Professor Robertson has unwittingly suggested the answer to his own argument. The distinction that he fails to recognize is that for the surrogate mother the ends and means *cannot* intertwine. She cannot treat the child as an end valued for himself alone if she is going to enter into a surrogate mother contract, while, conversely, with natural procreation it is *possible*[15] for the parents to treat their child as an end.

Furthermore, that natural parents commonly do have mixed motives for having children, valuing them for themselves, while at the same time expecting to derive pleasure from them, is not ethically impermissible, so long as the latter does not preclude the former. To use Kantian ideology, the pursuit of one's happiness and the performance of one's moral duty (to treat persons as ends) may coincide. For example, one may enter into a marriage expecting to enjoy conjugal relations, but to value one's husband solely as a means of sexual gratification is to turn him, in your mind, into a prostitute. One may enter into marriage expecting to receive financial support, aid, and succor, but to view one's wife solely as a means of support is to treat her, in your mind, as though she were a slave.

What is this treatment of the child as an end, that natural parents are capable of, but surrogate mothers cannot attain and still be surrogate mothers? It is to love the child simply for who he is, selflessly and unconditionally. It is not possible for the surrogate mother even to make a pretense of loving the child in this manner[16] when she would not have created him but for the dual assurances that someone else would take him off her hands at birth *and* make it worth her while.

Why Surrogate Mother Arrangements and Adoption Are Different

If this is true, how is it possible for adoption to be ethical?[17] How is it possible to voluntarily part with someone you truly love? You cannot, by definition,[18] if it is in exchange for something else; no, not even for good feelings. You can only do so if it is solely for the good of the one you love. In other words, only if it is a selfless act. The distinction between surrogate mother arrangements and adoption is that the latter can be a selfless act of love, while the former cannot be.[19]

The typical situations that give rise to the placement of a child for adoption are (1) the child was unintentionally conceived and his mother decides to bring him to term or (2) the parents desired to have a child, but because of some serious and unfortunate circumstances arising after conception decide that they cannot keep him. What is important for our discussion, however, is what does not happen in adoption. There, the child's mother does not conceive him for the purpose of giving him up. Adoption is an emergency: What will we do with the baby if the mother cannot keep him? Surrogate mother arrangements, on the other hand, are premeditated.

This results in a distinction of ethical importance. In adoption, the mother can make her decision on whether to keep the child or to place him for adoption on the basis of what is the best interests of the child, regardless of her own preferences. What she cannot legally do is sell the child. The surrogate mother, on the other hand, does not, and cannot, decide the question of the child's custody on the basis of what is in the child's best interests. That is what is expressly precluded by the very idea of surrogate parenting. She must have decided this issue on the basis of contract even before the child was conceived, and for reasons that suited her purposes.

Why the Love of the Adopting Parents Is Not Enough

But, it might be asked, why should it matter what the motivation of the surrogate mother is, when according to the surrogate mother arrangement it has been prearranged that the child will be taken by an adopting couple? Why isn't the love of the adopting couple a complete and adequate substitute for that of the surrogate mother?[20]

Parental love is not fungible. One wouldn't expect a child who is unloved by his father to find complete solace in his mother's devotion. To demur to a child's question of why his mother didn't love him enough to keep him, by saying that he needn't trouble himself seeking an answer to that question because someone else loves him, is not an emotionally adequate answer. If anything, our experience with adopted children should have taught us this: that children suffer terribly about the question of why they were given away. (And we are starting to see a similar manifestation of this phenomenon with children conceived through artificial insemination by donor.[21]) Parental love is not fungible any more than romantic love is. One does not comfort a person who has just lost his spouse with the thought that the "woods are full" of eligible persons of the opposite gender.

An adopted child deeply appreciates the love of his adopting family, but he feels the loss of his biological parents nevertheless. At least the adopted child—although still feeling the loss—can perhaps find some consolation in the explanation, if true, that his parents loved him but couldn't keep him. This explanation cannot be used to comfort the child conceived through a surrogate mother arrangement for the simple reason that the surrogate mother never wanted the child for herself.[22]

In surrogate mother arrangements it is only a deflection, not an answer, to tell a child that because some other people love him, it is unimportant that his mother did not love him enough to keep him. Such a response willfully misses the emotional point of the child's question. This inquiry is made all the more poignant because the surrogate mother's giving up of her baby was not unavoidable, which the child might otherwise eventually come to understand and forgive. Rather, it was the very essence of the deal, without which the child would never have been conceived. The child will come to learn that it was *only because* his mother had the assurance of a binding contract that she could give him up for the money for which she conceived him in the first place. That is, this child came into existence on order, as a custom-made commodity for a guaranteed purchaser. Can any child be expected to understand, much less forgive, that?

The Motivations of Adopting Parents

Why do the adopting parents enter into surrogate mother arrangements? Typically, those who are currently[23] seeking to utilize surrogate mother arrangements are, for the most part, infertile couples. They generally have gone to great lengths to remedy their infertility, and when that proved to be of no avail, they sought to adopt infants. Their attempts to adopt children proved unsatisfactory or frustrating to them either because they were turned down, or they were able to adopt children but were discouraged by the long wait (for white infants), or they were dissatisfied with the type of children available for immediate adoption (that is, older, "wrong race," handicapped, retarded). A few couples utilizing surrogate mother arrangements never sought to adopt. They are particularly attracted to the surrogate mother arrangement because it results in a child with a biological link to one of the adopting parents, which they find to be a highly desirable advantage in comparison with adoption. These couples would choose surrogate mother arrangements in preference to adoption.

What motivates the adopting parents is, for the most part, the desire to raise a child. So, what can be wrong with this desire? And, what can be wrong with the desire to procreate and raise a child of one's own blood in preference to adopting a child? Isn't that what almost all of us desire? Nothing is wrong with those desires per se. What is wrong is what is being done in utilizing surrogate mother arrangements in order to satisfy these desires. Surrogate mother arrangements are wrong because you should not purchase[24] people;[25] because a child should not be an item of manufacture, which you create to specifications as you would a car; and because persons do not *exist* for your pleasure or in order to fulfill your needs. And yet, this is precisely the type of thinking that surrogate mother arrangements necessarily encourage and inevitably entail.[26] The evil that surrogate mother arrangements do is to deprive the child of the dignity to which he is entitled as a person by treating him as a means. It matters not that the adopting parents' objective is worthy if their method of obtaining it is corrupt.

Commodification: The Result of Treating and Perceiving the Child as a Means Rather Than as an End

It is when children are thought of as existing in order to fulfill needs that they become, in our minds, commodities. Surrogate mother arrangements entail and embody this type of thinking in two related ways: first, simply by virtue of the fact that they are, in essence, contracts for the creation and custody of children; second, because they encourage and tempt the adopting parents to view children as items of manufacture.

The surrogate mother and the adopting couple enter into the surrogate mother contract for the same reason that any person contracts: because the subject matter of the contract is more highly valued by one party than its quid pro quo, and vice versa. A contract is thereby designed to maximize the satisfaction of the contracting parties, and the subject matter of the contract is seen as a means to this end. The interests of the thing traded (if such a notion has any meaning at all) is unimportant.[27]

One hundred years ago, if an expecting couple were asked whether they wanted a boy or a girl, it was largely an idle question. They took what they got. If they had a preference, which they very well might, there was very little they could do about it. It was not a preference about which they expected to be able to exercise control. Today, with the techniques of amniocentesis, ultrasound, and sperm centrifuge, one can choose the sex of one's children. And, as our knowledge of genetics and, equally important, our ability to manipulate and engineer results increases, the proponents of collaborative reproduction invite us in earnest to consider what type of baby we would like—even arguing that the parents have a "right" to so decide.[28] What they do not seem to consider is that what is being invited is also a change in our attitude toward children. Their viewpoint would move us away from a simple, loving, and grateful acceptance of the child we in fact receive and toward a critical consumerism of the "perfect" child we're entitled to, can afford, and therefore must have.[29]

The proffered *ability* to pick and choose builds expectations. It does with products. It will, and already has, with children.[30] Why does one buy a product? Because it fulfills a real or perceived need. How does one value a product? By how well it performs in fulfilling one's expectations. Defective and inferior products are those that disappoint us. What implications does this have for the child? If the parents have a right to a perfect baby of their own design, who has the correlative duty? Does it not become the baby's duty to please his parents and to meet their expectations? Is it any surprise that a recent study of 8,000 abortions performed at clinics in Bombay, India, reveals that 7,997 of them were of female fetuses?

That surrogate mother arrangements do encourage and tempt the adopting parents to think of the child born through that process as a means to their happiness is quite evident from the not so subtle language used by them and the proponents of surrogate mothering.[31] One magazine article quotes an

adopting couple as referring to their "right to have a normal newborn infant."[31] To speak as though your need and desire to have a child give rise to a
"right" to a child is wrong for the same reason it would be wrong to argue that
your loneliness entitles you to a spouse. It is neither your needs nor your
desires that provide the justification for another's existence. It is wrong to act
and talk as though another person's reason for being were to satisfy your
needs, to be the means to your happiness.

Does the Child Have Grounds to Complain?

Professor Robertson has argued that "[e]ven if there is a higher degree of
confusion, unhappiness, or maladjustment in donor-assisted reproduction, a
child would seem better off under this collaborative structure than not to exist
at all."[33] Be that as it may, one may agree that no human life is without value
and still find the practice of surrogate parenting to be unethical. By analogy,
although it might be both objectively true, and subjectively felt, that a life
without the use of one's legs is preferable to no life at all, that does not mean
that a person would not be wronged by someone intentionally setting forth to
manufacture him without legs in order to serve another's purposes.[34] By
Professor Robertson's logic, no black American could object that his ancestors were brought to this country as slaves, since otherwise he most probably
would not be living here today. That an evil act may have good consequences
as well as bad ones does not justify the act, allow the actor to take credit for
them, or erase the stain of their origin.

The fundamental mistake underlying Professor Robertson's argument is
that he addresses the wrong question. Even if the children born under surrogate mother arrangements are objectively "better off" in comparison with
non-existence, and even if we presume hypothetically that subjectively they
would prefer life with these impairments in preference to no life at all, this
does not mean that they were not wronged. The ethical issue is not resolved
simply by knowing that the impairments imposed by surrogate parenting
have not succeeded in depriving the child's life of all value, or even by
knowing whether the child would have consented if presented with the limited choice of having either an impaired existence or no existence at all.
Rather, we must also address the question of why, in the first place, the
parents should have a right to premeditatedly create a child with planned
and intended impairments.[35]

Viewed from this perspective the answer becomes clear. It is unethical for
parents to treat their children as things even if such acts do not succeed in
depriving their children's lives of all meaning. And, furthermore, it is not
right to treat persons as means, and not as ends, even if they grudgingly[36]
consent to being so treated. For example, I suppose one could also say that
sweatshop laborers are objectively "better off" than having no jobs at all, but
this would not make taking advantage of their plight by paying them less than
a fair wage ethically justifiable. Neither are blackmail or armed robbery justi-

fied because the victim chooses the subjectively less loathsome alternative presented to him. Indeed, we do not even hold the consent of the victim to be valid in such instances, and not because it didn't reflect the victim's true preference on the occasion of his choice, but rather, because we don't consider the person who forced the choice upon him as entitled to make the victim choose from such a limited menu. Simply stated, one is not entitled to purposely stack the deck with Hobson's choices and then plead consent as a justification for one's evil act.

Professor Robertson has discovered that children are largely at the mercy of their parents. This, however, should be a cause for heightened responsibility, not for exploitation. People do not have an obligation to create children. The choice is theirs, but that choice does not encompass the right to abuse them.[37]

Conclusion

Surrogate mother arrangements are unethical. They preclude the surrogate mother from treating the child as an end in himself, and they strongly encourage and tempt the adopting couple to do the same. What is at stake here, however, is more than some persnickety concern over moral tidiness. The children born from these surrogate mother arrangements are going to hurt for the same reasons you and I would hurt. The ethical concerns I have raised in this article are those born of a concern for their feelings.

Coda

It is reported that following the birth of a baby girl in April 1986, twenty-three-year-old Shannon Boff of Redford Township, Michigan, having twice been a surrogate mother, announced her retirement with these words: "Any more babies coming form me are going to be keepers."[38] The fundamental question the advocates of surrogate mother arrangements must answer is why any child should have to grow up with the knowledge that he was created in order to be "given" away, that *he* was not a keeper.

Notes

1. Many perhaps will dismiss this questioning as hypothetical and speculative. After all, who can know how anyone will feel in the future, and can't we expect that there will be a broad range of feelings on the part of these children? Generalization? Certainly. It is the general case that we want to inquire about: What will the typical child born of these surrogate mother arrangements feel? Yes, we can expect that different persons might exhibit a range of reactions to being orphaned, for example, but no one doubts that for the average orphan it must be a thoroughly miserable

feeling—a feeling that anyone who was once three years old and "lost" his mommy in the department store can relate to. (But see note 34, infra.) Speculation? Perhaps. But if so, it is one for which there is a strong basis in fact arising from the known experiences of adopted children, a schooled speculation based on what we have learned from past analogous experiences. The same rule that teaches me that if I wouldn't like something done to me, probably you won't like it done to you either. Perhaps we are engaging in speculation, but if so, it is what we had better do for the sake of these children.

2. J. Robertson, *Embryos, Families, and Procreative Liberty: The Legal Structure of the New Reproduction,* 59 S. Cal. L. Rev. 939, 1001 (1986) [hereinafter cited as Robertson (1986)].

3. For simplicity, I will refer hereafter in this article to the biological father and his wife as the "adopting parents."

4. See generally, A. Sorosky et al., *The Adoption Triangle* (1978); and see Testimony of Suzanne Rubin before the California Assembly Committee on Judiciary, Surrogate Parenting Contracts, Assembly Publication No. 962, pp. 72–75 (Nov. 19, 1982) (hereinafter cited as Rubin); C. Gorney, *For Love and Money,* California Magazine p. 88, at 151 (Oct. 1983) (hereinafter cited as Gorney).

5. Although I am in complete accord with Katha Pollitt's point that we should refer to the surrogate mother simply as the mother, since the term mother "describes the relationship of a woman to a child, not to the father of that child and his wife" (K. Pollitt, *The Strange Case of Baby M,* 244 The Nation 667, at 682–83 (May 23, 1987) (hereinafter cited as Pollitt), nevertheless, the term "surrogate mother" unfortunately has caught hold, and I have decided to continue to use it for the sake of clarity. But see *In re Baby M.,* 537 A. 2d 1227, 1234 (N.J., 1988).

6. See I. Kant, *Metaphysical Foundations of Morals* (1785) in C. Fredrich (ed.), The Philosophy of Kant, 176–78 (1949) (hereinafter cited as Kant).

7. There has been a lot of loose talk that surrogate mother arrangements are not baby bartering because the adopting parents are merely renting the services of the surrogate mother. See, e.g., *In re Baby M.,* 525 A.2d 1128, 1160 (N.J. Super. Ch., 1987), *rev'd,* 537 A.2d 1227 (N.J., 1988) (hereinafter cited as *In re Baby M.*—Ch. Ct. Opn.). The argument is a red herring. Surrogate mother arrangements are about procuring babies. The adopting couple want the end product and would dearly love to dispense with the services of the surrogate if they could. In general they have tried, having only come to surrogacy after attempting to acquire a baby by adoption. As has been pointed out by Professor Capron (L.A. Times, April 7, 1987, Sec. II, p. 5, col. 7) and others, most surrogate mother contracts only provide for compensation to the surrogate mother on delivery of a baby, no payment being made if the surrogate miscarries (i.e., renders the service but fails to deliver the product). But even the more sophisticated contracts currently being drafted, which provide for some compensation to the surrogate mother if she miscarries, do not change what these contracts are about. Surrogate mother contracts are not pure, or even primarily, service contracts. They are mixed contracts for both services and a product. If anything, the service portion is incidental to the expectations, and in the minds, of the adopting parents. . . . If the surrogate mother miscarries through no fault of her own—i.e., she performs the service—the adopting parents will be disappointed, and their disappointment will not relate to the service, but to the failure to get the product. . . .

8. In point of fact, surrogate mothers do not create these children merely for the sake of bringing them into existence. Were we to find such a person, however, would her actions be ethical? No, for the same reason that it is not ethical for the proverbial

sailor, acting solely of course in the interest of adding to human existence, to cheerfully bestow the "gift of life" on all naive females he can talk into it. To desire something to exist requires one to desire all those things that are necessary for its existence, and all those things that are essential elements of it or are inseparably connected with it. To desire a child is to desire the responsibilities that come with a child, for that is what a child is, a package. Separating the decision to procreate a child from the desire to have and raise that child fails to respect that child as an end in himself because that act is incompatible with loving him.

9. See, e.g., P. Parker, *Motivations of Surrogate Mothers: Initial Findings,* 140 Am. J. Psych. p. 117–18 (Jan. 1983) B. Kantrowitz et al., *Who Keeps 'Baby M'? Newsweek,* Jan. 19, 1987, pp. 44–49. at 47; M. Gladwell, *Surrogate Parenting Industry Goes into Legal Labor Pains,* Insight p. 20, at 21 (Sept. 22, 1986) Gorney.

10. Robertson (1986), at 1025.

11. Id.

12. Id. at 1025 n. 296.

13. A mere means, to use Kantian parlance.

14. See L.A. Times, April 17, 1979, Sec. I, p. 2, col. 1, reporting the case of parents who conceived a child for the purpose of having him serve as a bone marrow donor for his sister.

15. Kant did not say that it was easy to be good or to be free, only that it was possible. Kant, at 199.

16. I am not speaking here of love in the sense of an emotion (i.e., affection: *philia*), but rather in the sense of an act of will (*agapē*). And see Kant, at 147. For example, an antebellum slave owner might have had affection for some of his slaves, but his actions prove that he did not love them in the sense in which I am using the word.

17. I am not implying that all offerings of children for adoption are necessarily ethical. In order to be so they must be done in the best interests of the child. See H. Krimmel, *The Case Against Surrogate Parenting,* 13 Hastings Center Report 35, at 36 (Oct. 1983).

18. The fact remains that man is incapable of giving a nonreligious justification for his existence and essential worth. It is precisely for this reason that a secular society must treat persons as ends in themselves. No man is required to justify his existence, because no man can. To violate this "taboo" and challenge another's right to exist is to challenge one's own. To require a reason for a person's being is to treat him as a means, which makes his worth to depend both upon his ability to satisfy some end, and also upon the value of that end itself, and *that* is a pit from which no man can escape.

19. Surrogate mother arrangements and adoption also differ in their essential purposes and functions. The purpose of adoption is to provide good homes for existing children who need them. The purpose of surrogate mother arrangements is to create "desirable" children for people who want to be parents.

20. Using the term "surrogate mother" here, rather than "mother," especially brings home the truth of Katha Pollitt's point to which I have previously alluded.

21. See Rubin, at 72–75; L. Dusky, *Brave New Babies?* Newsweek p. 30 (Dec. 6, 1982); J. Hollinger, *From Coitus to Commerce: Legal and Social Consequences of Noncoital Reproduction,* 18 J. L. Reform 865, at 922–23 (1985).

22. Katha Pollitt's discussion of this point in her critique of the trial court's opinion in the *Baby M* case compels quotation:

> To be sure, there are worse ways of coming into the world, but not many, and none that are elaborately prearranged by sane people. Much is made of the so-called trauma of

adoption, but adoption is a piece of cake compared with contracting. Adoptive parents can tell their child, Your mother loved you so much she gave you up, even though it made her sad, because that was best for you. What can the father and adoptive mother of a contract baby say? Your mother needed $10,000? Your mother wanted to do something nice for us, so she made you? (Pollitt, at 688.)

23. There is nothing, however, inherent in the technology of surrogate parenting that limits its use to infertile couples. It has been suggested that surrogate parenting might be used by single men, by homosexual couples, by career women too busy to be pregnant, and even by models who want a baby but no stretch marks.

24. No one doubts that the adopting parents truly want a child. But in surrogate mother arrangements, as with the more traditional forms of baby bartering, paying for the child corrupts their good intentions. In this sense surrogate mother arrangements are like the sin of simony: attempting to purchase, and thereby corrupting, that which is given as a matter of grace.

25. In the Baby M case, the trial court judge, Harvey Sorkow, made quite a point of arguing that surrogate mother arrangements couldn't be baby buying because a father couldn't buy what was already his. *In re Baby M.*—Ch. Ct. Opn., at 1157. I believe that Judge Sorkow made a factual error, which led him into making a legal one. First, what is it that makes a baby yours? If it is the biological link, the surrogate mother's claim is equal, if not superior, to the father's. And indeed, if you are only claiming what is yours already, what is the need of paying anyone anything? What the adopting parents are paying for is the termination of the biological mother's custody rights in the child, and that is no different than paying off the co-owner of a piece of land because you want undisputed ownership of the whole. Second, parental agreements concerning custody rights are subject to court approval. If, in a divorce case, one spouse attempted to trade custody rights in children as a pawn in the marital property settlement, one wonders how Judge Sorkow would react, and how he would distinguish that from what happens in surrogate mother agreements. And, while we are on the subject, how would we expect a child to feel when he finds out his mother traded him for the house?

26. See, e.g., J. Robertson, *Procreative Liberty and the Control of Conception, Pregnancy, and Childbirth,* 69 Vir. L. Rev. 405 (1983) [hereinafter cited as Robertson (1983)], esp. at 408–09, 412, 424, 429–30.

27. Cf. E. Landes and R. Posner, *The Economics of the Baby Shortage,* 7 J. L. Stud. 323 (1978); J. Prichard, *A Market for Babies?* 34 Toronto L. J. 341 (1984).

28. See Robertson (1983), at 429–30.

29. The following exchange of letters in the Hastings Center Report is illustrative of the point:

[I]f the happiness of the infertile couple is genuine, what good reason is there to suppose that the child will not benefit by being loved, cared for, and provided with suitable surroundings for growth and happiness? [M. Goodman, *Correspondence,* 14 Hastings Center Report at 43 (June 1984).]

Goodman . . . asks rhetorically what good reason there would be to suppose that a couple made happy by the newborn would not reciprocate. There would be many, if the analysis begins, as does Goodman's, with the implicit assumption that it is somehow the infant's duty to make the *parents* happy, or even that there is some sort of mutual or equal measure of responsibility and expectations on that score. And yet, as Goodman unconsciously suggests to us, in the surrogate arrangement, there certainly will be. Those parents have contracted, at substantial fee, for that infant. Who among us willingly purchases damaged goods? Will a child with birth defects be as willingly and lovingly received from the surrogate as a "perfect" child? Will it? [Krimmel, *Correspondence*, 14 Hastings Center Report at 44 (June 1984).]

30. See, e.g., Robertson (1983), at 429–30, 430 n. 66.

31. See, e.g., Robertson (1983), esp. at 408–10, 412, 424, 429–436.

32. Gorney, at 155.

33. Robertson (1986), at 1000; and see *Surrogate Parenthood*, A.B.A.J. p. 39 (June 1, 1987).

34. Professor Robertson apparently would agree that his proposed right of procreational autonomy would not extend to "harming" the child. Robertson (1983), at 432. He believes, however, that "fabrication or manipulation alone is not harmful, or at least not harmful enough." Id. at 432 n. 76. Elsewhere (Robertson (1986), at 995–97), he suggests that posthumous conception of children even "fifty or one hundred years after the genetic source's death, would not necessarily subject offspring to a life worse than death." And to ban such a practice "might . . . interfere with the procreative liberty of the deceased person, who contemplated posthumous reproduction." Id. at 997. If planning an orphan doesn't count as harm, one must wonder how Professor Robertson defines the word.

35. It is precisely at this point that surrogate mother arrangements are distinguished from the problem posed by "wrongful life" cases such as *Gleitman v. Cosgrove*, 49 N.J. 22, 227 A. 2d 689 (1967). Although both surrogate mother arrangements and "wrongful life" cases involve the situation where the cause that results in a person's existence is inseparably connected to that cause that results in an injury to the person as well; they differ due to the dissimilar characters of their causal elements, i.e., the reasons why existence and damage are inseparably connected. Stated otherwise, "wrongful life" cases and surrogate mother arrangements are similar in that, in both, existence and injury *are* inseparably connected, but they differ from one another in *why* this is so. In a majority of jurisdictions, in "wrongful life" cases the child has not been allowed to sue for being born deformed because his deformity and existence are inseparably connected, and the courts, for the most part, are unwilling to say that there is such a thing as a life without value. Hence, the large majority of courts have concluded, the child was not wronged by being born deformed because he could not otherwise have been. See G. Tedeschi, *On Tort Liability for "Wrongful Life,"* 1 Israel L. Rev. 513 (1966). In "wrongful life" cases the injured child could not have been other than he was and still be. In this respect "wrongful life" cases and surrogate mother arrangements are indistinguishable. However, when we inquire in each of these situations into the *reason* for why there is a connection between existence and damage we see the distinction. In the case of "wrongful life," the reason for the connection between the child's existence and his deformity is not due to any choice his parents made, but rather is the result of some natural or accidental cause beyond human control. In surrogate parenting, however, the parents are only willing to create the child if he has the impairment (of being born under a surrogate mother arrangement). It is the parents' choice that forges the link between existence and impairment. The connection between these elements is due not to nature, but to human will. The child still is not damaged by being brought into existence, per se, but the premeditated planning of his parents to give him a substandard or limited existence is evil.

36. I am not implying that a freely given consent would alleviate the ethical difficulty here. For, neither is one entitled to treat one's self as a means, and not as an end. See Kant, at 178. The criminal law provides an interesting illustration of this

point. Both the common law and modern authorities concur in the principle that consent is not a defense to the crime of mayhem. See *Wright's Case,* Co. Lit. 127a (1604) (defendant complying with a beggar's request, cut off the beggar's hand in order to give him more "colour to begge."); *State v. Bass,* 255 N.C. 42, 120 S.E. 2d 580 (1961) (defendant assisted in his accomplice's scheme to cut off the latter's fingers in order to obtain insurance money).

37. Furthermore, Professor Robertson's argument proves too much. The implications of his logic go far beyond the situation posed by surrogate parenting. For if a child has no ethical complaint about the manner of his conception or the specifications of his manufacture, so long as these do not make his life "worthless," why couldn't parents using traditional methods of procreation strike similar deals? What, for example, would prevent them from saying: "We will conceive a child only on the condition that he serve as a serf on our farm until he reaches the age of 35"? Or, once the technology of cloning becomes available to humans, how could it then be ethically objectionable to clone a replicant only on the condition that he serve as your organ donor if needed. (Cf. supra note 14.) When it comes time to take the replicant's kidneys, might one say to him: "You didn't get such a bad deal. You got to live up until now, and besides, had I not wanted an organ donor, I never would have made you"? This argument, when coupled with the belief that human existence is of incomparable worth, becomes a variation on the theme: I created you; therefore, I own you, and you owe me everything. Under such a view, child abuse would be a theoretical impossibility.

38. N. Blodgett, *Who Is Mother?* 72 A.B.A.J. p. 18 (June 1, 1986).

Fertilization of Human Eggs in Vitro: A Defense

R. G. Edwards

The widespread debates arising from medical advances have become a familiar aspect of contemporary society, and the clinical application of man's increasing control over his physiological and biochemical systems is bound to stimulate further controversy. This review is concerned with the current debate on one of these novel advances—the fertilization of human oocytes in vitro, and their reimplantation as cleaving embryos in the uterus of the mother. The attitudes expressed here on social and ethical values will obviously reflect the viewpoint of the writer, a scientist engaged in initiating and continuing the research and its clinical application. . . .

Doctors, and occasionally scientists, are faced with decisions about the nature and social value of their work. An immediate issue with new clinical methods concerns the ethics of human experimentation, for if patients are to benefit, new methods have to be perfected, often with the collaboration of people unlikely to gain from the research. The impact of human research can obviously be wider than merely affecting patients and doctors, and many of the themes running through debates on fertilization in vitro also arise in connection with abortion, contraception and artificial insemination from a donor (AID). The idea of initiating human life in vitro will probably be unacceptable in principle to some people, even for the cure of infertility. This response is partly emotional and might be modified as the notion becomes more familiar and the benefits clearer, just as previous debates have led to the acceptance of new attitudes towards various other aspects of human reproduction and sexuality. Certain other well-known concepts stimulating a great deal of discussion concern the moment when human life begins and the "rights" of embryos, fetuses, and neonates, especially those growing in culture. . . . We will now consider these issues in turn.

From "Fertilization of Human Eggs In Vitro: Morals, Ethics, and the Law." *Quarterly Review of Biology* 49 (1974), 3–26. Copyright 1974, Stony Brook Foundation, Inc. Abridged. Reprinted with permission of the University of Chicago Press.

The Development of Clinical IVF

Like other new medical advances, studies on the cure of infertility by re-implanting cleaving embryos must pass through an initial phase where meth-ods are being established and the prospects are assessed. Volunteers who have had a chance of ultimately benefiting from the work have been involved while the methods were being developed. Demands on these volunteers were not excessive, for treatments with gonadotropins or clomiphene were in use by many doctors to alleviate amenorrhea, and the operational risks of laparos-copy in the cure of infertility were well known and minor. Aspirating oocytes from follicles is similar to the natural events of follicular rupture during ovula-tion, and the ovary recovers just as quickly. The reimplantation of embryos via the cervix would demand neither anesthetic nor operation and is simple, rapid, and free from dangers such as infection, while the risks of disorders such as perforation of the uterus seem very low. These procedures are now fully practiced and performed routinely.

The application of new methods in clinical medicine usually follows a certain amount of previous work done with animals. The data published on several animal species concerning fertilization in vitro, embryo culture and transfer, and the treatment of embryos with the various agents have shown the preimplantation embryo to be highly resistant to malformation. Attempts to repeat the work on the culture of embryos using nonhuman primates have been almost a total failure, and the clinical methods have outstripped experi-mental studies on these species. There is disagreement among teratologists and doctors about the necessity of including such primates among the three animal species to be used before clinical trials are carried out. Thus, primates were not tested before the clinical application of either kidney transplanta-tion, relevant data being obtained from pigs and dogs, or vasectomy. Recent data on the carcinogenetic effects of contraceptive pills have come from rats and mice, the results of studies on dogs and monkeys being yet unavailable. It is likely that all known human anomalies have been found in subprimates, including the effects of thalidomide, and in their response to some compounds the fetuses of nonhuman primates are less resistant than human fetuses. In view of the vast number of fetuses and offspring arising through embryo transfer in animals, without evidence of any increase in number or type of abnormality, there seems to be no point in delaying the clinical application of work on human infertility. This conclusion is supported by the evidence that the cleaving embryos of nonhuman primates are similar to those of sub-primates in resisting the teratogenic effects of agents applied in vivo. Many infertile couples and others with different problems would forfeit their chances of a cure if medical progress depended on verification in non-human primates.

Some prenatal diagnoses, especially the analysis of their chromosome com-plement, should be carried out on any fetuses arising from the reimplantation of cleaving human embryos. The chances of trisomy, i.e., individuals with an extra chromosome, arising as the result of fertilization in vitro have not been estimated because there are few mitoses in cleaving embryos, and vast numbers would be needed to carry out this study. There is likely to be nothing novel in this respect about fertilization in vitro, because many trisomies for every human chromosome group have now been found after natural conception, and as many as 5 percent or more of all fetuses are known to be imbalanced chromosomally at three months' gestation. The incidence at fertilization is likely to be much greater for the frequency of imbalanced embryos increases as embryos earlier in pregnancy are being examined. Almost all nondiploid human embryos fail to survive, and those that do develop can be identified at four months' gestation by using amniocentesis to collect fetal cells for chromosomal examination. Other types of prenatal diagnosis could also be applied to the fetuses. Measurements of heartbeat and fetal scanning by ultrasonics can detect anomalies of the head, limbs, and other organs, and further advances are possible with three-dimensional ultrasonic images of the fetus. Amniotic fluid can be used to identify fetuses with anencephaly and other malformations, and the chances of disorders such as choriocarcinoma are determined largely by the relationship between the blood groups of the parents. The risks of abnormal offspring following human embryo transfer should thus be very small.

Spin-Off Benefits

The accumulation of knowledge regarding human conception should prove of considerable value to other types of clinical studies. Some of the most important contraceptive methods in use today, e.g., the safe period and the "pill," involve an understanding of human ovulation, and studies on oocyte recovery have provided the first definite indication of the moment of human ovulation. New contraceptive or sterilization methods for suppressing implantation could arise from studies on the early differentiation of the human embryo, together with a clearer understanding of the mode of action of intrauterine devices in expelling the blastocyst from the uterus. Analyses concerning the origin of various inherited or induced human malformations are even more restricted to clinical work, as shown, for example, by the rare animal counterparts of trisomy due to aging. Some inherited diseases might one day be avoided or averted by sexing blastocysts or by making chimeras in cleavage stages, for some evidence indicates that the expression of recessive genes carried on one of the cell lines is modified in mouse chimeras. On the other hand, chimeras might suffer from the combined defects of both stem lines or from interactions between them, and any embryo known to be defective would be better discarded than subjected to such methods of salvage. Human chimeras have been created at full term by injecting thymus and other hemopoietic stem cells into newborn children, and their suffering from immunological deficiency diseases has thereby been alleviated.

Benefits to Infertile Patients

The reimplantation of cleaving embryos into the uterus is the only method to help many patients who are infertile through tubal occlusion. Estimates of the numbers of these patients vary widely, partly due to ethnic or other differences in the population under study. In the United Kingdom, approximately 2 percent of all women suffer from tubal occlusion. The reconstruction of damaged oviducts might help one-fifth of them. Other forms of infertility might also be treated, including endocrine disturbances or antibodies against spermatozoa in men and women and oligospermia in men. Artificial insemination using pooled ejaculates can help some men with oligospermia, and male infertility can obviously be bypassed by using AID, i.e., using semen taken from a donor, a method now being widely used despite the ethical and legal problems it evokes. A woman without her own occytes might be able to conceive through intercourse with her own husband if oocytes were placed in her oviduct, the similarities with AID being obvious. The recipient would carry the child through gestation, and hence both parents would help to establish their family. The legal and ethical issues involved in AID have been widely debated (Wolstenholme and Fitzsimons, 1973), and oocyte transfer should be as acceptable ethically and legally (Revillard, 1973; Stone, 1973) in the rare cases where it is needed. The number of women who lack oocytes and are still in their reproductive age is very small, and various difficulties might arise for some of them in establishing pregnancy. Congenital absence of the ovary can lead to maldevelopment of the oviduct and uterus, and some women with ovarian disorders arising in adult life have other contraindications for pregnancy. The transfer of embryos from one woman to another could alleviate infertility arising where both parents lack gametes, a very rare occurrence. There are many women, potentially fertile, who are advised against pregnancy, and the transfer of their embryos to a surrogate mother who would carry the fetus to full term would enable them to have their own children. The transfer of embryos from one woman to another is perhaps the only ethical issue requiring caution, and this form of treatment will be considered separately below.

There are clear arguments in favor of proceeding with the reimplantation of embryos into the mother for the cure of infertility, for to give a couple their own wanted child obviously needs no justification. The right to have children is stated in various international declarations on human rights. Infertility might lead to deprivation and the breakdown of a marriage, although the statistical methods supporting this view have been challenged. Adoption can satisfy the desires of some infertile couples, but fewer children are available today for adoption because of contraception, abortion, and the widespread acceptance of the illegitimate child, and many infertile couples have been unsuccessful in their attempts to adopt. The cure of infertility by reimplanting cleaving embryos does not impose intolerable treatments or surgery, or cause irreversible physical damage, and violates no canon of medical treatment. The cost is very small, if it should be thought an important point to judge the economics of the treatment. The cure of infertility would not raise the frequency of unsuitable genes, for only a few minor causes of infertility, such as congenital occlusion or absence of the vas deferens in man and some endocrine disturbances in women, have a genetic basis, and these conditions are very rare. Even if they were successfully treated, the increase in gene frequency would be insignificant, as with the cure of other rare disorders.

The problems of population growth might ultimately erode some privileges of parenthood, although most debates stress—correctly in our view—the voluntary nature of restricting family size. Yet objections to the reimplantation of embryos as a cure of infertility have been based on the mounting pressures of population. In numbers alone, such an attitude seems mistaken, for perhaps only a small proportion of the women who could benefit will accept the treatment. More serious objections can be raised to this attitude, which implies that all forms of infertility ought to remain uncured, leaving this unfortunate minority to their own devices. Doctors dealing with infertile patients should not, and almost certainly will not, be subject to such pressures to modify their diagnoses and treatment according to events outside their consulting rooms. Strictures and regulations about procreation, if ever needed, should apply to the population as a whole and as impartially as possible.

The Meaning of Medical Treatment

Some other comments on the treatment of infertile patients appear to be equally mistaken. One remarkable opinion holds that the reimplantation of embryos to cure infertility is not therapeutic in the accepted sense, for the patient remains infertile even if transfer results in live children. What is supposedly being treated is the desire of people to have children (Kass, 1971a). A great many medical advances depend on the replacement of a deficient compound or an organ. Examples include insulin, false teeth, and spectacles: the clinical condition itself remains, but treatment modifies its expression. Patients taking advantage of these three treatments are surely receiving the correct therapeutic measures, the doctors treating the desire to be nondiabetic or to see and eat properly. In fact, most medical treatment, particularly of constitutional or genetic disorders, is similarly symptomatic in nature. Exactly the same argument applies to the cure of infertility: should patients have their desired children, the treatment would have achieved its purpose. To state the opposite is nonsense.

"Thin End of the Wedge"

Another untenable proposition is the argument based on the "thin end of the wedge" or "camel's nose," suggesting that fertilization in vitro and reimplantation of embryos in the mother should be banned because they might lead to less desirable ends such as cloning (Kass, 1971a,b). The immediate appeal of this argument lies in its purported offer of a quick solution to difficult decisions, and in its instinctive appeal to those who are fearful or uncertain of the real issues. Its weaknesses include the pessimistic assumption that the worst will inevitably happen, and the uncritical rejection of good and bad alike. The whole edifice of the argument is fragile: thus, nuclear physics led inevitably to the atom bomb, electricity to the electric chair, air transport to bombers and hijackers, civil engineering to the gas chambers. The list is as long as the argument is fallacious for acceptance of the beginning does not imply embracing the undesirable ends.

Patients' Consent

Patients seeking treatments must be kept fully informed about the methods contemplated and the probability of success, just as in other forms of novel clinical methods. Many infertile couples urgently desire the work on fertilization and reimplantation to proceed, wish to help with it, and are fully capable of understanding their condition and the attempts to cure it. A significant proportion are doctors or the wives of doctors, scientists, solicitors, clerics, and other members of the community who are articulate, discriminating, and fully capable of analyzing and judging social and medical situations, although it is very important to avoid an "elitist" attitude in selecting patients. They are evidently aware, too, that the methods might not work, their infertility remain uncured, and that other women may be the ultimate beneficiaries of the developing methods. It is obviously hard to assess how much some patients understand; in follow-up studies after genetic counseling, one-half of the patients had fully grasped the nature of their problems, and their level of education was a significant factor in comprehension but not in their decision to limit their family. Perhaps a preferable alternative to the treatments designed to cure infertility is to persuade patients to accept their childlessness, but such advice assumes that a doctor or someone else is sufficiently authoritative to decide on the problems of the couple. Patients have the right to benefit from research, and there is no reason to believe that ethical advice from outsiders about their condition is sounder than their own judgment of it. The future child must be considered too, for there could be psychological or other problems in store for children conceived through fertilization in vitro. Most evidence would suggest an opposite conclusion: the children would give thanks to be alive, just as the rest of us do, for they would be the children of their own parents, born into a family where they are wanted for their own sake. If there is no undue risk of deformity additional to those in natural conception, and publicity is avoided, the children should grow and develop normally and be no more misfits than other children born today after some form of medical help.

Surrogate Motherhood

The only issue needing care seems to be the case of surrogate mothers for those women unable to carry their own children. This form of treatment could lead to conflicting claims on the child by the embryo donor and the uterine mother, and to the divided loyalty of the child itself. The surrogate mother might request an abortion or refuse to hand over the child, the donor might reject the child at birth, and the child might suffer on learning of the circumstances of its birth. Surrogate mothers could be used purely for the convenience of fertile women who wish to avoid the problems of pregnancy. At present this approach, and the use of surrogate mothers to help the infertile should, perhaps, be avoided until more consideration is given to the psychological demands on donor, host, and child, even though some existing situations do not differ greatly from this practice. Illegitimate children are often surrendered at birth, and some couples have deliberately conceived and carried babies to full term for those unable to have their own. Despite these examples, embryo transfer between women should not be encouraged until more can be deduced about the psychological relationships between parents, recipients, and children. . . .

The Beginning of Life

Contributions to debates on the more esoteric issues arising from fertilization in vitro have come from various quarters. Themes occurring repeatedly in these discussions include defining the moment when human life begins, the challenge of new methods of conception to established ideas on life and procreation, and the imminence of genetic engineering. The divergent viewpoints forming the basis of ethical judgements are perhaps best illustrated in attitudes expressed towards defining the moment when human life begins. Absolutists insist that full rights must be given from the instant of fertilization, partly on the grounds that the embryo is then a human being. This view is challenged on biological grounds. Fertilization is only incidental to the beginning of life, for the processes essential to development begin long before ovulation, and parthenogenetic fetuses can develop partially, and perhaps one day wholly through gestation. The potentiality for life must therefore reside in the unfertilized egg and all of its precursors. Nuclear transfer experiments are also held to weaken the absolutist case by showing that all nuclei can potentially sustain the development of an embryo. The assumption of full human rights at a single moment in a continuous developmental sequence obviously demands making arbitrary decisions that are unjustified biologically. Nevertheless, fertilization and implantation are two convenient points that are often suggested in debates on contraception and abortion, and legal guides have included quickening of the fetus and the earliest stage when neonates can survive independently (28 weeks). Granting full rights from fertilization on-

wards is sometimes combined with condoning the abortion of deformed fetuses, an outlook that is totally unrealistic, for it would lead to the justification
of infanticide or euthanasia for deformed adults.

Most of the contributions by theologians to debates on fertilization in vitro
and embryo transfer can be accepted and answered by laymen, for appeals
and allusions to earlier Church authorities or to a "revealed ethic" are largely
absent. There is no parallel between current scientific and clinical work and
earlier clerical situations, and the attitudes of different theologians probably
reflect their known stances on other issues, such as contraception and abortion. The Church, like other professions, represents a diverse body of opinion, even on religious issues, and will probably never give a unified decision
on embryo transfer; indeed, the differences in outlook among theologians are
as wide as among scientists, doctors, and others, as judged by a perusal of
their published opinions.

A strict denunciation was to be expected, and duly came, from the hierarchy of the Roman Catholic Church. Their initial ruling, based on papal pronouncements, was to declare fertilization in vitro "absolutely immoral." But
absolutes are not easy to define or uphold, especially in today's society, and
this ruling was not accepted by an ethical committee of Catholic doctors, who
wrote in one of their statements: (Guild of Catholic Doctors Ethical Committee, 1972, p. 242): "In vitro fertilization, with a view to transfer at an early
stage to the womb of the 'mother' is, in principle, acceptable. . . ." Many of
the views expressed in this document on other issues raised by embryo transfer coincide fairly closely with those of the present reviewer, but not the
tendency to define absolutes such as giving full human rights to a fertilized
egg. This belief is obviously rejected implicitly by many people, for IUDs
almost certainly expel unimplanted embryos from the uterus, and abortion is
legalized in many countries. The gradual acquisition of human rights during
development is tacitly accepted in other situations, and is clearly illustrated by
the prevalence of eugenic abortion, but not infanticide, in cases of inherited
anomalies.

Procreative Arts, Child's Consent, and Dehumanization

Some theologians still rely heavily on their own interpretations of biblical or
theological concepts in judging new clinical methods, and have been described by their colleagues as "a priorists" (Fletcher, 1971a; McCormick,
1972). Reimplanting embryos was judged as unacceptable because the nature
of procreation must remain as it is, divine and unchangeable. This view is
astonishingly held simultaneously with an acceptance of AID, provided the
sterile couple hold acts of procreation by performing intercourse (Ramsey,
1970)! It is challenged by several commentators (Guild of Catholic Doctors
Ethical Committee, 1972), as summed up by one of them who writes that
"these moral positions assume that only God can make a tree or a man. They
ignore the fact that God has shared with us His creative power so that we may

contribute to the ongoing task of creating man and nature" (Francouer, 1972, p. 438). In a more practical vein, reimplanting embryos for curing infertility is also judged to be unacceptable because the future child cannot consent before-hand to procedures that might entail risks for itself, an attitude that is un-realistic in practice because it leads to total negation—even to denying a mother a sleeping pill, a Caesarian section, or an amniocentesis for fear of disturbing the child. Every medical treatment, from eating aspirin to open-heart surgery, carries a risk for each patient, and fetuses are not asked before-hand about their own conception or even their abortion, hence this ethical stance is difficult to justify and seems to be one of the "cliches of an irrelevant ideology" (Fletcher, 1971b). Another review, in a similar vein (Kass, 1971b), dominated by a consideration of cloning and other improbable methods of genetic engineering, returns again to the supposed risks of reimplanting em-bryos and the immorality of discarding unimplanted embryos, and postulates that increasing control over conception would "dehumanize" mankind. The same attitude toward reimplanting embryos is surprising in a theologian (Mc-Cormick, 1972) who criticizes others for failing to discuss the proper ethical issues, but himself judges it as unethical because the marital relationship and essential links in family life are "debiologized" by removing procreation from the sphere of bodily love. Most bodily love is already removed from procre-ation by means of a battery of contraceptive methods, and how the notion of the family, which has survived abortion, divorce, sexual freedom, and rejec-tion of the parents by children, is to be preserved by withholding treatment from the infertile is not clear to the present writer. The raising of children will demand expression of high forms of love and duty. How surprising, then, to read of theologians withholding the procreative aspect of marriage from infer-tile couples because it "debiologizes" all the others! Far more disturbing, but perhaps to be expected from an extremist, is the hope half-offered by one theologian that the first child born through these methods will be abnormal and will be publicly displayed (Ramsey, 1972a,b). The wrath of the pulpit is obviously to be heaped on the heads of sinners! . . .

Motives and Decision Making

Some revealing attitudes are struck in these debates. According to one com-mentator, the developments and the benefits of new scientific advances should not be judged by "man the technician" but rather by minds that "grasp and transform reality." This view is allied with a feeling that secret experi-ments detrimental to human values—especially genetic engineering—are con-stantly occurring so that external controls should be imposed on scientists (Crotty, 1972). Two notable aspects of this contribution are its inherent suspi-cion of other people's motives—reinforced by allusions to the Nazis and Hiroshima—and the belief that "a pattern of behavior is more genuinely human . . . because [it] embodies greater human values than do alternative responses." How can anyone possibly disagree with such a fine quotation, but how far does it take us? The exact problem with many clinical advances is deciding where the great human values lie among a conflicting welter of attitudes and possibilities, and allusions to the Nazis, Hiroshima, and other cataclysms hardly helps to provide clarification. The subtleties involved in making decisions and judgments on scientific and clinical advances are well illustrated in recent symposia (Kunz and Fehr, 1972; Wolstenholme and Fitzsimons, 1973). Note, too, the attitude that "technology" (including science) is inferior to "humanity" (philosophy and theology) in helping to establish values. Some points derived from the word-centered concepts of the latter appear to be obvious and acceptable from simple reasoning; for example, the conclusion that human sexuality is an ambiguous basis for creating children, since it may be used in lust, selfishness, accident, or hatred (McNeill, 1972). McNeill considers that the ambiguity is removed by baptism, but surely love and commitment between two people are preferable. . . .

Responsibility in Biological and Clinical Research

Research is usually divided into basic and applied science, but the borderline between them is often blurred. The distinction between them becomes almost meaningless as new methods are put into practice, and responsibility changes from the demands imposed by scientific research to those involved in the conduct of clinical trials. The problems become oriented toward patients and hence more pressing as they move to the hospital. The responsibilities of scientists in "pure" research have been debated with respect to their role in developing chemical warfare and other issues, but the primary concern of the present review involves clinical medicine.

The responsibility for applying new research methods to patients has rested traditionally on the individual doctor, often working in collaboration with scientists who are regarded as auxiliaries. This may still be the best position to adopt today, although the increased participation of non-medical men in making decisions should be recognized. The ethical and legal complexities in clinical situations can sometimes be formidable, and some commentators have advocated making committee decisions—for example, with respect to the timing of the first transfer of a human embryo. This outlook seems to be unrealistic. There are the "rights" of the patient to consider. The selection of committees and their methods of making decisions also present difficulties. Would such decisions need to be unanimous, by a majority only, or subject to veto by any single member? Can ethics be decided by a majority vote? The questions at issue—euthanasia, existence, interference with inherited characteristics—are so much more complex than those usually dealt with by most councils, and relevant opinion can come from wide sources, artistic and philosophical in addition to those outlined in this review. The chance of a united ethical and moral stance on such questions seems remote.

Individual responsibility must now cover problems additional to those defined earlier. The necessity of obtaining the informed consent of patients and the establishment of clinical ethical committees in hospitals have obviously become widely accepted. Some responsibilities are novel. Doctors and scientists should understand the issues confronting each other, and both groups should familiarize themselves with the problems of the patients. Research of social significance should be published in widely read journals or articles, although the patients' privacy must be fully protected and publicity in the press avoided. Various organizations and courses have been established to study the ever-increasing ethical questions in biology and medicine . . . , and should extend informed debate provided any bias in their constitution is recognized. The mass media have a responsibility to publicize work of public concern, but attempts at widespread discussion are often compromised by sensational press reporting, so that the standards of different professions come into conflict as control of the ensuing debate passes from doctor to journalist. Constant recourse to the Press Council is ineffective, since the damage is difficult to repair.

This review has stressed some issues raised by fertilization in vitro and the reimplantation of embryos. Many of the points raised in it are equally valid in connection with research in other areas of scientific medicine. The increasing tempo of scientific advances is occurring at a time when earlier and accepted standards of society, and the value of many scientific and technological advances are being widely questioned. There is an obvious need for continuing the debate on the value of scientific and clinical novelty, even though too much discussion can stimulate needless concern. Social priorities in clinical medicine should perhaps be listed and supported accordingly, but new avenues of scientific and clinical research will probably arise "as the acts of creation of individual geniuses, either working alone or possibly as members of teams of research workers" (Zuckerman, 1972). The widespread publicity, desired or otherwise, that now accompanies scientific and clinical advances will call for such individuals to participate in debate on social values, and equally will call for considered judgments from other professional men. There may be pitfalls and problems in the application of new methods in clinical research, yet, encouragingly, members of diverse professions can arrive at similar conclusions on complex issues.

References

Crotty, N. 1972. The technological imperative: reflection on reflections. *Theological Studies*, 33: 440–449.
Fletcher, J. 1971a. Ethical aspects of genetic controls. *New Eng. J. Med.*, 285: 776–783.
———. 1971b. The "right" to live and the "right" to die. Vesper Exchange No. 7 (VE 1384).
Francouer, R. T. 1972. We can—we must; reflections on the technological imperative. *Theological Studies*, 33: 428–439.
Guild of Catholic Doctors Ethical Committee. 1972. In vitro fertilization. *Catholic Med. Quart.*, 24: 237–243.

Kass, L. 1971a. Babies by means of in vitro fertilization: unethical experiments on the unborn? *New. Eng. J. Med.*, 285: 1174–1179.

———. 1971b. The new biology: what price relieving man's estate? *Science,* 174: 779–788.

Kunz, R. M., and H. Fehr (eds.). 1972. *The Challenge of Life.* Section 1, Biomedical Frontiers. Birkhauser Verlag, Basel & Stuttgart.

McCormick, R. 1972. Genetic medicine: notes on the moral literature. *Theological Studies,* 32: 531–552.

McNeill, J. J. 1972. Freedom and the future. *Theological Studies,* 33: 503–530.

Ramsey, P. 1970. *Fabricated Man. The Ethics of Genetic Control.* Yale University Press, New Haven.

———. 1972a. Shall we "reproduce"? I. The medical ethics of in vitro fertilization. *J. Am. Med Assoc.,* 220: 1346–1350.

———. 1972b. Shall we "reproduce"? II. Rejoinders and future forecast. *J. Am. Med. Assoc.,* 220: 1480–1485.

Revillard, M. L. 1973. Legal aspects of artificial insemination and embryo transfer in French domestic law and private international law. In G. E. W. Wolstenholme and D. Fitzsimons (eds.). 1973. Ciba Foundation Symposium, *Law and Ethics of A.I.D. and Embryo Transfer,* pp. 77–90. Elsevier, Excerpta Medica, North Holland, Amsterdam.

Stone, O. M. 1973. English law in relation to AID and embryo transfer. In G. E. W. Wolstenholme and D. Fitzsimons (eds.). 1973. Ciba Foundation Symposium, *Law and Ethics of A.I.D. and Embryo Transfer,* pp. 69–76. Elsevier, Excerpta Medica, North Holland, Amsterdam.

Wolstenholme, G. E. W., and D. Fitzsimons (eds.). 1973. Ciba Foundation Symposium, *Law and Ethics of A.I.D. and Embryo Transfer.* Elsevier, Excerpta Medica, North Holland, Amsterdam.

Zuckerman, Lord. 1972. The doctor's dilemma. In R. M. Kunz and H. Fehr (eds.). *The Challenge of Life,* pp. 421–440. Birkhauser Verlag, Basel and Stuttgart.

Instruction on Respect for Human Life in Its Origin and on the Dignity of Procreation

Vatican, Congregation for the Doctrine of the Faith

Biomedical Research and the Teaching of the Church
The gift of life which God the Creator and Father has entrusted to man calls him to appreciate the inestimable value of what he has been given and to take responsibility for it: This fundamental principle must be placed at the center of one's reflection in order to clarify and solve the moral problems raised by artificial interventions on life as it originates and on the processes of procreation.

Thanks to the progress of the biological and medical sciences, man has at his disposal ever more effective therapeutic resources; but he can also acquire new powers, with unforeseeable consequences, over human life at its very beginning and in its first stages. Various procedures now make it possible to intervene not only in order to assist, but also to dominate the processes of procreation. These techniques can enable man to "take in hand his own destiny," but they also expose him "to the temptation to go beyond the limits of a reasonable dominion over nature."[1] They might constitute progress in the service of man, but they also involve serious risks. Many people are therefore expressing an urgent appeal that in interventions on procreation the values and rights of the human person be safeguarded. Requests for clarification and guidance are coming not only from the faithful, but also from those who recognize the church as "an expert in humanity"[2] with a mission to serve the "civilization of love"[3] and of life.

The church's magisterium [asserts] . . . the criteria of moral judgment as regards the applications of scientific research and technology, especially in relation to human life and its beginnings . . . to be the respect, defense and promotion of man, his "primary and fundamental right" to life,[4] his dignity as a person who is endowed with a spiritual soul and with moral responsibility and who is called to beatific communion with God. . . .

Anthropology and Procedures in the Biomedical Field
Which moral criteria must be applied in order to clarify the problems posed today in the field of biomedicine? The answer to this question presupposes a proper idea of the nature of the human person in his bodily dimension.

From *Origins* 16, no. 40 (March 19, 1987). Abridged.

For it is only in keeping with his true nature that the human person can achieve self-realization as a "unified totality";[5] and this nature is at the same time corporal and spiritual. By virtue of its substantial union with a spiritual soul, the human body cannot be considered as a mere complex of tissues, organs and functions, nor can it be evaluated in the same way as the body of animals; rather, it is a constitutive part of the person who manifests and expresses himself through it.

The natural moral law expresses and lays down the purposes, rights and duties which are based upon the bodily and spiritual nature of the human person. Therefore this law cannot be thought of as simply a set of norms on the biological level; rather, it must be defined as the rational order whereby man is called by the Creator to direct and regulate his life and actions and in particular to make use of his own body.

A first consequence can be deduced from these principles: An intervention on the human body affects not only the tissues, the organs and their functions, but also involves the person himself on different levels. It involves, therefore, perhaps in an implicit but nonetheless real way, a moral significance and responsibility. . . .

Applied biology and medicine work together for the integral good of human life when they come to the aid of a person stricken by illness and infirmity and when they respect his or her dignity as a creature of God. No biologist or doctor can reasonably claim, by virtue of his scientific competence, to be able to decide on people's origin and destiny. This norm must be applied in a particular way in the field of sexuality and procreation, in which man and woman actualize the fundamental values of love and life.

God, who is love and life, has inscribed in man and woman the vocation to share in a special way in his mystery of personal communion and in his work as Creator and Father. For this reason marriage possesses specific goods and values in its union and in procreation which cannot be likened to those existing in lower forms of life. Such values and meanings are of the personal order and determine from the moral point of view the meaning and limits of artificial interventions on procreation and on the origin of human life. These interventions are not to be rejected on the grounds that they are artificial. As such, they bear witness to the possibilities of the art of medicine. But they must be given a moral evaluation in reference to the dignity of the human person, who is called to realize his vocation from God to the gift of love and the gift of life.

Fundamental Criteria for a Moral Judgment

The fundamental values connected with the techniques of artificial human procreation are two: the life of the human being called into existence and the special nature of the transmission of human life in marriage. The moral judgment on such methods of artificial procreation must therefore be formulated in reference to these values.

Physical life, with which the course of human life in the world begins, certainly does not itself contain the whole of a person's value, nor does it represent the supreme good of man, who is called to eternal life. However it does constitute in a certain way the "fundamental" value of life precisely because upon this physical life all the other values of the person are based and developed. The inviolability of the innocent human being's right to life "from the moment of conception until death"[6] is a sign and requirement of the very inviolability of the person to whom the Creator has given the gift of life.

By comparison with the transmission of other forms of life in the universe, the transmission of human life has a special character of its own, which derives from the special nature of the human person. "The transmission of human life is entrusted by nature to a personal and conscious act and as such is subject to the all-holy laws of God: immutable and inviolable laws which must be recognized and observed. For this reason one cannot use means and follow methods which could be licit in the transmission of the life of plants and animals."[7]

Advances in technology have now made it possible to procreate apart from sexual relations through the meeting *in vitro* of the germ cells previously taken from the man and the woman. But what is technically possible is not for that very reason morally admissible. Rational reflection on the fundamental values of life and of human procreation is therefore indispensable for formulating a moral evaluation of such technological interventions on a human being from the first stages of his development. . . .[8]

I. Respect for Human Embryos

What respect is due to the human embryo, taking into account
his nature and identity?
The human being must be respected—as a person—from the very first instant of
his existence. . . .

This congregation is aware of the current debates concerning the beginning of human life, concerning the individuality of the human being and concerning the identity of the human person. The congregation recalls the teachings found in the Declaration on Procured Abortion:

"From the time that the ovum is fertilized, a new life is begun which is neither that of the father nor of the mother; it is rather the life of a new human being with his own growth. It would never be made human if it were not human already. To this perpetual evidence . . . modern genetic science brings valuable confirmation. It has demonstrated that, from the first instant, the program is fixed as to what this living being will be: a man, this individual man with his characteristic aspects already well determined. Right from fertilization is begun the adventure of a human life, and each of its great capacities requires time . . . to find its place and to be in a position to act."[9]

This teaching remains valid and is further confirmed, if confirmation were needed, by recent findings of human biological science which recognize that in the zygote (the cell produced when the nuclei of the two gametes have fused) resulting from fertilization the biological identity of a new human individual is already constituted.

Certainly no experimental datum can be in itself sufficient to bring us to the recognition of a spiritual soul; nevertheless, the conclusions of science regarding the human embryo provide a valuable indication for discerning by the use of reason a personal presence at the moment of this first appearance of a human life: How could a human individual not be a human person? The magisterium has not expressly committed itself to an affirmation of a philosophical nature, but it constantly reaffirms the moral condemnation of any kind of procured abortion. This teaching has not been changed and is unchangeable.

Thus the fruit of human generation from the first moment of its existence, that is to say, from the moment the zygote has formed, demands the unconditional respect that is morally due to the human being in his bodily and spiritual totality. The human being is to be respected and treated as a person from the moment of conception and therefore from that same moment his rights as a person must be recognized, among which in the first place is the inviolable right of every innocent human being to life.

This doctrinal reminder provides the fundamental criterion for the solution of the various problems posed by the development of the biomedical sciences in this field: Since the embryo must be treated as a person, it must also be defended in its integrity, tended and cared for, to the extent possible, in the same way as any other human being as far as medical assistance is concerned. . . .

How is one to evaluate morally research and experimentation on human embryos and fetuses?

Medical research must refrain from operations on live embryos, unless there is a moral certainty of not causing harm to the life or integrity of the unborn child and the mother, and on condition that the parents have given their free and informed consent to the procedure. It follows that all research, even when limited to the simple observation of the embryo, would become illicit were it to involve risk to the embryo's physical integrity or life by reason of the methods used or the effects induced.

As regards experimentation, and presupposing the general distinction between experimentation for purposes which are not directly therapeutic and experimentation which is clearly therapeutic and experimentation which is clearly therapeutic for the subject himself, in the case in point one must also distinguish between experimentation carried out on embryos which are still alive and experimentation carried out on embryos which are dead. *If the embryos are living, whether viable or not, they must be respected just like any other human person; experimentation on embryos which is not directly therapeutic is illicit.*

No objective, even though noble in itself such as a foreseeable advantage to science, to other human beings or to society, can in any way justify experimentation on living human embryos or fetuses, whether viable or not, either inside or outside the mother's womb. The informed consent ordinarily required for clinical experimentation on adults cannot be granted by the parents, who may not freely dispose of the physical integrity or life of the unborn child. Moreover, experimentation on embryos and fetuses always involves risk, and indeed in most cases it involves the certain expectation of harm to their physical integrity or even their death.

To use human embryos or fetuses as the object or instrument of experimentation constitutes a crime against their dignity as human beings having a right to the same respect that is due to the child already born and to every human person. . . .

In the case of experimentation that is clearly therapeutic, namely, when it is a matter of experimental forms of therapy used for the benefit of the embryo itself in a final attempt to save its life and in the absence of other reliable forms of therapy, recourse to drugs or procedures not yet fully tested can be licit.

The corpses of human embryos and fetuses, whether they have been deliberately aborted or not, must be respected just as the remains of other human beings. In particular, they cannot be subjected to mutilation or to autopsies if their death has not yet been verified and without the consent of the parents or of the mother. Furthermore, the moral requirements must be safeguarded that there be no complicity in deliberate abortion and that the risk of scandal be avoided. Also, in the case of dead fetuses, as for the corpses of adult persons, all commercial trafficking must be considered illicit and should be prohibited.

How is one to evaluate morally the use for research purposes of embryos obtained by fertilization "in vitro?"
Human embryos obtained *in vitro* are human beings and subjects with rights: Their dignity and right to life must be respected from the first moment of their existence. *It is immoral to produce human embryos destined to be exploited as disposable "biological material."*

In the usual practice of *in vitro* fertilization, not all of the embryos are transferred to the woman's body; some are destroyed. Just as the church condemns induced abortion, so she also forbids acts against the life of these human beings. *It is a duty to condemn the particular gravity of the voluntary destruction of human embryos obtained "in vitro" for the sole purpose of research, either by means of artificial insemination or by means of "twin fission." By acting in this way the researcher usurps the place of God; and, even though he may be unaware of this, he sets himself up as the master of the destiny of others inasmuch as he arbitrarily chooses whom he will allow to live and whom he will send to death and kills defenseless human beings.*

Methods of observation or experimentation which damage or impose grave and disproportionate risks upon embryos obtained *in vitro* are morally illicit for the same reasons. Every human being is to be respected for himself and cannot be reduced in worth to a pure and simple instrument for the advantage of others. *It is therefore not in conformity with the moral law deliberately to expose to death human embryos obtained "in vitro."* In consequence of the fact that they have been produced *in vitro,* those embryos which are not transferred into the body of the mother and are called "spare" are exposed to an absurd fate, with no possibility of their being offered safe means of survival which can be licitly pursued.

What judgment should be made on other procedures of manipulating embryos connected with the "techniques of human reproduction?"
Techniques of fertilization *in vitro* can open the way to other forms of biological and genetic manipulation of human embryos, such as attempts or plans for fertilization between human and animal gametes and the gestation of human embryos in the uterus of animals, or the hypothesis or project of constructing artificial uteruses for the human embryo. *These procedures are contrary to the human dignity proper to the embryo, and at the same time they are contrary to the right of every person to be conceived and to be born within marriage and from marriage.*[10] *Also, attempts or hypotheses for obtaining a human being without any connection with sexuality through "twin fission," cloning or parthenogenesis are to be considered contrary to the moral law, since they are in opposition to the dignity both of human procreation and of the conjugal union.*

The freezing of embryos, even when carried out in order to preserve the life of an embryo—cryopreservation—*constitutes an offense against the respect due to human beings* by exposing them to grave risks of death or harm to their physical integrity and depriving them, at least temporarily, of maternal shelter and gestation, thus placing them in a situation in which further offenses and manipulation are possible.

Certain attempts to influence chromosomic or genetic inheritance are not therapeutic, but are aimed at producing human beings selected according to sex or other predetermined qualities. These manipulations are contrary to the personal dignity of the human being and his or her integrity and identity. . . .

II. Interventions upon Human Procreation

. . . A preliminary point for the moral evaluation of [*in vitro* fertilization and artificial insemination] is constituted by the consideration of the circumstances and consequences which those procedures involve in relation to the respect due the human embryo. Development of the practice of *in vitro* fertilization has required innumerable fertilizations and destructions of human embryos. Even today, the usual practice presupposes a hyperovulation on the part of the woman: A number of ova are withdrawn, fertilized and then cultivated *in vitro* for some days. Usually not all are transferred into the genital tracts of the woman; some embryos, generally called "spare," are destroyed or frozen. On occasion, some of the implanted embryos are sacrificed for various eugenic, economic or psychological reasons. Such deliberate destruction of human beings or their utilization for different purposes to the detriment of their integrity and life is contrary to the doctrine on procured abortion already recalled.

The connection between *in vitro* fertilization and the voluntary destruction of human embryos occurs too often. This is significant: Through these procedures, with apparently contrary purposes, life and death are subjected to the decision of man, who thus sets himself up as the giver of life and death by decree. This dynamic of violence and domination may remain unnoticed by those very individuals who, in wishing to utilize this procedure, become subject to it themselves. The facts recorded and the cold logic which links them must be taken into consideration for a moral judgment on *in vitro* fertilization and embryo transfer: The abortion mentality which has made this procedure possible thus leads, whether one wants it or not, to man's domination over the life and death of his fellow human beings and can lead to a system of radical eugenics. . . .

A. Heterologous* Artificial Fertilization

Why must human procreation take place in marriage?
Every human being is always to be accepted as a gift and blessing of God. However, from the moral point of view a truly responsible procreation vis-a-vis the unborn child must be the fruit of marriage.

For human procreation has specific characteristics by virtue of the personal dignity of the parents and of the children: The procreation of a new person, whereby the man and the woman collaborate with the power of the Creator, must be the fruit and the sign of the mutual self-giving of the spouses, of their love and of their fidelity. *The fidelity of the spouses in the unity of marriage involves reciprocal respect of their right to become a father and a mother only through each other.*

The child has the right to be conceived, carried in the womb, brought into the world and brought up within marriage: It is through the secure and recognized relationship to his own parents that the child can discover his own identity and achieve his own proper human development.

The parents find in their child a confirmation and completion of their reciprocal self-giving: The child is the living image of their love, the permanent sign of their conjugal union, the living and indissoluble concrete expression of their paternity and maternity.

By reason of the vocation and social responsibilities of the person, the good of the children and of the parents contributes to the good of civil society; the vitality and stability of society require that children come into the world within a family and that the family be firmly based on marriage.

The tradition of the church and anthropological reflection recognize in marriage and in its indissoluble unity the only setting worthy of truly responsible procreation.

Does heterologous artificial fertilization conform to the dignity of the couple and to the truth of marriage?
Through *in vitro* fertilization and embryo transfer and heterologous artificial insemination, human conception is achieved through the fusion of ga-

---

* [Heterologous: involving sperm and egg from a man and woman who are not married to each other.]

metes of at least one donor other than the spouses who are united in marriage. *Heterologous artificial fertilization is contrary to the unity of marriage, to the dignity of the spouses, to the vocation proper to parents, and to the child's right to be conceived and brought into the world in marriage and from marriage.*

Respect for the unity of marriage and for conjugal fidelity demands that the child be conceived in marriage; the bond existing between husband and wife accords the spouses, in an objective and inalienable manner, the exclusive right to become father and mother solely through each other. Recourse to the gametes of a third person in order to have sperm or ovum available constitutes a violation of the reciprocal commitment of the spouses and a grave lack in regard to that essential property of marriage which is its unity.

Heterologous artificial fertilization violates the rights of the child; it deprives him of his filial relationship with his parental origins and can hinder the maturing of his personal identity. Furthermore, it offends the common vocation of the spouses who are called to fatherhood and motherhood: It objectively deprives conjugal fruitfulness of its unity and integrity; it brings about and manifests a rupture between genetic parenthood, gestational parenthood and responsibility for upbringing. Such damage to the personal relationships within the family has repercussions on civil society: What threatens the unity and stability of the family is a source of dissension, disorder and injustice in the whole of social life.

These reasons lead to a negative moral judgment concerning heterologous artificial fertilization: Consequently, fertilization of a married woman with the sperm of a donor different from her husband and fertilization with the husband's sperm of an ovum not coming from his wife are morally illicit. Furthermore, the artificial fertilization of a woman who is unmarried or a widow, whoever the donor may be, cannot be morally justified.

The desire to have a child and the love between spouses who long to obviate a sterility which cannot be overcome in any other way constitute understandable motivations; but subjectively good intentions do not render heterologous artificial fertilization conformable to the objective and inalienable properties of marriage or respectful of the rights of the child and of the spouses.

Is "surrogate" motherhood morally licit?
No, for the same reasons which lead one to reject heterologous artificial fertilization: For it is contrary to the unity of marriage and to the dignity of the procreation of the human person. . . .

B. Homologous* Artificial Fertilization

Since heterologous artificial fertilization has been declared unacceptable, the question arises of how to evaluate morally the process of homologous artificial

---

* [Homologous: involving sperm and egg from a man and woman who are married to each other.]

fertilization: *in vitro* fertilization and embryo transfer and artificial insemination between husband and wife. First a question of principle must be clarified.

What connection is required from the moral point of view between procreation and the conjugal act?
a) The church's teaching on marriage and human procreation affirms the "inseparable connection, willed by God and unable to be broken by man on his own initiative, between the two meanings of the conjugal act: the unitive meaning and the procreative meaning. Indeed, by its intimate structure the conjugal act, while most closely uniting husband and wife, capacitates them for the generation of new lives according to laws inscribed in the very being of man and of woman." . . .[11] "By safeguarding both these essential aspects, the unitive and the procreative, the conjugal act preserves in its fullness the sense of true mutual love and its ordination toward man's exalted vocation to parenthood."[12]

The same doctrine concerning the link between the meanings of the conjugal act and between the goods of marriage throws light on the moral problem of homologous artificial fertilization, since "it is never permitted to separate these different aspects to such a degree as positively to exclude either the procreative intention or the conjugal relation."[13]

Contraception deliberately deprives the conjugal act of its openness to procreation and in this way brings about a voluntary dissociation of the ends of marriage. Homologous artificial fertilization, in seeking a procreation which is not the fruit of a specific act of conjugal union, objectively effects an analogous separation between the goods and the meanings of marriage.

Thus . . . *from the moral point of view procreation is deprived of its proper perfection when it is not desired as the fruit of the conjugal act, that is to say, of the specific act of the spouses' union.*

b) The moral value of the intimate link between the goods of marriage and between the meanings of the conjugal act is based upon the unity of the human being, a unity involving body and spiritual soul. Spouses mutually express their personal love in the "language of the body," which clearly involves both "spousal meanings" and parental ones. The conjugal act by which the couple mutually express their self-gift at the same time expresses openness to the gift of life. It is an act that is inseparably corporal and spiritual. It is in their bodies and through their bodies that the spouses consummate their marriage and are able to become father and mother. In order to respect the language of their bodies and their natural generosity, the conjugal union must take place with respect for its openness to procreation; and the procreation of a person must be the fruit and the result of married love. The origin of the human being thus follows from a procreation that is "linked to the union, not only biological but also spiritual, of the parents, made one by the bond of marriage."[14] Fertilization achieved outside the bodies of the couple remains by this very fact deprived of the meanings and the values which are expressed in the language of the body and in the union of human persons.

c) Only respect for the link between the meanings of the conjugal act and respect for the unity of the human being make possible procreation in conformity with the dignity of the person. In his unique and irrepeatable origin, the child must be respected and recognized as equal in personal dignity to those who give him life. The human person must be accepted in his parents' act of union and love; the generation of a child must therefore be the fruit of that mutual giving which is realized in the conjugal act wherein the spouses cooperate as servants and not as masters in the work of the Creator, who is love.

In reality, the origin of a human person is the result of an act of giving. The one conceived must be the fruit of his parents' love. He cannot be desired or conceived as the product of an intervention of medical or biological techniques; that would be equivalent to reducing him to an object of scientific technology. No one may subject the coming of a child into the world to conditions of technical efficiency which are to be evaluated according to standards of control and dominion.

The moral relevance of the link between the meanings of the conjugal act and between the goods of marriage, as well as the unity of the human being and the dignity of his origin, demand that the procreation of a human person be brought about as the fruit of the conjugal act specific to the love between spouses. . . .

Is homologous "in vitro" fertilization morally licit?

The answer to this question is strictly dependent on the principles just mentioned. Certainly one cannot ignore the legitimate aspirations of sterile couples. For some, recourse to homologous *in vitro* fertilization and embryo transfer appears to be the only way of fulfilling their sincere desire for a child. The question is asked whether the totality of conjugal life in such situations is not sufficient to ensure the dignity proper to human procreation. It is acknowledged that *in vitro* fertilization and embryo transfer certainly cannot supply for the absence of sexual relations and cannot be preferred to the specific acts of conjugal union, given the risks involved for the child and the difficulties of the procedure. But it is asked whether, when there is no other way of overcoming the sterility which is a source of suffering, homologous *in vitro* fertilization may not constitute an aid, if not a form of therapy, whereby its moral licitness could be admitted.

The desire for a child—or at the very least an openness to the transmission of life—is a necessary prerequisite from the moral point of view for responsible human procreation. But this good intention is not sufficient for making a positive moral evaluation of *in vitro* fertilization between spouses. The process of *in vitro* fertilization and embryo transfer must be judged in itself and cannot borrow its definitive moral quality from the totality of conjugal life of which it becomes part nor from the conjugal acts which may precede or follow it. . . .

[E]ven in a situation in which every precaution were taken to avoid the death of human embryos, homologous *in vitro* fertilization and embryo transfer dissociates from the conjugal act the actions which are directed to human fertilization. For this reason the very nature of homologous *in vitro* fertilization and embryo transfer also must be taken into account, even abstracting from the link with procured abortion.

Homologous *in vitro* fertilization and embryo transfer is brought about outside the bodies of the couple through actions of third parties whose competence and technical activity determine the success of the procedure. Such fertilization entrusts the life and identity of the embryo into the power of doctors and biologists and establishes the domination of technology over the origin and destiny of the human person. Such a relationship of domination is in itself contrary to the dignity and equality that must be common to parents and children.

Conception *in vitro* is the result of the technical action which presides over fertilization. *Such fertilization is neither in fact achieved nor positively willed as the expression and fruit of a specific act of the conjugal union. In homologous "in vitro" fertilization and embryo transfer, therefore, even if it is considered in the context of de facto existing sexual relations, the generation of the human person is objectively deprived of its proper perfection: namely, that of being the result and fruit of a conjugal act* in which the spouses can become "cooperators with God for giving life to a new person." . . .[15]

Although the manner in which human conception is achieved with *in vitro* fertilization and embryo transfer cannot be approved, every child which comes into the world must in any case be accepted as a living gift of the divine Goodness and must be brought up with love.

How is homologous artificial insemination to be evaluated from the moral point of view?

Homologous artificial insemination within marriage cannot be admitted except for those cases in which the technical means is not a substitute for the conjugal act but serves to facilitate and to help so that the act attains its natural purpose. . . .

"In its natural structure, the conjugal act is a personal action, a simultaneous and immediate cooperation on the part of the husband and wife, which by the very nature of the agents and the proper nature of the act is the expression of the mutual gift which, according to the words of Scripture, brings about union 'in one flesh.' "[16] Thus moral conscience "does not necessarily proscribe the use of certain artificial means destined solely either to the facilitating of the natural act or to ensuring that the natural act normally performed achieves its proper end."[17] If the technical means facilitates the conjugal act or helps it to reach its natural objectives, it can be morally acceptable. If, on the other hand, the procedure were to replace the conjugal act, it is morally illicit.

Artificial insemination as a substitute for the conjugal act is prohibited by reason of the voluntarily achieved dissociation of the two meanings of the conjugal act. Masturbation, through which the sperm is normally obtained, is another sign of this dissociation: Even when it is done for the purpose of procreation the act remains deprived of its unitive meaning: "It lacks the sexual relationship called for by the moral order, namely the relationship which realizes 'the full sense of mutual self-giving and human procreation in the context of true love.' " . . .[18]

What moral criterion can be proposed with regard to medical intervention in human procreation?

The medical act must be evaluated not only with reference to its technical dimension, but also and above all in relation to its goal, which is the good of persons and their bodily and psychological health. The moral criteria for medical intervention in procreation are deduced from the dignity of human persons, of their sexuality and of their origin.

Medicine which seeks to be ordered to the integral good of the person must respect the specifically human values of sexuality. The doctor is at the service of persons and of human procreation. He does not have the authority to dispose of them or to decide their fate. A medical intervention respects the dignity of persons when it seeks to assist the conjugal act either in order to facilitate its performance or in order to enable it to achieve its objective once it has been normally performed.

On the other hand, it sometimes happens that a medical procedure technologically replaces the conjugal act in order to obtain a procreation which is neither its result nor its fruit. In this case the medical act is not, as it should be, at the service of conjugal union, but rather appropriates to itself the procreative function and thus contradicts the dignity and the inalienable rights of the spouses and of the child to be born.

The humanization of medicine, which is insisted upon today by everyone, requires respect for the integral dignity of the human person first of all in the act and at the moment in which the spouses transmit life to a new person. It is only logical therefore to address an urgent appeal to Catholic doctors and scientists that they bear exemplary witness to the respect due to the human embryo and to the dignity of procreation. The medical and nursing staff of Catholic hospitals and clinics are in a special way urged to do justice to the moral obligations which they have assumed, frequently also, as part of their contract. Those who are in charge of Catholic hospitals and clinics and who are often religious will take special care to safeguard and promote a diligent observance of the moral norms recalled in the present instruction.

The suffering caused by infertility in marriage.

The suffering of spouses who cannot have children or who are afraid of bringing a handicapped child into the world is a suffering that everyone must understand and properly evaluate.

On the part of the spouses, the desire for a child is natural: It expresses the vocation to fatherhood and motherhood inscribed in conjugal love. This desire can be even stronger if the couple is affected by sterility which appears incurable. Nevertheless, marriage does not confer upon the spouses the right to have a child, but only the right to perform those natural acts which are per se ordered to procreation.

A true and proper right to a child would be contrary to the child's dignity and nature. The child is not an object to which one has a right nor can he be considered as an object of ownership: Rather, a child is a gift, "the supreme gift" and the most gratuitous gift of marriage, and is a living testimony of the mutual giving of his parents. For this reason, the child has the right as already mentioned, to be the fruit of the specific act of the conjugal love of his parents; and he also has the right to be respected as a person from the moment of his conception.

Nevertheless, whatever its cause or prognosis, sterility is certainly a difficult trial. The community of believers is called to shed light upon and support the suffering of those who are unable to fulfill their legitimate aspiration to motherhood and fatherhood. Spouses who find themselves in this sad situation are called to find in it an opportunity for sharing in a particular way in the Lord's cross, the source of spiritual fruitfulness. Sterile couples must not forget that "even when procreation is not possible, conjugal life does not for this reason lose its value. Physical sterility in fact can be for spouses the occasion for other important services to the life of the human person, for example, adoption, various forms of educational work and assistance to other families and to poor or handicapped children." . . .[19]

III. Moral and Civil Law

The Values and Moral Obligations That Civil Legislation Must Respect and Sanction in This Matter

The inviolable right to life of every innocent human individual and the rights of the family and of the institution of marriage constitute fundamental moral values because they concern the natural condition and integral vocation of the human person; at the same time they are constitutive elements of civil society and its order.

For this reason the new technological possibilities which have opened up in the field of biomedicine require the intervention of the political authorities and of the legislator, since an uncontrolled application of such techniques could lead to unforeseeable and damaging consequences for civil society. Recourse to the conscience of each individual and to the self-regulation of researchers cannot be sufficient for ensuring respect for personal rights and public order. . . .

The intervention of the public authority must be inspired by the rational principles which regulate the relationships between civil law and moral law. The task of the civil law is to ensure the common good of people through the recognition of and the defense of fundamental rights and through the promotion of peace and of public morality. . . .

As a consequence of the respect and protection which must be ensured for the unborn child from the moment of his conception, the law must provide appropriate penal sanctions for every deliberate violation of the child's rights. The law cannot tolerate—indeed it must expressly forbid—that human beings, even at the embryonic stage, should be treated as objects of experimentation, be mutilated or destroyed with the excuse that they are superfluous or incapable of developing normally.

The political authority is bound to guarantee to the institution of the family, upon which society is based, the juridical protection to which it has a right. From the very fact that it is at the service of people, the political authority must also be at the service of the family. Civil law cannot grant approval to techniques of artificial procreation which, for the benefit of third parties (doctors, biologists, economic or governmental powers), take away what is a right inherent in the relationship between spouses; and therefore civil law cannot legalize the donation of gametes between persons who are not legitimately united in marriage.

Legislation must also prohibit, by virtue of the support which is due to the family, embryo banks, post-mortem insemination and "surrogate motherhood." . . .

Notes

Submitted and signed by Cardinal Joseph Ratzinger, Prefect, and Archbishop Alberto Bovone, Secretary, and approved by Pope John Paul II.

1. Pope John Paul II, Discourse to those taking part in the 81st Congress of the Italian Society of Internal Medicine and the 82nd Congress of the Italian Society of General Surgery, Oct. 27, 1980: AAS 72 (1980) 1126.

2. Pope Paul VI, Discourse to the General Assembly of the United Nations, Oct. 4, 1965: AAS 57 (1965) 878; encyclical *Populorum Progressio,* 13: AAS 59 (1967) 263.

3. Ibid., Homily During the Mass Closing the Holy Year, Dec. 25, 1975: AAS 68 (1976) 145; Pope John Paul II, encyclical *Dives in Misericordia,* 30: AAS 72 (1980) 1224.

4. Pope John Paul II, Discourse to those taking part in the 35th General Assembly of the World Medical Association, Oct. 29, 1983; AAS 76 (1984) 390.

5. *Familiaris Consortio,* 11.

6. Pope John Paul II, Discourse to those taking part in the 35th General Assembly of the World Medical Association, Oct. 29, 1983: AAS 76 (1984) 390.

7. Pope John XXIII, encyclical *Mater et Magistra,* III: AAS 53 (1961) 447.

8. Cf. *Gaudium et Spes,* 51: "When it is a question of harmonizing married love with the responsible transmission of life, the moral character of one's behavior does not depend only on the good intentions and the evaluation of the motives: The objective criteria must be used, criteria drawn from the nature of the human person and human acts, criteria which respect the total meaning of mutual self-giving and human procreation in the context of true love."

9. Congregation for the Doctrine of the Faith, Declaration on Procured Abortion, 12–13.

10. No one, before coming into existence, can claim a subjective right to begin to exist; nevertheless, it is legitimate to affirm the right of the child to have a fully human origin through conception in conformity with the personal nature of the human being. Life is a gift that must be bestowed in a manner worthy both of the subject receiving it and of the subjects transmitting it. This statement is to be borne in mind also for what will be explained concerning artificial human procreation.

11. *Humanae Vitae,* 12.

12. Ibid.

13. Pope Pius XII, Discourse to those taking part in the Second Naples World Congress on Fertility and Human Sterility, May 19, 1956: AAS 48 (1956) 470.

14. Pope John Paul II, Discourse to those taking part in the 35th General Assembly of the World Medical Association, Oct. 29, 1983: AAS 76 (1984) 393.

15. *Familiaris Consortio,* 14: AAS 74 (1982) 96.

16. Pope Pius XII, Discourse to the Italian Catholic Union of Midwives, Oct. 29, 1951: AAS 43 (1951) 850.

17. Ibid. Discourse to those taking part in the Fourth International Congress of Catholic Doctors, Sept. 29, 1949: AAS 41 (1949) 560.

18. Congregation for the Doctrine of the Faith, Declaration on Certain Questions Concerning Sexual Ethics, 9 AAS 68 (1976) 86, which quotes *Gaudium et Spes,* 51. . . .

19. *Familiaris Consortio,* 14.

The Meaning of Life—In the Laboratory

Leon Kass

People will not look forward to posterity who never look backward to
their ancestors.

EDMUND BURKE, *Reflections on the Revolution in France*

What's a nice embryo like you doing in a place like this?

TRADITIONAL

The readers of Aldous Huxley's novel, like the inhabitants of the society it
depicts, enter into the Brave New World through "a squat gray building . . .
the Central London Hatchery and Conditioning Centre," beginning, in fact,
in the Fertilizing Room. There, three hundred fertilizers sit bent over their
instruments, inspecting eggs, immersing them "in a warm bouillon containing
free-swimming spermatozoa," and incubating the successfully fertilized eggs
until they are ripe for bottling (or Bokanovskification).[1] Here, most emphatically, life begins with fertilization—in the laboratory. Life in the laboratory is
the gateway to the Brave New World.

We stand today fully on the threshold of that gateway. How far and how
fast we travel through this entrance is not a matter of chance or necessity but
rather a matter of human decision—*our* human decision. Indeed, it seems to
be reserved to the people of this country and this century, by our conduct and
example, to decide also this important question.

Should we allow or encourage the initiation and growth of human life in
the laboratory [as in development and use of *in vitro* fertilization]? . . . .

The Meaning of the Question: The Question of Meaning

How should one think about such ethical questions, here and in general? There
are many possible ways, and it is not altogether clear which way is best. For

From *Toward a More Natural Science: Biology and Human Affairs,* Chapter Four. New York: The
Free Press, 1985, 1988 (paperback), pp. 99–127, a revised version of "Making Babies Revisited,"
The Public Interest 54 (1979). Abridged. Reprinted with permission of *The Public Interest* and the
author.

some people, ethical issues are immediately matters of right and wrong, of purity and sin, of good and evil. For others, the critical terms are benefits and harms, risks and promises, gains and costs. Some will focus on so-called rights of individuals or groups (e.g., a right to life or childbirth); still others will emphasize so-called goods for society and its members, such as the advancement of knowledge and the prevention and cure of disease. My own orientation here is somewhat different. I wish to suggest that before deciding what to do, one should try to understand the implications of doing or not doing. The first task, it seems to me, is not to ask "moral or immoral?" or "right or wrong?" but to try to understand fully the meaning and significance of the proposed actions.

This concern with significance leads me to take a broad view of the matter. For we are concerned here not only with some limited research project . . . and the narrow issues of safety and informed consent . . . ; we are concerned also with a whole range of implications, including many that are tied to definitely foreseeable consequences of this research and its predictable extensions—and touching even our common conception of our own humanity. As most of us are at least tacitly aware, more is at stake than in ordinary biomedical research or in experimenting with human subjects at risk of bodily harm. At stake is the *idea* of the *humanness* of our human life and the meaning of our embodiment, our sexual being, and our relation to ancestors and descendants. In thinking about necessarily particular and immediate decisions . . . we must be mindful of the larger picture and must avoid the great danger of trivializing the matter for the sake of rendering it manageable.

The Status of Extracorporeal Life

The meaning of "life in the laboratory" turns in part on the nature and meaning of the human embryo, isolated in the laboratory and separate from the confines of a woman's body. What is the status of a fertilized human egg (i.e., a human zygote) and the embryo that develops from it? How are we to regard its being? How are we to regard it morally (i.e., how are we to behave toward it)? These are, alas, all too familiar questions. At least analogous, if not identical, questions are central to the abortion controversy and are also crucial in considering whether and what sort of experimentation is properly conducted on living but aborted fetuses. Would that it were possible to say that the matter is simple and obvious, and that it has been resolved to everyone's satisfaction!

But the controversy about the morality of abortion continues to rage and divide our nation. Moreover, many who favor or who do not oppose abortion do so despite the fact that they regard the previable fetus as a living human organism, even if less worthy of protection than a woman's desire not to give it birth. Almost everyone senses the importance of this matter for the decision about laboratory culture of and experimentation with human embryos. Thus, we are obliged to take up the question of the status of the embryo in our search for the outlines of some common ground on which many of us can stand. To the best of my knowledge, the discussion that follows is not informed by any particular sectarian or religious teaching, though it may perhaps reveal that I am a person not devoid of reverence and the capacity for awe and wonder, said by some to be the core of the religious sentiment.

I begin by noting that the circumstances of laboratory-grown blastocysts (i.e., three-to-six-day-old embryos) and embryos are not identical with those of the analogous cases of (1) living fetuses facing abortion and (2) living aborted fetuses used in research. First, the fetuses whose fates are at issue in abortion are unwanted, usually the result of so-called accidental conception. Here, the embryos are wanted, and deliberately created, despite a certain knowledge that many of them will be destroyed or discarded. Moreover, the fate of these embryos is not in conflict with the wishes, interests, or alleged rights of the pregnant women. Second, though the federal guidelines governing fetal research permit studies conducted on the not-at-all viable aborted fetus, such research merely takes advantage of available "products" of abortions not themselves undertaken for the sake of the research. No one has proposed and no one would sanction the deliberate production of live fetuses to be aborted for the sake of research, even very beneficial research.[2] In contrast, we are here considering the deliberate production of embryos for the express purpose of experimentation.

The cases may also differ in other ways. Given the present state of the art, the largest embryo under discussion is the blastocyst, a spherical, relatively undifferentiated mass of cells, barely visible to the naked eye. In appearance it does not look human; indeed, only the most careful scrutiny by the most experienced scientist might distinguish it from similar blastocysts of other mammals. If the human zygote and blastocyst are more like the animal zygote and blastocyst than they are like the twelve-week-old human fetus (which already has a humanoid appearance, differentiated organs, and electrical activity of the brain), then there would be a much diminished ethical dilemma regarding their deliberate creation and experimental use. Needless to say, there are articulate and passionate defenders of all points of view. Let us try, however, to consider the matter afresh.

First of all, the zygote and early embryonic stages are clearly alive. They metabolize, respire, and respond to changes in the environment; they grow and divide. Second, though not yet organized into distinctive parts or organs, the blastocyst is an organic whole, self-developing, genetically unique and distinct from the egg and sperm whose union marked the beginning of its career as a discrete, unfolding being. While the egg and sperm are alive as cells, something new and alive *in a different sense* comes into being with fertilization. The truth of this is unaffected by the fact that fertilization takes time and is not an instantaneous event. For after fertilization is *complete,* there exists a new individual, with its unique genetic identity, fully potent for the self-initiated development into a mature human being, if circumstances are cooperative. Though there is some sense in which the lives of egg and sperm are continuous with the life of the new organism (or, in human terms, that the parents live on in the child-to-be [or child]), in the decisive sense there is a discontinuity, a new beginning, with fertilization. *After* fertilization, there is continuity of subsequent development, even if the locus of the new living being alters with implantation (or birth). Any honest biologist must be impressed by these facts, and must be inclined, at least on first glance, to the view that a human life begins at fertilization.[3] Even Dr. Robert Edwards had apparently stumbled over this truth, perhaps inadvertently, in his remark about Louise Brown, his first successful test-tube baby: "The last time I saw *her, she* was just eight cells in a test-tube. *She* was beautiful *then,* and she's still beautiful *now!*"[4]

Granting that a human life begins at fertilization, and comes to be via a continuous process thereafter, surely—one might say—the blastocyst itself can hardly be considered a human being. I myself would agree that a blastocyst is not, in a *full* sense, a human being—or what the current fashion calls, rather arbitrarily and without clear definition, a person. It does not look like a human being, nor can it do very much of what human beings do. Yet, at the same time, I must acknowledge that the human blastocyst is (1) human in origin and (2) *potentially* a mature human being, if all goes well. This, too, is beyond dispute; indeed it is precisely because of its peculiarly human potentialities that people propose to study *it* rather than the embryos of other mammals. The human blastocyst, even the human blastocyst *in vitro,* is not humanly nothing; it possesses a power to become what everyone will agree is a human being.

Here it may be objected that the blastocyst *in vitro* has today no such power, because there is now no *in vitro* way to bring the blastocyst to that much later fetal stage in which it might survive on its own. There are no published reports of culture of human embryos beyond the blastocyst stage (though this has been reported for mice). The *in vitro* blastocyst, like the twelve-week-old aborted fetus, is *in this sense* not viable (i.e., it is at a stage of maturation before the stage of possible independent existence). But if we distinguish, among the *not*-viable embryos, between the *pre*viable and the *not-at-all* viable—on the basis that the former, though not yet viable is capable of *becoming* or *being made* viable[5]—we note a crucial difference between the blastocyst and the twelve-week-old abortus. Unlike an aborted fetus, the blastocyst is possibly salvageable, and hence potentially viable, *if it is transferred to a woman for implantation.* It is not strictly true that the *in vitro* blastocyst is *necessarily* not viable. Until proven otherwise, by embryo transfer and attempted implantation, we are right to consider the human blastocyst *in vitro* as potentially a human being and, in this respect, not fundamentally different from a blastocyst *in utero.* To put the matter more forcefully, the blastocyst *in vitro* is more viable, in the sense of more salvageable, than aborted fetuses at most later stages, up to say twenty weeks.

This is not to say that such a blastocyst is therefore endowed with a so-called right to life, that failure to implant it is negligent homicide, or that experimental touchings of such blastocysts constitute assault and battery. (I myself tend to reject such claims, and indeed think that the ethical questions are not best posed in terms of rights.) But the blastocyst is not nothing; it is *at least* potential humanity, and as such it elicits, or ought to elicit, our feelings of awe and respect. In the blastocyst, even in the zygote, we face a mysterious and awesome power, a power governed by an immanent plan that may produce an indisputably and fully human being. It deserves our respect not because it has rights or claims or sentience (which it does not have at this stage), but because of what it is, now *and* prospectively.

Let us test this provisional conclusion by considering intuitively our response to two possible fates of such zygotes, blastocysts, and early embryos. First, should such an embryo die, will we be inclined to mourn its passing? When a woman we know miscarries, we are sad—largely for *her* loss and disappointment, but perhaps also at the premature death of a life that might have been. But we do not mourn the departed fetus, nor do we seek ritually to dispose of the remains. In this respect, we do not treat even the fetus as fully one of us.

On the other hand, we would, I suppose, recoil even from the thought, let alone the practice—I apologize for forcing it upon the reader—of eating such embryos, should someone discover that they would provide a great delicacy, a "human caviar." The human blastocyst would be protected by our taboo against cannibalism, which insists on the humanness of human flesh and does not permit us to treat even the flesh of the dead as if it were mere meat. *The human embryo is not mere meat; it is not just stuff; it is not a "thing."*[6] Because of its origin and because of its capacity, it commands a higher respect.

How much more respect? As much as for a fully developed human being? My own inclination is to say probably not, but who can be certain? Indeed, there might be prudential and reasonable grounds for an affirmative answer, partly because the presumption of ignorance ought to err in the direction of never underestimating the basis for respect of human life (not least, for our own self-respect), partly because so many people feel very strongly that even the blastocyst is protectably human. As a first approximation, I would analogize the early embryo *in vitro* to the early embryo *in utero* (because both are potentially viable and human). On this ground alone, the most sensible policy is to *treat the early embryo as a previable fetus, with constraints imposed on early embryo research at least as great as those on fetal research.*

To some this may seem excessively scrupulous. They will argue for the importance of the absence of distinctively humanoid appearance or the absence of sentience. To be sure, we would feel more restraint in invasive procedures conducted on a five-month-old or even a twelve-week-old living fetus than on a blastocyst. But this added restraint on inflicting suffering on a look-alike, feeling creature in no way denies the propriety of a prior restraint, grounded in respect for individuated, living, potential humanity. Before I would be persuaded to treat early embryos differently from later ones, I would insist on the establishment of a reasonably clear, naturally grounded boundary that would separate "early" and "late," and provide the basis for respecting the "early" less than the "late." This burden must be accepted by proponents of experimentation with human embryos *in vitro* if a decision to permit the creation of embryos for such experimentation is to be treated as ethically responsible.

The Treatment of Extracorporeal Embryos

Where does the above analysis lead in thinking about treatment of human embryos in the laboratory? I indicate, very briefly, the lines toward a possible policy, though that is not my major intent.

The *in vitro* fertilized embryo has four possible fates: (1) implantation, in the hope of producing from it a child; (2) death, by active killing or disaggregation, or by a "natural" demise; (3) use in manipulative experimentation—embryological, genetic, etc.; and (4) use in attempts at perpetuation *in vitro,* beyond the blastocyst stage, ultimately, perhaps, to viability. Let us consider each in turn.

On the strength of my analysis of the status of the embryo, and the respect due it, no objection would be raised to implantation. *In vitro* fertilization and embryo transfer to treat infertility, as in the case of Mr. and Mrs. Brown, is perfectly compatible with a respect and reverence for human life, including potential human life. Moreover, no disrespect is intended or practiced by the mere fact that several eggs are removed to increase the chance of success. Were it possible to guarantee successful fertilization and normal growth with a single egg, no more would need to be obtained. Assuming nothing further is done with the unimplanted embryos, there is nothing disrespectful going on. The demise of the unimplanted embryos would be analogous to the loss of numerous embryos wasted in the normal *in vivo* attempts to generate a child. It is estimated that over 50 percent of eggs successfully fertilized during unprotected sexual intercourse fail to implant, or do not remain implanted, in the uterine wall, and are shed soon thereafter, before a diagnosis of pregnancy could be made. Any couple attempting to conceive a child tacitly accepts such embryonic wastage as the perfectly acceptable price to be paid for the birth of a (usually) healthy child. Current procedures to initiate pregnancy with laboratory fertilization thus differ from the natural process in that what would normally be spread over four or five months *in vivo* is compressed into a single effort, using all at once a four or five months' supply of eggs.[7]

Parenthetically, we should note that the natural occurrence of embryo and fetal loss and wastage does not necessarily or automatically justify all deliberate, humanly caused destruction of fetal life. For example, the natural loss of embryos in early pregnancy cannot in itself be a warrant for deliberately aborting them or for invasively experimenting on them *in vitro,* any more than stillbirths could be a justification for newborn infanticide. There are many things that could happen naturally that we ought not do deliberately. It is curious how the same people who deny the relevance of nature as a guide for evaluating human interventions into human generation, and who deny that the term "unnatural" carries any ethical weight, will themselves appeal to "nature's way" when it suits their purposes. Still, in this present matter, the closeness to natural procreation—the goal is the same, the embryonic loss is unavoidable and not desired, and the amount of loss is similar—leads me to believe that we do no more intentional or unjustified harm in one case than in the other and practice no disrespect.

But must we allow the unimplanted *in vitro* embryos to die? Why should they not be either transferred for adoption into another infertile woman or else used for investigative purposes, to seek new knowledge, say about gene action? The first option raises questions about lineage and the nature of parenthood to which I will return. But even on first glance, it would seem likely to raise a large objection from the first couple who were seeking a child of their own, and not the dissemination of their children for prenatal adoption.

But what about experimentation on such blastocysts and early embryos? Is that compatible with the respect they deserve? This is the hard question. On balance, I would think not. Invasive and manipulative experiments involving such embryos very likely presume that they are things or mere stuff, and deny the fact of their possible viability. Certain observational and noninvasive experiments might be different. But on the whole, I would think that the respect for human embryos for which I have argued—I repeat, not their so-called right to life—would lead one to oppose most potentially interesting and useful experimentation. This is a dilemma, but one which cannot be ducked or defined away. Either we accept certain great restrictions on the permissible uses of human embryos or we deliberately decide to override—though I hope not deny—the respect due to the embryos.

I am aware that I have pointed toward a seemingly paradoxical conclusion about the treatment of the unimplanted embryos: leave them alone, and do not create embryos for experimentation only. To let them die naturally would be the most respectful course, grounded on a reverence, generically, for their potential humanity, and a respect, individually, for their being the seed and offspring of a particular couple, who were themselves seeking only to have a child of their own. An analysis that stressed a right to life, rather than respect, would, of course, lead to different conclusions. Only an analysis of the status of the embryo that denies both its so-called rights or its worthiness of all respect would have no trouble sanctioning its use in investigative research, donation to other couples, commercial transactions, and other activities of these sorts.

I have to this point ignored the fourth and future fate of life in the laboratory: perpetuation in the bottle beyond the blastocyst stage, ultimately, perhaps, to viability. As a practical matter, this repugnant Huxleyan prospect probably need not concern us much for the time being. But as a thought experiment, it permits us to test further our intuitions about the meaning of life in the laboratory, and to discover thereby the limitations of the previous analysis. For these unimplanted and cultivated embryos raise even more profound difficulties. Bad as it may now be to discard or experiment upon them in these primordial stages, it will be far worse once we learn how to perpetuate them to later stages in their laboratory existence—especially when the technology arrives that can bring them to viability *in vitro*. For how long and up to what stage of development will they be considered fit material for experimentation? When ought they to be released from the machinery and admitted into the human fraternity or, at least, into the premature nursery? The need for a respectable boundary defining protectable human life cannot be overstated. The current boundaries, gerrymandered for the sake of abortion—namely, birth or viability—may now satisfy both women's liberation and the United States Supreme Court, and may someday satisfy even a future pope, but they will not survive the coming of more sophisticated technologies for growing life in the laboratory.

But what if perpetuation in the laboratory were to be sought not for the sake of experimentation but in order to produce a healthy living child—say, one with all the benefits of a scientifically based gestational nourishment and care? Would such treatment of a laboratory-grown embryo be compatible with the respect it is owed? If we consider only what is owed to its vitality and potential humanity *as an individuated human being,* then the laboratory growth of an embryo into a viable full-term baby (i.e., ectogenesis) would be perfectly compatible with that requisite respect. (Indeed, for these reasons one would guess that the right to life people, who object even to the destruction of blastocysts, would find infinitely preferable any form of their preservation and perpetuation to term, in the bottle if necessary.) But the practice of ectogenesis would be incompatible with the *further* respect owed to our humanity on account of *the bonds of lineage, kinship, and descent.* To be human means not only to have human form and powers; it means also to have a human context and to be humanly connected. The navel, no less than speech and the upright posture, is a mark of our being. It is for these sorts of reasons that we find the Brave New World's Hatcheries dehumanizing. . . .

Questions of Lineage and Parenthood, Embodiment and Gender

. . . Our society is dangerously close to losing its grip on the meaning of some fundamental aspects of human existence. In reviewing the problem of the disrespect shown to embryonic and fetal life in our efforts to master them, we noted a tendency—we shall meet it again shortly—to reduce certain aspects of human being to mere body, a tendency opposed most decisively in the nearly universal prohibition of cannibalism. Here, in noticing our growing casualness about marriage, legitimacy, kinship, and lineage, we discover how our individualistic and willful projects lead us to ignore the truths defended by the equally widespread prohibition of incest (especially parent-child incest). Properly understood, the largely universal taboo against incest, and also the prohibitions against adultery, defend the integrity of marriage, kinship, and especially the lines of origin and descent. These time-honored restraints implicitly teach that clarity about who your parents are, clarity in the lines of generation, clarity about who is whose, are the indispensable foundations of a sound family life, itself the sound foundation of civilized community. Clarity about your origins is crucial for self-identity, itself important for self-respect. It would be, in my view, deplorable public policy to erode further such fundamental beliefs, values, institutions, and practices. This means, concretely, no encouragement of embryo adoption or especially of surrogate pregnancy. While it would perhaps be foolish to try to proscribe or outlaw such practices, it would not be wise to support or foster them.

The existence of human life in the laboratory, outside the confines of the generating bodies from which it sprang, also challenges the meaning of our embodiment. People like Mr. and Mrs. Brown, who seek a child derived from their flesh, celebrate in so doing their self-identity with their own bodies, and acknowledge the meaning of the living human body by following its pointings to its own perpetuation. For them, their bodies contain the seeds of their own self-transcendence and enable them to strike a blow for the enduring goodness of the life in which they participate. Affirming the gift of their embodied life, they show their gratitude by passing on that gift to their children. Only the body's failure to serve the transmission of embodiment has led them—and only temporarily—to generate beyond its confines. But life in the laboratory also allows other people—including those who would donate or sell sperm, eggs, or embryos; or those who would bear another's child in surrogate pregnancy; or even those who will prefer to have their children rationally manufactured entirely in the laboratory—to declare themselves independent of their bodies, in this ultimate liberation. For them the body is a mere tool, ideally an instrument of the conscious will, the sole repository of human dignity. Yet this blind assertion of will against our bodily nature—in contradiction of the meaning of the human generation it seeks to control—can only lead to self-degradation and dehumanization.

In this connection, the case of surrogate wombs bears a further comment. While expressing no objection to the practice of foster pregnancy itself, some people object that it will be done for pay, largely because of their fear that poor women will be exploited by such a practice. But if there were nothing wrong with foster pregnancy, what would be wrong with making a living at it? Clearly, this objection harbors a tacit understanding that to bear another's child for pay is in some sense a degradation of oneself—in the same sense that prostitution is a degradation primarily because it entails the loveless surrender of the body to serve another's lust, and only derivatively because the woman is paid. It is to deny the meaning and worth of one's body to treat it as a mere incubator, divested of its human meaning. It is also to deny the meaning of the bond among sexuality, love, and procreation. The buying and selling of human flesh and the dehumanized uses of the human body ought not to be encouraged. To be sure, the practice of womb donation could be engaged in for love, not money, as it apparently has been in some cases, including the original case in Michigan. A woman could bear her sister's child out of sisterly love. But to the degree that she escapes in this way from the degradation and difficulties of the sale of human flesh and bodily services and the treating of the body as undignified stuff (the problem of cannibalism), once again she approaches instead the difficulties of incest and near incest.

To this point we have been examining the meaning of the presence of human life in the laboratory, but we have neglected the meaning of putting it there in the first place, that is, the meaning of extracorporeal fertilization *as such*. What is the significance of divorcing human generation from human sexuality, precisely for the meaning of our bodily natures as male and female, as both gendered and engendering? To be male or to be female derives its deepest meaning only in relation to the other, and therewith in the gender-mated prospects for generation through union. Our separated embodiment prevents us as lovers from attaining that complete fusion of souls that we as lovers seek; but the complementarity of gender provides a bodily means for transcending separateness through the children born of sexual union. As the navel is our bodily mark of lineage, pointing back to our ancestors, so our genitals are the bodily mark of linkage, pointing ultimately forward to our descendants. Can these aspects of our being be fulfilled through the rational-ized techniques of laboratory sexuality and fertilization? Does not the scientist-partner produce a triangle that somehow subverts the meaning of "two"? Even in the best of cases, do we not pay in coin of our humanity for electing to generate sexlessly? . . .

Future Prospects

. . . I can here do no more than identify a few kinds of questions that must be considered in relation to possible coming control over human heredity and reproduction: questions about the wisdom required to engage in such prac-tices; questions about the goals and standards that will guide our interven-tions; questions about changes in the concepts of being human, including embodiment, gender, love, lineage, identity, parenthood, and sexuality; ques-tions about the responsibility of power over future generations; questions about awe, respect, humility; questions about the kind of society we will have if we follow along our present course.

Though I cannot discuss these questions now, I can and must face a serious objection to considering them at all. Most people would agree that the pro-jected possibilities raise far more serious questions than do simple fertilization of a few embryos, their growth *in vitro* to the blastocyst stage, and their subsequent use in experimentation or possible transfer to women for gesta-tion. Why burden present policy with these possibilities? Future abuses, it is often said, do not disqualify present uses (though these same people often say that "future benefits justify present practices, even questionable ones"). More-over, there can be no certainty that *A* will lead to *B*. This thin-edge-of-the-wedge argument has been open to criticism.

But such criticism misses the point for two reasons. First, critics often misunderstand the wedge argument, which is not primarily an argument of prediction, that *A* will lead to *B*, say on the strength of the empirical analysis of precedent and an appraisal of the likely direction of present research. It is primarily an argument about the logic of justification. Do not the principles of justification *now* used to justify the current research proposal already justify *in advance* the further developments? Consider some of these principles:

1. It is desirable to learn as much as possible about the processes of fertilization, growth, implantation, and the differentiation of human embryos and about human gene expression and its control.
2. It would be desirable to acquire improved techniques for enhancing conception and implantation, for preventing conception and implantation, for the treatment of genetic and chromosomal abnormalities, etc.
3. In the end, only research using *human* embryos can answer these questions and provide these techniques.
4. There should be no censorship or limitation of scientific inquiry or research.

This logic knows no boundary at the blastocyst stage or, for that matter, at any later stage. For these principles *not* to justify future extensions of current work, some independent additional principles (e.g., a principle limiting such justification to particular stages of development) would have to be found. (Here, the task is to find such a biologically defensible distinction that could be respected as reasonable and not arbitrary, a difficult—perhaps impossible— task, given the continuity of development after fertilization.) Perhaps even more important than any present decision to encourage bringing human life into the laboratory will be the reasons given to support that decision. We will want to know *precisely* what grounds our policymakers will give for endorsing such research and whether their principles have not already sanctioned future developments. If they do give such wedge-opening justifications, let them do so deliberately, candidly, and intentionally.

A better case to illustrate the wedge logic is the principle offered for the embryo transfer procedure as treatment for infertility. Will we support the use of *in vitro* fertilization and embryo transfer because it provides a child of one's own, in a strict sense of "one's own," to a married couple? Or will we support the transfer because it is treatment of involuntary infertility, which deserves treatment in or out of marriage, hence endorsing the use of any available technical means (that would produce a healthy and normal child), including surrogate wombs or even ectogenesis?

Second, logic aside, the opponents of the wedge argument do not counsel well. It would be simply foolish to ignore what might come next, and to fail to make the best possible assessment of the implications of present action (or inaction). Let me put the matter very bluntly: The decisions we must now make may very well help to determine whether human beings will eventually be produced in laboratories. I say this not to shock—and I do not mean to beg the question of whether that would be desirable or not. I say this to make sure that we and our policymakers face squarely the full import and magnitude of this decision. Once the genies let the babies into the bottle, it may be impossible to get them out again.

What Should We Do? The Question of Federal Funding

So much, then, for the meanings of initiating, housing, and manipulating human embryos in the laboratory. We are now better prepared to consider the original practical question: Should we allow or encourage these activities? The foregoing reflections still make me doubt the wisdom of proceeding with these practices, both in research and in their clinical application, notwithstanding that valuable knowledge might be had by continuing the research and identifiable suffering might be alleviated by using it to circumvent infertility. To doubt the wisdom of going ahead makes one at least a fellow traveler of the opponents of such research, but it does not, either logically or practically, require that one join them in trying to prevent it, say by legal prohibition. Not every folly can or should be legislated against. Attempts at prohibition here would seem to be both ineffective and dangerous, ineffective because impossible to enforce, dangerous because the costs of such precedent-setting interference with scientific research might be greater than the harm it prevents. To be sure, we already have legal restrictions on experimentation with human subjects, restrictions that are manifestly not incompatible with the progress of modern science. Neither is it true that science cannot survive if it must take some direction from the law. Nor is it the case that all research, because it is research, is or should be absolutely protected. But it does not seem to me that *in vitro* fertilization and growth of human embryos or embryo transfer deserve, at least at present, to be treated as sufficiently dangerous for legislative interference.

But if to doubt the wisdom does not oblige one to seek to outlaw the folly, neither does a decision to permit require a decision to encourage or support. A researcher's freedom to do *in vitro* fertilization, or a woman's right to have a child with laboratory assistance, in no way implies a public (or even a private) obligation to pay for such research or treatment. A right *against* interference is not an entitlement *for* assistance. The question before the Department of Health and Human Services is not whether such research should be permitted or outlawed, but only whether the Federal government should fund it. This is the policy question that needs to be discussed.

I propose to discuss it here, and at some length, not because it is itself timely or relatively important—it is neither—but because it is exemplary. Policy questions regarding controversial new biomedical technologies and practices—as well as other morally and politically charged matters on the border between private and public life (e.g., abortion, racial discrimination, developing the artificial heart, or affirmative action)—frequently take the form of arguments over Federal support. Social control and direction of new developments is often given not in terms of yes and no, but rather, how much, how fast, or how soon? Thus, much of the present analysis . . . can be generalized and made applicable to other developments in the field and to the field as a whole.

The arguments in favor of Federal support are well known. First, the research is seen as continuous with, if not quite an ordinary instance of, the biomedical research that the Federal government supports handsomely; roughly two-thirds of the money spent on biomedical research in the United States comes from Uncle Sam. Why is this research different from all other research? Its scientific merit has been attested to by the normal peer review process of [the National Institutes of Health]. For some, that is a sufficient reason to support it.

Second, there are specific practical fruits expected from the anticipated successes of this new line of research. Besides relief for many cases of infertility, the research promises new birth-control measures based upon improved understanding of the mechanisms of fertilization and implantation, which in turn could lead to techniques for blocking these processes. Also, studies on early embryonic development hold forth the promise of learning how to prevent some congenital malformations and certain highly malignant tumors (e.g., hydatidiform mole) that derive from aberrant fetal tissue.

Third, as he who pays the piper calls the tune, Federal support would make easy Federal regulation and supervision of this research. For the government to abstain, so the argument runs, is to leave the control of research and clinical application in the hands of profit-hungry, adventurous, insensitive, reckless, or power-hungry private physicians, scientists, or drug companies, or, on the other hand, at the mercy of the vindictive, mindless, and superstitious civic groups that will interfere with this research through state and local legislation. Only through Federal regulation—which, it is said, can only follow with Federal funding—can we have reasonable, enforceable, and uniform guidelines.

Fourth is the chauvinistic argument that the United States should lead the way in this brave new research, especially as it will apparently be going forward in other nations. Indeed, one witness testifying before the Ethics Advisory Board deplored the fact that the first test-tube baby was British and not American, and complained, in effect, that the existing moratorium on Federal support has already created what one might call an "*in vitro* fertilization gap." The preeminence of American science and technology, so the argument implies, is the center of our preeminence among the nations, a position that will be jeopardized if we hang back out of fear.

Let me respond to these arguments, in reverse order. Conceding—even embracing—the premise of the importance of American science for American strength and prestige, it is far from clear that failure to support *this* research would jeopardize American science. Certainly the use of embryo transfer to overcome infertility, though a vital matter for the couples involved, is hardly a matter of vital national interest—at least not unless and until the majority of American women are similarly infertile. The demands of international competition, admittedly often a necessary evil, should be invoked only for things that really matter; a missile gap and an embryo-transfer gap are chasms apart. In areas not crucial to our own survival, there will be many things we should allow other nations to develop, if that is their wish, without feeling obliged to join them. Moreover, one should not rush into potential folly to avoid being the last to commit it.

The argument about governmental regulations has much to recommend it. But it fails to consider that there are other safeguards against recklessness, at least in the clinical applications, known to the high-minded as the canons of medical ethics and to the cynical as liability for malpractice. Also, Federal regulations attached to Federal funding will not in any case regulate research done with private monies, say by the drug companies. Moreover, there are enough concerned practitioners of these new arts who would have a compelling interest in regulating their own practice, if only to escape the wrath and interference of hostile citizen's groups in response to unsavory goings-on. The available evidence does not convince me that a sensible practice of *in vitro* experimentation requires regulation by the Federal government.

In turning to the argument about anticipated technological powers, we face difficult calculations of unpredictable and more-or-less likely costs and benefits, and the all-important questions of priorities in the allocation of scarce resources. Here it seems useful to consider separately the techniques for generating children and the anticipated techniques for birth control or for preventing developmental anomalies and malignancies.

First, accepting that providing a child of their own to infertile couples is a worthy goal—and it is both insensitive and illogical to cite the population problem as an argument for ignoring the problem of infertility—one can nevertheless question its rank relative to other goals of medical research. One can even wonder whether it is indeed a *medical* goal, or a worthy goal for *medicine,* that is, whether alleviating infertility, especially in this way, is part of the art of healing.[8] Just as abortion for genetic defect is a peculiar innovation in medicine (or in preventive medicine) in which a disease is treated by eliminating the patient (or, if you prefer, a disease is prevented by "preventing" the patient), so laboratory fertilization is a peculiar treatment for oviduct obstruction in that it requires the creation of new life to "heal" an existing one. All this simply emphasizes the uniqueness of the reproductive organs in that their proper function involves other people and calls attention to the fact that infertility is not a disease, like heart disease or stroke, even though obstruction of a normally patent tube or vessel is the proximate cause of each.

However this may be, there is a more important objection to this approach to the problem. It represents yet another instance of our thoughtless preference for expensive, high-technology, therapy-oriented approaches to disease and dysfunctions. What about spending this money on discovering the causes of infertility? What about the prevention of tubal obstruction? We complain about rising medical costs, but we insist on the most spectacular and the most technological—and thereby often the most costly—remedies.

The truth is that we do know a little about the causes of tubal obstruction, though much less than we should or could. For instance, it is estimated that at least one third of such cases are the aftermath of pelvic inflammatory disease, caused by that uninvited venereal guest, gonococcus. Leaving aside any question about whether it makes sense for a Federally funded baby to be the wage of aphrodisiac indiscretion, one can only look with wonder at a society that will have "petri-dish babies" before it has found a vaccine against gonorrhea.

True, there are other causes of blocked oviducts, and blocked oviducts are not the only cause of female infertility. True, it is not logically necessary to choose between prevention and cure. But *practically* speaking, with money for research as limited as it is, research funds targeted for the relief of infertility should certainly go first to epidemiological and preventive measures—especially where the costs of success in the high-technology cure are likely to be great.

What about these costs? I have already explored some of the non-financial costs, in discussing the meaning of this research for our images of humanness. Let us, for now, consider only the financial costs. How expensive was Louise Brown? We do not know, partly because Drs. Edwards and Steptoe did not tell us how many failures preceded their success, how many procedures for egg removal and for fetal monitoring were performed on Mrs. Brown, and so on. To the costs of laparoscopy, fertilization and growth *in vitro,* and transfer, one must add the costs of monitoring the baby's development to check on her "normality" and, should it come, the costs of governmental regulation. A conservative estimate might place the cost of a successful pregnancy of this kind to be between $5,000 and $10,000. If we use the conservative figure of 500,000 for estimating the number of infertile women with blocked oviducts in the United States whose *only* hope of having children lies *in vitro* fertilization, we reach a conservative estimated cost of $2.5 to $5 billion. Is it really even fiscally wise for the Federal government to start down this road?

Clearly not, if it is also understood that the costs of providing the service, rendered possible by a successful technology, will also be borne by the taxpayers. Nearly everyone now agrees that the kidney machine legislation, obliging the Federal government to pay an average of $25,000 to $30,000 per patient per year for kidney dialysis for anyone in need (cost to the taxpayers in 1983 was over $1 billion), is an impossible precedent—notwithstanding that individual lives have been prolonged as a result. But once the technique of *in vitro* fertilization and embryo transfer is developed and available, how should the baby-making be paid for? Should it be covered under medical insurance? If a National Health Insurance program is enacted, will and should these services be included? (Those who argue that they are part of medicine will have a hard time saying no.) Failure to do so will make this procedure available only to the well-to-do, on a fee-for-service basis. Would that be a fair alternative? Perhaps, but it is unlikely to be tolerated. Indeed, the principle of equality—equal access to equal levels of medical care—is the leading principle in the press for medical reform. One can be certain that efforts will be forthcoming to make this procedure available equally to all, independent of ability to pay, under Medicaid or National Health Insurance or in some other way. (Only a few years ago, an egalitarian Boston-based group concerned with infertility managed to obtain private funding to pay for artificial insemination for women on welfare!)

Much as I sympathize with the plight of infertile couples, I do not believe that they are entitled to the provision of a child at public expense, especially now, especially at this cost, especially by a procedure that also involves many moral difficulties. Given the many vexing dilemmas that will surely be spawned by laboratory-assisted reproduction, the Federal government should not be misled by compassion to embark on this imprudent course.

In considering the Federal funding of such research for its other anticipated technological benefits, independent of its clinical use in baby-making, we face a more difficult matter. In brief, as is the case with all basic research, one simply cannot predict what kinds of techniques and uses it will yield. But here, also, I think good sense would at present say that before one undertakes *human in vitro* fertilization to seek new methods of birth control (e.g., by developing antibodies to the human egg that would physically interfere with its fertilization) one should make adequate attempts to do this in animals. One simply can't get large-enough numbers of human eggs to do this pioneering research well—at least not without subjecting countless women to additional risks not for their immediate benefit. Why not test this conceit first in the mouse or rabbit? Only if the results were very promising—and judged also to be relatively safe in practice—should one consider trying such things in humans. Likewise, the developmental research can and should be first carried out in animals, especially in primates. Though *in vitro* fertilization has yet to be achieved in monkeys, embryo transfer of *in vivo* fertilized eggs has been accomplished, thus permitting the relevant research to proceed. Purely on scientific grounds, the Federal government ought not *now* to be investing its funds in this research for its promised technological benefits—benefits that, in the absence of pilot studies in animals, must be regarded as mere wishful thoughts in the imaginings of scientists.

There does remain, however, the first justification: research for the sake of knowledge itself—knowledge about cell cleavage, cell-cell and cell-environment interactions, and cell differentiation; knowledge of gene action and gene regulation; knowledge of the effects and mechanisms of action of various chemical and physical agents on growth and development; knowledge of the basic processes of fertilization and implantation. This is all knowledge worth having, and though much can be learned using animal sources—and these sources have barely begun to be sufficiently exploited—the investigation of these matters in *man* would, sooner or later, require the use of human-embryonic material. Here again, there are questions of research priority about which there is room for disagreement, among scientists and laymen alike. But there is also a more fundamental matter.

Is such research consistent with the ethical standards of our community? The question turns in large part on the status of the early human embryo. If, as I have argued, the early embryo is deserving of respect because of what it is, now and potentially, it is difficult to justify submitting it to invasive experiments, and especially difficult to justify *creating* it solely for the purpose of experimentation. The reader should test this conclusion against his or her reaction to imagining the Fertilizing Room of the Central London Hatchery or, more modestly, to encountering an incubator or refrigerator full of living human embryos.

But even if this argument fails to sway our policymakers, another one should. For their decision, I remind you, is not whether *in vitro* fertilization should be permitted in the United States, but whether our tax dollars should encourage and foster it. One cannot, therefore, ignore the deeply held convictions of a sizeable portion of our population—it may even be a majority on this issue—that regards the human embryo as protectable humanity, not to be experimented upon except for its own benefit. Never mind if these beliefs have a religious foundation—as if that should ever be a reason for dismissing them! The presence, sincerity, and depth of these beliefs, and the grave importance of their subject, is what must concern us. The holders of these beliefs have been very much alienated by the numerous court decisions and legislative enactments regarding abortion and research on fetuses. Many who by-and-large share their opinions about the humanity of prenatal life have with heavy heart gone along with the liberalization of abortion, out of deference to the wishes, desires, interests, or putative rights of pregnant women. But will they go along here with what they can only regard as gratuitous and willful assaults on human life, or at least on potential and salvageable human life, and on human dignity? We can ill afford to alienate them further, and it would be unstatesmanlike, to say the least, to do so, especially in a matter of so little importance to the national health and one so full of potential dangers.

Technological progress can be but one measure of our national health. Far more important is the affection and esteem in which our citizenry holds its laws and institutions. No amount of relieved infertility is worth the further disaffection and civil contention that the lifting of the moratorium on Federal funding is likely to produce. People opposed to abortion and people grudgingly willing to permit women to obtain elective abortion, but at their own expense, will not tolerate having their tax money spent on scientific research requiring what they regard as at best cruelty, at worst murder. A prudent and wise secretary of health and human services should take this matter most seriously and continue to refuse to lift the moratorium—at least until he is persuaded that public opinion will overwhelmingly support him. Imprudence in this matter may be the worst sin of all.

An Afterword

This has been for me a long and difficult exposition. Many of the arguments are hard to make. It is hard to get confident people to face unpleasant and future prospects. It is hard to get people to take seriously such "soft" matters as lineage, identity, respect, and self-respect when they are in tension with such "hard" matters as a cure for infertility or new methods of contraception. It is hard to claim respect for human life in the laboratory from a society that does not respect human life in the womb. It is hard to talk about the meaning of sexuality and embodiment in a culture that treats sex increasingly as sport and has trivialized the significance of gender, marriage, and procreation. It is hard to oppose Federal funding of baby-making in a society that increasingly expects the Federal government to satisfy all demands, and that—contrary to so much evidence of waste, incompetence, and corruption—continues to believe that only Uncle Sam can do it. And, finally, it is hard to speak about restraint in a culture that seems to venerate very little above man's own attempt to master all. Here, I am afraid, is the biggest question and one which we perhaps can no longer ask or face: the question about the reasonableness of the desire to become masters and possessors of nature, human nature included.

Here we approach the deepest meaning of *in vitro* fertilization. Those who have likened it to artificial insemination are only partly correct. With *in vitro* fertilization, the human embryo emerges for the first time from the natural darkness and privacy of its own mother's womb, where it is hidden away in mystery, into the bright light and utter publicity of the scientist's laboratory, where it will be treated with unswerving rationality, before the clever and shameless eye of the mind and beneath the obedient and equally clever touch of the hand. What does it mean to hold the beginning of human life before your eyes, in your hands—even for five days (for the meaning does not depend on duration)? Perhaps the meaning is contained in the following story.

Long ago there was a man of great intellect and great courage. He was a remarkable man, a giant, able to answer questions that no other human being could answer, willing boldly to face any challenge or problem. He was a confident man, a masterful man. He saved his city from disaster and ruled it as a father rules his children, revered by all. But something was wrong in his city. A plague had fallen on generation; infertility affected plants, animals, and human beings. The man confidently promised to uncover the cause of the plague and to cure the infertility. Resolutely, confidently, he put his sharp mind to work to solve the problem, to bring the dark things to light. No secrets, no reticences, a full public inquiry. He raged against the representatives of caution, moderation, prudence, and piety, who urged him to curtail his inquiry; he accused them of trying to usurp his rightfully earned power, to replace human and masterful control with submissive reverence. The story ends in tragedy: He solved the problem but, in making visible and public the dark and intimate details of his origins, he ruined his life and that of his family. In the end, too late, he learned about the price of presumption, of overconfidence, of the overweening desire to master and control one's fate. In symbolic rejection of his desire to look into everything, he punished his eyes with self-inflicted blindness.

Sophocles seems to suggest that such a man is always in principle—albeit unwittingly—a patricide, a regicide, and a practitioner of incest. These are the crimes of the tyrant, that misguided and vain seeker of self-sufficiency and full autonomy, who loathes being reminded of his dependence and neediness and who crushes all opposition to the assertion of his will, and whose incest is symbolic of his desire to be even the godlike source of his own being. His character is his destiny.

We men of modern science may have something to learn from our philosophical forebear Oedipus. It appears that Oedipus, being the kind of man an Oedipus is (the chorus call him a paradigm of man), had no choice but to learn through suffering. Is it really true that we, too, have no other choice?

Notes

1. Aldous Huxley, *Brave New World,* New York: Torchbooks, Harper and Row, 1965, pp. 1–3.

2. Though perhaps a justifiable exception would be a universal plague that fatally attacked all fetuses *in utero.* To find a cure for the end of the species may entail deliberately "producing" (and aborting) live fetuses for research.

3. The truth of this is not decisively affected by the fact that the early embryo may soon divide and give rise to identical twins or by the fact that scientists may disaggregate and reassemble the cells of the early embryos, even mixing in cells from different embryos in the reaggregation. These unusual and artificial cases do not affect the natural norm, or the truth that *a* human life begins with fertilization—and does so always, if nothing abnormal occurs.

4. Quoted in Peter Gwynne, "Was the Birth of Louise Brown Only a Happy Accident?" *Science Digest,* October 1978, pp. 7–12, at p. 9. Emphasis added.

5. For the supporting analysis of the concept of viability, see my article "Determining Death and Viability in Fetuses and Abortuses," prepared for the National Commission for the Protection of Human Subjects of Biomedical and Behavioral Research, and published in *Appendix: Research on the Fetus,* Washington, D.C.: U.S. Department of Health, Education, and Welfare, DHEW Publ. No. (OS) 76-128, 1975.

6. Some people have suggested that the embryo be regarded in the same manner as a vital organ, salvaged from a newly dead corpse, usable for transplantation or research, and that its donation by egg and sperm donors be governed by the Uniform Anatomical Gift Act, which legitimates premortem consent for organ donation upon death. But though this acknowledges that embryos are not "things," it is a mistake to treat embryos as mere organs, thereby overlooking that they are early stages of a complete, whole human being. The Uniform Anatomical Gift Act does not apply to, nor should it be stretched to cover, donation of gonads, gametes (male sperm or female eggs) or—especially—zygotes and embryos.

7. There is a good chance that the problem of surplus embryos may be avoidable, for purely technical reasons. Some researchers believe that the uterine receptivity to the transferred embryo might be reduced during the particular menstrual cycle in which the ova are obtained because of the effects of the hormones given to induce superovulation. They propose that the harvested eggs be frozen and then defrosted one at a time each month for fertilization, culture, and transfer, until pregnancy is achieved. By refusing to fertilize all the eggs at once—not placing all one's eggs in one uterine cycle—there will not be surplus embryos, but at most only surplus eggs. This change in the procedure would make the demise of unimplanted embryos exactly analogous to the "natural" embryonic loss in ordinary reproduction.

8. See Chapter 2 [of Leon Kass, *Toward a More Natural Science,* New York: Free Press, 1985,] "Making Babies—the New Biology and the 'Old' Morality," especially pp. 44–45. See also Chapter 6, "The End of Medicine and the Pursuit of Health," especially pp. 157–164 and 177–179.

Progeny, Progress, and Primrose Paths

Samuel Gorovitz

. . . Let us pursue the debate about *in vitro* fertilization by imagining a woman who desperately wants to have a child of her own, for whom IVF is the only possibility. She is deeply religious, totally committed to doing the morally right thing, aware that there is controversy about the morality of IVF, and unsure what to do. She asks her gynecologist for advice, but the physician is also unsure what to do. She and her colleagues have been asked by a number of patients to make the service available through their practice, either directly or by referral to another clinic. The patient and the physician agree to survey the literature, assess the arguments they find, and try to reach agreement about whether such technologically aided reproduction is an appropriate option. What are the discussions like that they will find?

Slippery Slope Arguments

Laced through the literature of objection to abortion, IVF therapy and research is an argument variously called the primrose path argument, the thin edge of the wedge argument, and the camel's nose in the tent argument. Its structure is familiar: Once one starts sliding down a slippery slope, things get out of control. There is no stopping; disaster awaits us. No skier thinks the argument is generally good; fortunately it is often possible to start down a slippery slope and then to stop.

Paul Ramsey—a prominent Protestant theologian and a leading critic of the use of modern technology in clinical medicine—assures us of disaster in his discussions of such matters, relying heavily, as we shall see, on arguments of this kind. He claims that such measures as artificial insemination and *in vitro* fertilization are the first steps down the primrose path, and there is, in his apocalyptic view, no slowing up, no turning back short of social disaster.[1] Whether or not that view is reasonable is an empirical question. Some processes, like nuclear chain reactions or the spreading of an epidemic, once

From *Doctors' Dilemmas: Moral Conflict and Medical Care,* Chapter 10. New York: Oxford University Press, 1985, pp. 164–178, 223–224. Abridged; headings added. © Samuel Gorovitz 1982. Used with permission.

begun are difficult or impossible to stop. Others are not. It is always an empirical question what sort of process we are dealing with in any particular instance.

I will not attempt to ski the Schilthorn—though I have seen it done—because my descent, once begun on that insanely precipitous slope, would surely end in cataclysm below. I might as well attempt to ski to safety from a plane in flight. In view of my ability, the argument against my attempting that slope is conclusive. Yet I can handle slopes that beginning skiers properly shun. It is a question of control and judgment.

Is the slippery slope argument against IVF a good one? It is not enough to show that disaster awaits if the process is not controlled. A man walking east in Omaha will drown in the Atlantic—if he does not stop. The argument must also rest on evidence about the likelihood that judgment and control will be exercised responsibly. Here Ramsey's position collapses; he describes disaster and rests his argument on the unduly pessimistic assumption that such unhappy outcomes as are possible will surely occur. But Ramsey sells us short. Collectively we have significant capacity to exercise judgment and control. We have not always done well, especially in areas like foreign policy or energy planning. But our record has been rather good in regard to medical treatment and research.

Consider the vexatious problem of abortion as a case in point. Some opponents of a liberal law have argued that once we allow the killing of fetuses, nothing can stop the slide. If we sanction abortion, they fear, even where amniocentesis reveals a defect like trisomy 21 (Down's syndrome), we will sanction capricious infanticide as well. If we would abort a fetus on the ground that it is going to be seriously defective, why not allow infanticide on the ground that the child actually has the dreaded defect? Further, such infanticide is just a short skid away from the killing of those judged socially useless, so that if one sanctions early-term abortions even in cases of demonstrable defect, one has irretrievably opened the floodgates to the selective slaughter of anyone in social disfavor.

No such disaster has ensued. Through a process of social policy determination, the society has exercised judgment. That judgment has made a lot of people on both sides unhappy, but it is nonetheless a judgment that makes clear that we can stop a process once we have begun it. Anyone who has ever had a haircut should know that. . . .

Note that with regard to IVF applications, we do not face any single slippery slope argument. Rather, there are several. There are arguments that clinical IVF poses a threat to marriage and the family and to mankind's self-image. There is a separate argument that IVF research will lead to experimentation of an ethically undesirable sort on late-stage fetuses. Each such consideration involves an empirical assessment of the likelihood that sound judgment will prevail, as well as an assessment of the magnitude of the disaster if it does not.

It is important here to recognize that the likelihood of the subsequent exercise of judgment and restraint may largely depend on the principles that are used to justify first steps. If early-term abortion were justified by the principle that parents enjoy absolute dominion over their issue, the adoption of that principle would already have constituted a sanctioning of infanticide, and there would be no basis for stopping the slide down the slippery slope. If IVF research on embryos is justified by the principle that prenatal fetal life is of no moral importance, there will be no basis for restraint in regard to research on later-stage fetuses. So it can matter decisively how the justification of first steps is formulated.

There has been considerable speculation about the impact of clinical IVF on marriage and the family. Some of the predictions based on slippery slope arguments are dire. Such prospects as the use of surrogate mothers have been especially disturbing to some writers. . . . Hellegers and McCormick warn of such outcomes, toward which they see IVF as leading: "We see in these procedures grave assaults on marriage and the family, to say nothing of the subtle devaluation of sexual intimacy that clings to them."[2] But whereas they raise concerns and call for "a serious public discussion," Ramsey speaks of "what the manipulation of embryos will surely do to ourselves and our progeny."[3] He goes on to invoke the chilling images of a Huxleyan world so sterile that "there is no poetry."[4]

These issues are of the first importance. But it is necessary not to lose sight, in the glare of that importance, of the need to examine the evidence. What reason is there to give credence to such portents of familial disaster? Much of the case seems based on concern about the separation of reproduction from sexual intercourse. But artificial insemination, with husbands' and with donors' sperm, has been practiced widely, if not very visibly, for decades. There has been no discernible deleterious effect on marriage or the family. More important, the wide availability of inexpensive and effective birth control means that for the first time in human history, sex and reproduction have already been separated. The impact on social structure will surely be astounding; no doubt it will transcend our current understanding. So it is a wholly idle worry that IVF will separate sex and procreation.

It is worth remembering, moreover, that IVF involves hospitalization and surgery, and it is a very small percentage of the population that is in any position to benefit from it. The traditional method of conception will remain the method of choice. It is inexpensive, can be performed at home, takes little time, training, or skill, and is a great deal of fun. I do not see it in serious jeopardy.

Further, we are only beginning to document what we have known all along: that there is no substitute for early parent-child interaction.[5] As we learn more fully how the family works when it is working well, I suspect that our appreciation of it and of its special capacity for nurturing will grow. Hellegers and McCormick are right; we should take the long view and look at societal consequences, not simply at individual needs, in evaluating IVF. But I do not see the family under grave assault because of IVF. Indeed, it is often a respect for family, lineage, and the traditional parental role that prompts the request for clinical IVF in the first place.

Finally, mankind's image of what it is to be human may well involve a sense of lineage and parenting, and that image may undergo some perturbation from the few cases in which procreation has a heavy dose of technology added. But mankind's sense of what it is to be human is threatened far more seriously on other fronts. Recent work on primate language acquisition, notwithstanding debate about its significance, has challenged the belief that we alone have the capacity for abstraction or to communicate to others a sense of self-awareness, and in the process the sharpness of the distinction between humans and the higher primates has been blunted.[6] Recent work in artificial intelligence has produced machines with awesome cognitive capacities, and the sharpness of the distinction between people and machines has also been challenged.[7] We have ample reason to reflect seriously about what we are. The prospects for IVF add little to the case.

Senses of "Natural"

Like the slippery slope argument, the concept of what is natural plays a frequent role in the writings of those who are troubled by IVF. Ramsey, for example, writes:

> Today many are testifying to the spiritual autonomy of all natural objects and to arrogance over none; to the scheme of things in which man has his place. But there is as yet no discernible evidence that we are recovering a sense of man as a natural object, too, toward whom a like form of "natural piety" is appropriate. . . . [P]rocreation, parenthood, is certainly one of those "courses of action" natural to man, which cannot without violation be disassembled and put back together again—any more than we have the wisdom or the right impiously to destroy the environment of which we are a part rather than working according to its lineaments, according to the functions we discover to be the case in the whole assemblage of natural objects.[8]

He then goes on to advocate the position that "the proper objective of medicine is to serve and care for man as a natural object, to help in all our natural 'courses of action,' to tend the garden of our creation."[9] It is time this sort of argument was laid permanently to rest. That something is natural has, by itself, absolutely no moral force.

We can distinguish three senses in which an action or process can be said to be natural:

1. It conforms to the laws of nature; the contrast, I presume, is with the impossible or with the supernatural. But *everything* we do or could do—the good and bad alike—is natural in this sense. No moral distinctions can be based on it.

2. It is free of human intervention; the contrast is with processes influenced by mankind's efforts to manipulate its environment. But *nothing* we do is natural in this sense, for our action is itself the mark of the unnatural. The

practice of medicine itself is a clear example of human efforts to manipulate the playing out of events, as when we deliberately destroy "natural" life forms and terminate a "natural" process by using antibiotics to cure an infection. No moral distinctions can be based on this sense of what is natural either.

3. It conforms to some natural moral law or other code or set or principles of value; the contrast here is with what is wrong, what is a violation of principles about how one ought to act. In this interpretation the concept of what is natural has moral force, but only because it is based on some prior judgment about what is right and what is wrong—a judgment then reflected in the choice of what to call natural and artificial.

The passage from Ramsey suggests that he employs the third sense of *natural;* that he sees certain processes, such as normal procreation, as desirable; and that he extols their naturalness without thereby suggesting that medical intervention is typically a violation of nature.

The claim of naturalness is thus a moral *conclusion,* not evidence that can be offered in a moral argument. Ramsey sees atypical reproduction as undesirable but says little about why. His invocation of the concept of the natural only obscures the point that there are morally desirable and morally undesirable actions, and we must strive to discern the difference between them on reasonable grounds, not on purported grounds of naturalness. I do not understand why this confusion about the moral significance of the concept of what is natural persists as widely and tenaciously as it does.

The Status of the Embryo

The most central issue in the debate about IVF, however, as in the debate about abortion, is the question of the status of the embryo. In approaching this question, we must recall the crucial distinction between facts we seek to discover and decisions we need to make. If we wish to know a fact, we seek to discover it through appropriate research. Contrast that with the question of when a young person becomes an adult. Whether a person warrants classification as an adult at thirteen, eighteen, or twenty-one is not a fact to discover through research in biology, physiology, psychology, or anything else. It is social policy, a decision of the body politic. This distinction between discoveries and decisions seems straightforward, yet sometimes the two become confused. Much discussion about death, for example, proceeds on the misconception that the criterion of death is a fact to discover. Yet . . . the appropriate criterion of death in clinical situations is not a fact to discover; it is a social policy to make. (That is one reason why the results of such discussions are somewhat unstable, why the criterion of death is a subject of ongoing dispute; the factors that go into justifying a social policy decision are always open to review and to argument.)

What, then, of the embryo—the embryo that is implanted and the embryo that is dealt with otherwise? Inevitably there arise questions of whether or not such embryos are persons or are the bearers of rights. These are not questions of fact but instead require the setting of social policy. To say that a question is a question of policy is not to say that the answers are unconstrained. There are clear cases of life and death; the question arises—and a policy is needed— only in cases at the margin where some physiological systems still function while others are irretrievably lost. So the range within which decisions can be made is rather narrow. Similarly, the questions of what to count as a person and what to count as a bearer of rights require decision only within a circum- scribed range—the cases at the margins of personhood. Such cases are of various sorts—the anencephalic newborn, the linguistically proficient pri- mate, the embryo.

I will not rehearse the extensive debate about the personhood of embryos and fetuses, a debate fueled by intense division of sentiment about abortion. Rather, I will sketch the conclusions that seem to me to provide the most reasonable basis for judgment.

Surely the concept of a person involves in some fundamental way the capacity for sentience, for an awareness of sensations at the very least. In the normal case there is much more. There is self-awareness, capacity for reflec- tion, a sense of others and of relationships between self and others. So the condition of sentience is very weak, a necessary condition for personhood but far from a sufficient condition.

No one seriously contends that embryos are sentient, that they are capable of even the slightest awareness of pleasure or pain. Of course, if all goes well, they will develop into people, and it is on that potential that the case for their personhood largely rests. The idea of potential is tricky. We often hear enco- miums to it: Individuals should have the opportunity to fulfill their potential, it is somehow grounds for disappointment when someone fails to live up to his potential, and the like. But that is careless talk, for some potentials are desirable and some are not. He who has the potential to be Sherlock Holmes has the potential to be a master criminal; she who has the manual dexterity for neurosurgery perhaps has the potential to be a leading pickpocket as well. Further, he who has the potential to be a swimmer and to be a ballet dancer must choose between them; what advances one potential interferes with the other. So aphorisms about potential do little to advance the debate. Mainly what they come to is that it is good to advance those potentials that it is good to advance.

Even though *people* should be encouraged in living up to some of their more desirable potentials, we cannot use that principle to defend a claim that *embryos* have personhood or rights since the principle is about the potentials of persons—and whether or not embryos should be accorded that status is precisely the point in question. It is not obvious that rights should accrue to an object just because it has the potential, assuming that all goes well, to become a person at some later time. Indeed, the unfertilized human egg, like the embryo, has the potential to become a person if all goes well—when all going well includes getting fertilized. And no one has argued that each unfertilized egg or each spermatozoon be accorded personhood or rights.

One does hear it said of the embryo that it has the potential to become a *particular* adult person. Its genetic identity is complete; it is already a unique individual. That does distinguish it from spermatozoa and ova in isolation (apart from the possibility of twinning), but not from identified, though un- joined, pairs of sperm and egg. That no union has yet occurred does not alter the fact that any pair of sperm and egg has the potential, if all goes well, to become a genetically specific adult person. The point of conception may be, for some, a convenient place to draw the line, but there should be no mistake about the fact that it is drawn there for convenience. That is no less "arbi- trary" a choice than the choice to draw the line later, which I believe it makes better sense to do. Indeed, it is a myth that conception is itself instantaneous. Even one who seeks to avoid the problem of "drawing a line" by choosing conception as an unproblematic point is in reality selecting a temporal region within which a process takes place over time. That we did not know this fact before it was possible to monitor the process of conception at the microscopic level does not make it any the less important a fact.

At the other end of fetal development we are struck by the similarity between infants and late-stage fetuses. Indeed, not only is the late-stage fetus clearly sentient, reacting to stimuli in its environment, but in most cases it already holds a place, as a specific, though unseen, individual in a network of human emotions and expectations. In most respects it is like a child and utterly unlike an embryo.

For my part, the onset of the capacity for sentience marks a qualitative change in fetal development. From that point forward what we do may cause it, as a present actuality, to suffer. Surely that is a morally significant factor, though not the only one. It is an empirical question of neurological develop- ment when that change occurs; it happens sometime prior to quickening but well after the embryonic stage. That we have no word for this stage in the series of events that includes conception, quickening, and birth reflects only the fact that we have not historically invested it with much significance or until recently had much understanding of the development of which it is a part. It is not necessarily less significant for that.

The later it is in its development, the more seriously we should take a fetus as a person in the making. I see no reason for, and no possibility of, holding to a clear-cut distinction between the nonperson and the person as if personhood somehow snaps into place in an instant, instead of emerging organically out of a developmental process. That emergence, I suggest, begins to have moral force with the onset of fetal sentience. In any case, I know of no persuasive arguments for the position that the most reasonable social policy is to accord the embryo the status of a person.

Leon Kass, a physician and persuasive commentator on ethical issues in medicine, has argued forcefully that the human embryo is an entity of moral significance:

> The human blastocyst, even the blastocyst *in vitro,* is not hu- manly nothing; it possesses a power to become what everyone will agree is a human being. . . . [T]he blastocyst is not nothing, it is *at*

least potential humanity, and as such it elicits, or ought to elicit, our
feelings of awe and respect. In the blastocyst, even in the zygote, we
face a mysterious and awesome power. . . . *The human embryo is
not mere meat, it is not just stuff; it is not a thing.* Because of its origin
and because of its capacity, it commands a higher respect.[10]

I agree that the human blastocyst is not humanly nothing. So, too, however, do all the advocates of IVF. It is *precisely* the human blastocyst's potential to become a human being that makes it an object of particular research
interest and that accounts for the possibility of clinical IVF. From the fact that
it is not humanly nothing, no conclusion directly follows about what should or
should not be done.

Of course, the force of Kass's argument is intended to rest not merely on
the fact that the human blastocyst has some human status but on its mysterious and awesome power, its capacity to engender awe and respect. But it is
not the *human* character of the blastocyst that accounts for its splendor. Any
strand of DNA confronts us with a mysterious and awesome power; any
mammalian embryo embodies an "immanent plan" that dwarfs our understanding; any acorn is, as much as anything ever is, miraculous; and even the
lowly hydrogen atom, reflected on with reverent disposition, is humbling in its
beauty, power, and complexity. And so are cathedrals, symphonies, great
literary works, and the minds of great scientists.

Surely, one might claim, I miss the point. Human blastocysts are not
uniquely grounds for awe, but they do command, as Kass puts it, a "higher
respect." He is not explicit, however, in the comparison; higher than what,
one wonders. The context suggests an answer: higher than the respect commanded by "mere meat," by that which is "just stuff." But two problems of
interpreting the point arise. First, Kass nowhere explains what he means by
respect. He has merely *invoked* the notion of the respect due the embryo,
much as Ramsey invoked the notion of the natural. Second, Kass does not
consider the respect due to other objects than the embryo. That omission is
what gives plausibility to his argument that since human blastocysts are due
respect, they ought not be the subjects of research or clinical manipulation.
Kass, I am certain, would agree that human cadavers should be treated with
respect; they are not mere meat, not humanly nothing, not unrelated to a
network of emotional attachments and deeply felt values that constrain how
we treat the bodily remains of former persons. Yet Kass does not protest the
use of cadavers in medical education or the practice of transplanting organs
from someone who has just died. To be sure, there is a difference between
using cadavers and abusing them, and it is to this difference that the concept
of respect is relevant. It is simply a mistake to assume that if an object is due
respect, it is therefore wrong to make practical use of it.

Finally, Kass speaks freely of the appropriateness of experimenting on animals, including primates. But are animals also not due respect? They are sentient creatures whose development and behavior are proper grounds for awe
and wonder, they participate in social communities, and in some cases their

communicative capacity is far greater than we had until recently imagined. The homocentricity of Kass's position enables him to make respect sound like a barrier to use. In fact, it is a barrier only to abuse. If we can justifiably experiment on animals under some circumstances, and if we can justifiably make use of human remains, despite the fact that they are not humanly nothing, I see no reason based on the concept of respect why we cannot, respectfully, make justifiable clinical and research use of human blastocysts.

The Function of Medicine

Both Kass and R. G. Edwards, in reply to Kass, have discussed the proper function of medicine and whether IVF is defensible in terms of it. There are serious issues here. Kass argues:

> Just as infertility is not a disease, so providing a child by artificial means to a woman with blocked oviducts is not treatment. . . . What is being "treated" is her desire—a perfectly normal and unobjectionable desire—to bear a child.[11]

Ramsey voices a similar concern:

> The important line lies between doctoring desires . . . and seeking to correct a medical condition if it is possible to do so. . . . [M]edical practice loses its way into an entirely different human activity—manufacture . . . if it undertakes either to produce a child without curing infertility as a condition or to produce simply the desired sort of child.[12]

Edwards replies:

> A great many medical advances depend on the replacement of a deficient compound or an organ. Examples include insulin, false teeth, and spectacles: the clinical condition itself remains, but treatment modifies its expression. Patients taking advantage of these three treatments are surely receiving the correct therapeutic measures, the doctors treating the desire to be nondiabetic or to see and eat properly. . . . Exactly the same argument applies to the cure of infertility: should patients have their desired children, the treatment would have achieved its purpose.[13]

We need not rely on the idea of prosthetic devices to make Edwards's point that treatment does often leave the initial condition unaltered while responding to a patient's desire to transcend the limitations imposed by that condition. The administration of tranquilizers, sleeping pills, and analgesics are examples of medical treatments which do not correct physiological deficiencies but respond, in a sense, to a patient's desires. Edwards's defense seems adequate; treating some desires is a traditional and appropriate part of medical practice.

But the problem runs deeper, for it may not be appropriate to treat all medically treatable desires. First, there is the question of the distribution of costs, a question that has heightened impact if we consider the use of public funds to pay for medical treatment. It is one thing to provide insulin, dialysis, or dentures to a patient. But should we provide cosmetic surgery when the desire does not arise out of injury or illness but rather is simply a wish to be more youthfully attractive? Perhaps such treatment is unexceptionable if the costs are borne wholly by the patient. But other desires arising out of vanity seem less legitimate. Should surgical treatment have been available to those women who, in the 1950s, had their little toes amputated in order to fit their feet into narrower and hence, in their benighted judgment, more fashionable shoes? Or is the provision of such treatment a misuse of medical skills, a perversion of the privilege that the right to practice medicine signifies? I submit that this is the case and that the underlying reason is that the treatment of a desire for self-mutilation in the service of a whimsical vanity is not the sort of desire that legitimately warrants treatment.

As [I have argued elsewhere[14]], value-free medicine is not fully possible. Some judgments about which desires are properly treatable, and which not, must be made. We cannot oppose clinical IVF on the ground that it is the treatment of a desire, nor can we simply approve it on the ground, as Edwards suggests, that the treatment of desires is medically legitimate. Rather, we must face directly the question of whether the desire to have a child of one's own, when IVF is the only available means, is one of the desires that warrants medical response.

At this point our hypothetical patient and physician, if they agree with me, will conclude that there is no adequate argument against the clinical use of IVF as a response to inoperable infertility. But they may remain troubled by some of the dangers to which critics like Ramsey, Hellegers, McCormick, and Kass call our attention, despite the weaknesses in their arguments. For there remains something discomforting about the notion of raising embryos in the laboratory for use as research subjects, notwithstanding the useful knowledge that might result. And there remains something discomforting about the growing incidence of surrogate motherhood arrangements that have already begun to lead us into uncharted waters of litigation, as when the surrogate mother decides during the pregnancy to try to keep the child she had agreed to incubate for someone else. But these problems must be faced on their own, and the judgments we make in response to them should remain distinguishable from the judgments we make about more straightforward uses of IVF as a clinical therapy. We need not consider all possible uses of IVF as parts of one inseparable package any more than we need endorse an absolutist position on abortion. There is no good reason why we cannot separate justifiable from unjustifiable instances on the basis of where the best arguments lie.

We have considered a number of issues relating to clinical decisions that raise questions of public policy. Abortion is a paradigm case since there is ongoing public debate about how the law should limit the range within which clinical and personal judgments are made. Many other aspects of clinical medicine are touched by the outcome of public policy debates regarding the legal definition of death, the collection and allocation of transplantable organs, the use of public funds to underwrite the costs of medical services, and the like. It is time we considered the question of how public policy should be determined in respect to such morally disputed matters.

Notes

1. Paul Ramsey, "Shall We 'Reproduce'?" *Journal of the American Medical Association* 220 (June 12, 1972), p. 1484.
2. Andre Hellegers and Richard McCormick, "Unanswered Questions on Test Tube Life," *America* (August 19, 1978), p. 77.
3. Ramsey, "Shall We 'Reproduce'?" p. 1485.
4. Paul Ramsey, "Manufacturing Our Offspring: Weighing the Risks," *The Hastings Center Report* 8, no. 5 (October 1979), p. 9.
5. See, for example, M. Klaus and J. Kennell, "Mothers Separated from Their Newborn Infants," *Pediatric Clinics of North America* 17 (1970), pp. 1015–37.
6. See, for example, P. Jenkins, "Ask No Questions," *The Guardian,* London (July 10, 1973), excerpted under the title "Teaching Chimpanzees to Communicate," in *Animal Rights and Human Obligations,* edited by T. Regan and P. Singer (Englewood Cliffs, N.J.: Prentice-Hall, 1976), pp. 85–92.
7. See, for example, B. G. Buchanan, "Scientific Theory Formulation by Computers," in *Computer Oriented Learning Processes,* edited by J. C. Simon (Leyden: Noordhoff, 1976).
8. Ramsey, "Shall We 'Reproduce'?" p. 1484.
9. Ibid.
10. Leon Kass, "Ethical Issues in Human *In Vitro* Fertilization, Embryo Culture and Research, and Embryo Transfer," in Ethics Advisory Board, DHEW, *Appendix, HEW Support of Research Involving Human* In Vitro *Fertilization and Embryo Transfer* (Washington, D.C.: U.S. Government Printing Office, 1979), pp. 6–8, emphases in original.
11. Leon Kass, "Babies by Means of *In Vitro* Fertilization: Unethical Experiments on the Unborn?" *New England Journal of Medicine* 285 (November 18, 1971), p. 1177.
12. Ramsey, "Shall We 'Reproduce'?" p. 1482.
13. R. G. Edwards, "Fertilization of Human Eggs *In Vitro:* Morals, Ethics and the Law," *Quarterly Review of Biology* 49 (1974), pp. 3–26.
14. [In *Doctors' Dilemmas: Moral Conflict and Medical Care,* chapter 6, New York: Oxford University Press, 1985.]

III

WHY HAVE CHILDREN?
MEANING AND SIGNIFICANCE

The primary motivation for development and use of reproductive technology is the desire to have children. Only to the extent that we understand precisely what it is about having children that is and should be valued can we have a solid foundation for answering normative questions about reproductive technology. It might be thought that we understand these matters well enough without philosophical analysis. Yet, disagreement and lack of clarity about these issues, and in particular about the significance of the separation of genetic, gestational, and social relations between parents and children, were at the heart of many of the unresolved debates introduced in Part II. The articles in the present part examine these issues more closely.

The passages from the ancient Greek philosopher Aristotle, though brief, present a developed conception of the relationship between parents and children, identifying and relating key elements of production, identity, emotional attachment, intention, and natural process. The essence of Aristotle's account is that in virtue of the parents' production of the child, the child is an actualization, and so a part, of the parents. The parents consequently love the child as a part of themselves. Aristotle illustrates his position through an analogy between parents and children, on the one hand, and craftsmen and the objects they produce, on the other.

In examining Aristotle's view, a number of issues should be raised. Taking Aristotle in his own terms, in what sense do parents actually produce their child? Do they design them? Do they make their children in the way that a cobbler cuts and assembles the pieces of a shoe? Do parents even necessarily comprehend the processes through which their child comes to be or actively participate in them? How do the differences between being a mother and being a father matter? Pressing Aristotle's analogy further, shouldn't producing a child in the laboratory through technological manipulations, since that would be more like being a producer or craftsperson, establish a more significant relationship than is established by generating the child through our bodies by natural processes?

The analogy of production may initially be appealing, but much remains to be worked out.[1] The other two articles in this part, as well as those by Corea and Tong, address many of the issues raised by Aristotle, and the article by O'Donovan, below, addresses precisely the relationship between production and procreation.

The next article in this part, from Simone de Beauvoir's classic *The Second Sex,* draws attention to the fact that having a child is not just "there being a child in existence," but also a *process* and an experience, the process and experience of *maternity.* De Beauvoir's account of having a child might be contrasted with what might be considered a more male-oriented view that focuses on the formal relations between parent and child (such as the pattern of their genes) rather than on the process through which that and other relations come about.

When we turn to the processes of having children, other problems emerge. According to de Beauvoir, maternity is an equivocal experience. While some women may experience only the emotions and fulfillment of a romantic notion of pregnancy, other women experience varying degrees of emancipation and subjugation, enrichment and injury, completeness (in giving life) and diminution (in sexual attractiveness). These attitudes and experiences, de Beauvoir holds, are an expression of a deeper struggle between immanence and transcendence (between what one is and "Otherness" that one can become or participate in). The value of the process of having a child is no simple thing to judge. De Beauvoir is determined to avoid cultural stereotypes. She clearly rejects the idea (such as presented in the Vatican statement above) that bearing children is a sacred and uniquely fulfilling role of women. Indeed, de Beauvoir's view may be further contrasted with Aristotle's in that she conceives of a parent (the mother) less as a producer or craftsperson than as a passive host to a potentially alienating process that proceeds independently of her will and control. For significantly different views on the nature and significance of maternity, see, again, the articles by Corea and Tong below.

The article by Kenneth Alpern examines the desire to have children. He argues that a felt desire to have a child may often be better understood in the context of desires for other things such as loving relationships, communal relations, status, and power, which the having of a child may be only one way to satisfy. Digging deeper, the article analyzes the idea of having one's *own* child, in the sense in which biological, but not adopted, children are held to be "really one's own." The relevance of this issue is that many reproductive technologies are attractive in part because they appear to offer one or both members of a couple a chance to have a child that is "really their own" or "more their own" than an adopted child would be. At the heart of the matter is the claim, criticized by Alpern, that the essence of having one's own child and of satisfying the desire for children is the existence of a child who has one's genes. In the end, Alpern's article does not argue for a definitive answer to questions of the meaning and significance of having children but does seek to advance the debate.

Notes

1. In considering Aristotle's views in his own terms, it may be helpful to draw on his "Doctrine of the Four Causes" (*Physics,* Book 2, chapters 3 and 7). There he identifies four ways in which one thing may be responsible for the existence and nature of another: the one thing can provide the *material* for the other thing, provide its *form,* be its *cause* (in a sense akin to our modern notion of causation), or provide the *end* or purpose for which the thing exists (in a sense of purpose that does not require a purposive agent, as when we speak of the purpose of the heart being to pump blood). These relations, then, can be used to characterize the nature and significance of various connections of parents to their child in natural and aided reproduction: providing material for it, providing its form (e.g., providing its genes), causally bringing it into existence, and having reproduction as their conscious intention or natural end. For remarks in this vein, see the fourth section of the article by Alpern.

On the Relationship of Parents and Children

Aristotle

Natural Affection

Nature seems to wish to implant in animals a sense of care for their young: in the inferior animals this lasts only to the moment of giving birth; in others it continues till they are perfect; in all that are more intelligent, during the bringing up of the young also. In those which have the greatest portion in intelligence we find familiarity and love shown also toward the young when perfected, as with men and some quadrupeds. . . . [From *Generation of Animals*, Book 3, chapter 2.]

The Child Is a Part of the Parents

The friendship of kinsmen itself, while it seems to be of many kinds, appears to depend in every case on paternal friendship; for parents love their children as being a part of themselves, and children their parents as being something originating from them. Now parents know their offspring better than their children know that they are their children, and the originator is more attached to his offspring than the offspring to their begetter; for the product belongs to the producer (e.g. a tooth or hair or anything else to him whose it is), but the producer does not belong to the product, or belongs in a less degree. And the length of time produces the same result; parents love their children as soon as these are born, but children love their parents only after time has elapsed and they have acquired understanding or perception. From these considerations it is also plain why mothers love more than fathers do. Parents, then, love their children as themselves (for their issue are by virtue of their separate existence a sort of other selves), while children love their parents as being born of them. . . . And children seem to be a bond of union (which is the reason why childless people part more easily); for children are a good common to both and what is common holds them together. [From *Nicomachean Ethics*, Book 8, chapter 12.]

Love for One's Product

Benefactors are thought to love those they have benefited more than those who have been well treated love those that have treated them well, and this is discussed as though it were paradoxical. Most people think it is because the latter are in the position of debtors and the former of creditors; and therefore as, in the case of loans, debtors wish their creditors did not exist, while creditors actually take care of the safety of their debtors, so it is thought that benefactors wish the objects of their action to exist since they will then get their gratitude, while the beneficiaries take no interest in making this return. Epicharmus would perhaps declare that they say this because they "look at things on their bad side," but it is quite like human nature; for most people are forgetful, and are more anxious to be well treated than to treat others well. But the cause would seem to be more deeply rooted in the nature of things; the case of those who have lent money is not even analogous. For they have no friendly feeling to their debtors, but only a wish that they may be kept safe with a view to what is to be got from them; while those who have done a service to others feel friendship and love for those they have served even if these are not of any use to them and never will be. This is what happens with craftsmen too; every man loves his own handiwork better than he would be loved by it if it came alive; and this happens perhaps most of all with poets; for they have an excessive love for their own poems, doting on them as if they were their children. This is what the position of benefactors is like; for that which they have treated well is their handiwork, and therefore they love this more than the handiwork does its maker. The cause of this is that existence is to all men a thing to be chosen and loved, and that we exist by virtue of activity (i.e. by living and acting), and that the handiwork *is* in a sense, the producer in activity; he loves his handiwork, therefore, because he loves existence. And this is rooted in the nature of things; for what he is in potentiality his handiwork manifests in activity. . . .

Further, love is like activity, being loved like passivity; and loving and its concomitants are attributes of those who are the more active.

Again, all men love more what they have won by labor; e.g. those who have made their money love it more than those who have inherited it; and to be well treated seems to involve no labor, while to treat others well is a laborious task. These are the reasons, too, why mothers are fonder of their children than fathers; bringing them into the world costs them more pains, and they know better that the children are their own. This last point, too, would seem to apply to benefactors. [From *Nicomachean Ethics,* Book 9, chapter 7.]

Seeking Eternity Through One's Offspring

. . . [F]or any living thing that has reached its normal development and which is unmutilated, and whose mode of generation is not spontaneous, the most natural act is the production of another like itself, an animal producing an animal, a plant a plant, in order that, as far as its nature allows, it may partake of the eternal and the divine. That is the goal toward which all things strive, that for the sake of which they do whatsoever their nature renders possible. The phrase "for the sake of which" is ambiguous; it may mean either the end to achieve which, or the being in whose interest, the act is done. Since then no living thing is able to partake in what is eternal and divine by uninterrupted continuance (for nothing perishable can for ever remain one and the same), it tries to achieve that end in the only way possible to it, and success is possible, in varying degrees; so it remains not indeed as the self-same individual but continues its existence in something like itself—not numerically but specifically one. [From *De Anima,* Book 2, chapter 4.]

The Mother

Simone de Beauvoir

It is in maternity that woman fulfills her physiological destiny; it is her natural "calling," since her whole organic structure is adapted for the perpetuation of the species. But we have seen already that human society is never abandoned wholly to nature. And for about a century the reproductive function in particular has no longer been at the mercy solely of biological chance; it has come under the voluntary control of human beings. . . .

During childhood and adolescence . . . woman passes through several phases in her attitude toward maternity. To the little girl it is a miracle and a game, the doll representing a future baby to possess and domineer; to the adolescent girl maternity seems a threat to the integrity of her precious person, sometimes savagely repudiated. Sometimes she at once fears and longs for it, with hallucinations of pregnancy and all sorts of anxieties. Some girls enjoy exercising a maternal authority over children in their care, without being disposed to assume all its responsibilities. And some women have this attitude throughout life, fearing pregnancy for themselves and becoming midwives, nurses, governesses, and devoted aunts. Others, not repelled by maternity, are too much preoccupied with love-life or career to undertake it. Or they fear the burden a child would be for them or their husbands. . . .

. . . During pregnancy the woman's childbirth dreams and adolescent anxieties reappear; it is experienced in very diverse ways according to the relations that exist between the subject and her mother, her husband, and herself.

Becoming a mother in her turn, the woman in a sense takes the place of her own mother: it means complete emancipation for her. If she sincerely desires it, she will be delighted with her pregnancy and will have the courage to go through with it by herself; but if she is still under maternal domination, and willingly, she, on the contrary, puts herself in her mother's hands; her newborn child will seem to her like a brother or sister rather than her own offspring. If she at once wishes yet does not dare to free herself, she is apprehensive lest the child, instead of saving her, will bring her again under the yoke, and this anxiety may even bring on a miscarriage. Guilt feelings in regard to a mother hated in childhood may also affect pregnancy more or less unfavorably.

Not less important is the relation between the woman and the father of her child. An already mature, independent woman may want to have a child belonging wholly to herself. I have known one whose eyes lighted up at the sight of a fine male, not with sexual desire but because she judged him a good begetter; such are the maternally minded amazons who are enthusiastic over the miraculous possibilities of artificial insemination. If a woman of this type is married to the father of her child, she denies him any rights in their offspring; she endeavors (like Paul's mother in Lawrence's *Sons and Lovers*) to develop an exclusive association between herself and their common progeny. But in most cases the woman needs masculine support in accepting her new responsibilities; she will gladly devote herself to her newborn only if a man devotes himself to her. . . .

If she loves her husband, a wife will often model her feelings on his: she accepts pregnancy and maternity with delight or the contrary according to his attitude of pride or annoyance. Sometimes the child is wished for to fortify a liaison or a marriage, the strength of the mother's attachment to her baby depends on the success or failure of her plans. If she is hostile to her husband, the situation is still different: she may devote herself fiercely to her child and withhold it from her husband or, on the contrary, hate it as being the offspring of the man she detests. . . .

But pregnancy is above all a drama that is acted out within the woman herself. She feels it as at once an enrichment and an injury; the fetus is a part of her body, and it is a parasite that feeds on it; she possesses it, and she is possessed by it; it represents the future and, carrying it, she feels herself vast as the world; but this very opulence annihilates her, she feels that she herself is no longer anything. A new life is going to manifest itself and justify its own separate existence, she is proud of it; but she also feels herself tossed and driven, the plaything of obscure forces. It is especially noteworthy that the pregnant woman feels the immanence of her body at just the time when it is in transcendence: it turns upon itself in nausea and discomfort; it has ceased to exist for itself and thereupon becomes more sizable than ever before. The transcendence of the artisan, of the man of action, contains the element of subjectivity; but in the mother-to-be the antithesis of subject and object ceases to exist; she and the child with which she is swollen make up together an equivocal pair overwhelmed by life. Ensnared by nature, the pregnant woman is plant and animal, a stock-pile of colloids, an incubator, an egg; she scares children proud of their young, straight bodies and makes young people titter contemptuously because she is a human being, a conscious and free individual, who has become life's passive instrument.

Ordinarily life is but a condition of existence; in gestation it appears as creative; but that is a strange kind of creation which is accomplished in a contingent and passive manner. There are women who enjoy the pleasures of pregnancy and suckling so much that they desire their indefinite repetitions;

as soon as a baby is weaned these mothers feel frustrated. Such women are not so much mothers as fertile organisms, like fowls with high egg-production. And they seek eagerly to sacrifice their liberty of action to the functioning of their flesh: it seems to them that their existence is tranquilly justified in the passive fecundity of their bodies. If the flesh is purely passive and inert, it cannot embody transcendence, even in a degraded form; it is sluggish and tiresome; but when the reproductive process begins, the flesh becomes root-stock, source, and blossom, it assumes transcendence, a stirring toward the future, the while it remains a gross and present reality. The disjunction previously suffered by the woman in the weaning of an earlier child is compensated for; she is plunged anew into the mainstream of life, reunited with the wholeness of things, a link in the endless chain of generations, flesh that exists by and for another fleshly being. The fusion sought in masculine arms—and no sooner granted than withdrawn—is realized by the mother when she feels her child heavy within her or when she clasps it to her swelling breasts. She is no longer an object subservient to a subject; she is no longer a subject afflicted with the anxiety that accompanies liberty, she is one with that equivocal reality: life. Her body is at last her own, since it exists for the child who belongs to her. Society recognizes her right of possession and invests it, moreover, with a sacred character. Her bosom, which was previously an erotic feature, can now be freely shown, for it is a source of life; even religious pictures show us the Virgin Mother exposing her breast as she beseeches her Son to save mankind. With her ego surrendered, alienated in her body and in her social dignity, the mother enjoys the comforting illusion of feeling that she is a human being *in herself,* a *value.*

But this is only an illusion. For she does not really make the baby, it makes itself within her; her flesh engenders flesh only, and she is quite incapable of establishing an existence that will have to establish itself. Creative acts originating in liberty establish the object as value and give it the quality of the essential, whereas the child in the maternal body is not thus justified; it is still only a gratuitous cellular growth, a brute fact of nature as contingent on circumstances as death and corresponding philosophically with it. A mother can have *her* reasons for wanting *a* child, but she cannot give to *this* independent person, who is to exist tomorrow, his own reasons, his justification, for existence; she engenders him as a product of her generalized body, not of her individualized existence. . . .

In a sense the mystery of the Incarnation repeats itself in each mother; every child born is a god who is made man: he cannot find self-realization as a being with consciousness and freedom unless he first comes into the world; the mother lends herself to this mystery, but she does not control it; it is beyond her power to influence what in the end will be the true nature of this being who is developing in her womb. She gives expression to this uncertainty in two contradictory fantasies: every mother entertains the idea that her child will be a hero, thus showing her wonderment at the thought of engendering a being with consciousness and freedom; but she is also in dread of giving birth to a defective or a monster, because she is aware to what a frightening extent the welfare of the flesh is contingent upon circumstances—and this embryo dwelling within her is only flesh. There are cases in which one or the other of the myths bemuses her; but frequently the woman oscillates between the two. She also feels another ambiguity. Caught up in the great cycle of the species, she affirms life in the teeth of time and death: in this she glimpses immortality; but in her flesh she feels the truth of Hegel's words: "The birth of children is the death of parents." The child, he says, again, is "the very being of their love which is external to them," and, inversely, the child will attain his own being "in separating from its source, a separation in which that source finds its end." This projection of herself is also for the woman the foreshadowing of her death. She expresses this truth in the fear she feels when she thinks of childbirth: she fears that it will mean the loss of her own life.

The significance of pregnancy being thus ambiguous, it is natural that woman should assume an ambivalent attitude toward it; moreover her attitude changes with the various stages in fetal development. It should first be emphasized that at the beginning of the process the baby is not present; it has as yet only an imaginary existence; the mother-to-be can muse upon the little being who is to be born some months hence and busy herself with the preparation of his cradle and layette; she experiences concretely no more than the disturbing organic phenomena taking place within her. . . . [When she learns that she is pregnant,] she knows that her body is destined to transcend itself; day after day a growth arising from her flesh but foreign to it is going to enlarge within her; she is the prey of the species, which imposes its mysterious laws upon her, and as a rule this subjection to strange outer forces frightens her, her fright being manifested in morning sickness and nausea. These are in part brought on by modification of the gastric secretions produced at this time; but if this reaction, unknown in other mammals, is an important one in woman, the cause of it is psychic; it expresses the sharpness that at this time marks the conflict, in the human female, between the species and the individual. Even if the woman deeply desires to have a child, her body vigorously revolts when obliged to undergo the reproductive process. . . .

Women who are treated with most concern, or who are most concerned with themselves, are the ones who show the greatest number of morbid symptoms. Those who undergo the ordeal of pregnancy with greatest ease are, on the one hand, the matrons who are wholly consecrated to their reproductive function, and, on the other, those mannish women who are not particularly fascinated by the adventures of their bodies and are quite ready and willing to go through them without fuss: Mme de Staël carried on a pregnancy as readily as a conversation.

While pregnancy advances, the relation between mother and fetus changes. The latter is firmly settled in the mother's womb; the two organisms are mutually adapted, and between them biological exchanges take place that enable the woman to regain her balance. She no longer feels herself possessed by the species; it is she who possesses the fruit of her body. During the first months she was an ordinary woman, and none the worse for the secret activity going on within her; later she is recognizably a mother-to-be, and her infirmities are but the other side of her glory. As her weakness becomes more pronounced, it excuses everything. Many women find in their later pregnancy a marvelous peace: they feel justified. Previously they had always felt a desire to observe themselves, to scrutinize their bodies; but they had not dared to indulge this interest too freely, from a sense of social propriety. Now it is their right; everything they do for their own benefit they are doing also for the child. They are no longer called upon for work or effort; they no longer have to think of others; the dreams of the future they cherish lend meaning to the present moment; they have only to let themselves live; they are on vacation.

The pregant woman's raison d'être is there, in her womb, and gives her a perfect sense of rich abundance. . . . Thus fulfilled, the woman has also the satisfaction of feeling that she is "interesting," something that has been her deepest wish since adolescence; as wife she suffered from her dependency with regard to man; now she is no longer in service as a sexual object, but she is the incarnation of the species, she represents the promise of life, of eternity. Her entourage respects her; her very caprices become sacred, and this, as we have seen, is what encourages her to invent "longings." As Helene Deutsch says, "Pregnancy permits woman to rationalize performances which otherwise would appear absurd." Justified by the presence of another in her womb, she at last enjoys the privilege of being wholly herself. . . .

Colette tells us that one of her friends called this pleasant pregnancy "a man's pregnancy." And in fact she seems typical of those women who bear their condition valiantly because they are not absorbed in it. At the same time she continued her work as a writer. "The baby indicated that he would be finished first, and I put the cap on my fountain pen."

Other women feel the weight of it more; they muse endlessly on their new importance. With the slightest encouragement they revive in their own cases the masculine myths: against the light of the mind they oppose the fecund darkness of Life; against the clarity of consciousness, the mysteries of inwardness; against productive liberty, the weight of this belly growing there enormously without human will. The mother-to-be feels herself one with soil and sod, stock and root; when she drowses off, her sleep is like that of brooding chaos with worlds in ferment. Some, those more forgetful of self, are delighted above all with the living treasure growing within them. . . .

On the other hand, women who are primarily interested in pleasing men, who see themselves essentially as erotic objects, who are in love with their own bodily beauty, are distressed to see themselves deformed, disfigured, incapable of arousing desire. Pregnancy seems to them no holiday, no enrichment at all, but rather a diminution of the ego. . . .

In the last stage of pregnancy there are indications of the break between mother and child. Women perceive the child's first movement with varied feelings, this kick delivered at the portals of the world, against the uterine wall that shuts him off from the world. One woman is lost in wonder at this signal announcing the presence of an independent being; another may feel repugnance at containing a stranger. Once more the union of fetus and maternal body is disturbed: the uterus descends, the woman has sensations of pressure, tension, and difficult breathing. She is now in the possession not of the species in general but of this infant who is about to be born; up to this time he has been only a mental image, a hope; now he becomes a solid, present reality, and his reality creates new problems. Every transition is fraught with anxiety: childbirth appears especially terrifying. When the woman approaches her term, all her childish terrors come to life again; if through feelings of guilt she believes she is under her mother's curse, she persuades herself that she is going to die or that the child will die. In *War and Peace* Tolstoy depicts in the young Lise one of these infantile women who see childbirth as a sentence of death; and in fact she does die.

The significance of childbirth varies greatly in different cases: the mother desires at the same time to retain the precious flesh that is a treasured portion of her ego and to rid herself of an intruder; she wants to have her dream actually in her hands at last, but she dreads the new responsibilities that this material realization is going to create. Either desire may predominate, but she is often torn between them. It frequently happens, also, that she is of two minds in her approach to the agonizing ordeal: she means to prove to herself and to her entourage—to her mother, to her husband—that she can weather the storm without assistance; but at the same time she bears a grudge against the world, against life, against her family, for the sufferings inflicted upon her, and in protest she remains passive. Women of independent character—matrons or mannish women—are disposed to play an active part just before and even during the birth; those of very childish nature are passive in [the] hands of midwife or mother; some take pride in making no outcry; others refuse to obey any directions.

On the whole we may say that in this crisis women give expression to their fundamental attitude toward the world in general and toward their own maternity in particular: they may be stoical, resigned, demanding, domineering, rebellious, passive, or tense. . . . It is significant that woman—like the females of certain domesticated animals—requires help in performing the function assigned to her by nature; there are peasants living in harsh circumstances and shamefaced unmarried mothers who give birth alone, but their being alone at this time often results in death for the baby or incurable illness for the mother. At just the time when woman attains the realization of her feminine destiny, she is still dependent: proof again that in the human species nature and artifice are never wholly separated. In natural circumstances the conflict between the interest of the feminine individual and that of the species is so acute that it often brings about the death of either the mother or the child: it is human intervention, medical or surgical, that has considerably reduced—and even almost eliminated—the formerly frequent mishaps. Anesthetic techniques are doing much to nullify the Biblical pronouncement: "In sorrow thou shalt bring forth children. . . .[1]" It is difficult to determine just how much relief from suffering woman obtains through these methods. The fact that the duration of delivery may vary from twenty-four to two or three hours forbids generalization. For some women childbirth is a martydom. . . . Some women, on the contrary, consider the ordeal a relatively easy one to bear. A few find sensual pleasure in it. . . .

There are some women who say that childbirth gives them a sense of creative power; they have really accomplished a voluntary and productive task. Many, at the other extreme, have felt themselves passive—suffering and tortured instruments.

The first relations of the mother with her newborn child are equally variable. Some women suffer from the emptiness they now feel in their bodies: it seems to them that their treasure has been stolen. . . .

At the same time, however, there is an amazed curiosity in every young mother. It is strangely miraculous to see and to hold a living being formed within oneself and issued forth from oneself. But just what part has the mother had in the extraordinary event that brings into the world a new existence? She does not know. The newborn would not exist had it not been for her, and yet he leaves her. There is an astonished melancholy in seeing him outside, cut off from her. And almost always disappointment. The woman would like to feel the new being as surely *hers* as is her own hand; but everything he experiences is shut up inside him; he is opaque, impenetrable, apart; she does not even recognize him because she does not know him. She has experienced her pregnancy without him: she has no past in common with this little stranger. She expected that he would be at once familiar; but no, he is a newcomer, and she is surprised at the indifference with which she receives him. In the reveries of her pregnancy he was a mental image with infinite possibilities, and the mother enjoyed her future maternity in thought; now he is a tiny, finite individual, and he is there in reality—dependent, delicate, demanding. Her quite real joy in his finally being there is mingled with regret to find him no more than that.

Many young mothers regain through nursing an intimate animal relationship with their infants after the birth separation has occurred; it is more tiring than pregnancy, but it enables the nursing mother to prolong the state of being on vacation, in peace and plenitude, enjoyed in pregnancy. . . .

But there are women who cannot nurse and whose first surprised indifference continues until they find definite new bonds with the infant. This was the case with Colette, for one, who was unable to nurse her baby daughter and who describes her first maternal feeling with her customary sincerity in *L'Etoile Vesper:*

> . . . Yet I shall recover my serenity only when intelligible language comes from her sweet lips, when consciousness, mischievousness, and even affection make a baby like any other into a daughter, and *a* daughter into *my* daughter!

There are also many mothers who are alarmed at their new responsibilities. During her pregnancy such a woman had only to abandon herself to her flesh; no initiative was called for. Now she is confronted by a person who has rights to be considered. There are some women who, still gay and carefree, gaily pet their babies while still in the hospital, but on returning home begin to regard them as burdensome. Even nursing affords such a woman no pleasure; on the contrary, she is apprehensive of ruining her bosom; she resents feeling her nipples cracked, the glands painful; suckling the baby hurts; the infant seems to her to be sucking out her strength, her life, her happiness. It inflicts a harsh slavery upon her and it is no longer a part of her: it seems a tyrant; she feels hostile to this little stranger, this individual who menaces her flesh, her freedom, her whole ego.

Many other factors are involved. The woman's relations with her mother retain all their importance. . . . Her relations with the baby's father and his own feelings in the matter also exert a large influence. A whole complex of economic and sentimental considerations makes the baby seem either a burden and a hindrance or a jewel, a means of liberation and security. There are cases in which hostility becomes open hatred, expressed by extreme neglect or bad treatment. Usually the mother, mindful of her duty, tries to combat this hostility; the remorse she feels gives rise to anxiety states in which the apprehensions of pregnancy are continued. . . .

What is in any case remarkable and distinguishes this relation of mother and baby from all other human relations is the fact that at first the baby itself takes no active part in it: its smiles, its babble, have no sense other than what the mother gives them; whether it seems charming and unique, or tiresome, commonplace, and hateful, depends upon her, not upon the baby. . . .

These examples all show that no maternal "instinct" exists: the word hardly applies, in any case, to the human species. The mother's attitude depends on her total situation and her reaction to it. As we have just seen, this is highly variable.

But the fact remains that unless the circumstances are positively unfavorable the mother will find her life enriched by her child. Concerning one young mother Colette Audry remarks that her child was like a proof of the reality of her own existence, through him she had a hold on things in general and on herself to begin with. . . .

If certain women who are fecund rather than motherly lose interest in their offspring at weaning or at birth and desire only a new pregnancy, many, on the contrary, feel that the separation is what gives them the child; it is no longer an indistinguishable part of themselves but a portion of the outer world; it no longer vaguely haunts their bodies, but can be seen and touched. . . .

It has been asserted time and again that woman is pleased to acquire in the infant an equivalent of the penis, but this is by no means an exact statement. The fact is that the grown man no longer sees in his penis a wonderful toy as in childhood; the value it has for the adult lies in the desirable objects it enables him to possess. Similarly, the adult woman envies the male the prey he takes possession of, not the instrument by which he takes it. The infant satisfies that aggressive eroticism which is not fully satisfied in the male embrace: the infant corresponds, for the woman, to the mistress whom she leaves to the male and whom he does not represent for her. The correspondence is not exact, of course; every relation is *sui generis,* unique; but the mother finds in her infant—as does the lover in his beloved—a carnal plenitude, and this not in surrender but in domination; she obtains in her child what man seeks in woman: an other, combining nature and mind, who is to be both prey and *double.* The baby incarnates all nature. . . .

Maternity takes on a new aspect when the child grows older; at first it is only a baby like any other, it exists only in its generality, one example of a class; then little by little it takes on individuality. Women of very domineering or very sensual disposition then grow cool toward the child; and at this time, on the contrary, certain others—like Colette—begin to take a real interest in their offspring. The relation of mother to child becomes more and more complex: the child is a double, an *alter ego,* into whom the mother is sometimes tempted to project herself entirely, but he is an independent subject and therefore rebellious; he is intensely real today, but in imagination he is the adolescent and adult of the future. He is a rich possession, a treasure, but also a charge upon her, a tyrant. The mother's joy in him is one of generosity; she must find her pleasure in serving, giving, making him happy. . . .

Like the woman in love, the mother is delighted to feel herself necessary; her existence is justified by the wants she supplies; but what gives mother love its difficulty and its grandeur is the fact that it implies no reciprocity; the mother has to do not with man, a hero, a demigod, but with a small, prattling soul, lost in a fragile and dependent body. The child is in possession of no values, he can bestow none, with him the woman remains alone; she expects no return for what she gives, it is for her to justify it herself. This generosity merits the laudation that men never tire of conferring upon her; but the distortion begins when the religion of Maternity proclaims that all mothers are saintly. For while maternal devotion may be perfectly genuine, this, in fact, is rarely the case. Maternity is usually a strange mixture of narcissism, altruism, idle daydreaming, sincerity, bad faith, devotion, and cynicism.

The great danger which threatens the infant in our culture lies in the fact that the mother to whom it is confided in all its helplessness is almost always a discontented woman: sexually she is frigid or unsatisfied; socially she feels herself inferior to man; she has no independent grasp on the world or on the future. She will seek to compensate for all these frustrations through her child. When it is realized how difficult woman's present situation makes her full self-realization, how many desires, rebellious feelings, just claims she nurses in secret, one is frightened at the thought that defenseless infants are abandoned to her care. Just as when she coddled and tortured her dolls by turns, her behavior is symbolic; but symbols become grim reality for her child. A mother who whips her child is not beating the child alone; in a sense she is not beating it at all: she is taking her vengeance on a man, on the world, or on herself. Such a mother is often remorseful and the child may not feel resentment, but it feels the blows. . . .

Another common attitude, and one not less ruinous to the child, is masochistic devotion, in which the mother makes herself the slave of her offspring to compensate for the emptiness of her heart and to punish herself for her unavowed hostility. Such a mother is morbidly anxious, not allowing her child out of her sight; she gives up all diversion, all personal life, thus assuming the role of victim; and she derives from these sacrifices the right to deny her child all independence. This renunciation on the mother's part is easily reconciled with a tyrannical will to domination; the *mater dolorosa* forges from her sufferings a weapon that she uses sadistically; her displays of resignation give rise to guilt feelings in the child which often last a lifetime: they are still more harmful than her displays of aggression. Tossed this way and that, baffled, the child can find no defensive position: now blows, now tears, make him out a criminal.

The main excuse of the mother is that her child by no means provides that happy self-fulfillment which has been promised her since her own childhood; she blames him for the deception of which she has been the victim and which he innocently exposes. She did as she pleased with her dolls; when she helped a sister or a friend with a baby, the responsibility was not hers. But now society, her husband, her mother, and her own pride hold her to account for that little strange life, as if it were all her doing. . . .

For the great difficulty is to bring within preconceived patterns an existence as mysterious as that of an animal, as turbulent and disorderly as natural forces, and yet human. . . .

The mother's relation with her children takes from within the totality of her life; it depends upon her relations with her husband, her past, her occupation, herself; it is an error as harmful as it is absurd to regard the child as a universal panacea. This is also Helene Deutsch's conclusion in the [*Psychology of Women*], in which she examines the phenomena of maternity in the light of her psychiatric experience. She gives this function a high importance, believing that through it woman finds complete self-realization—but on condition that it is freely assumed and *sincerely* wanted; the young woman must be in a psychological, moral, and material situation that allows her to bear the effort involved; otherwise the consequences will be disastrous. . . . Only the woman who is well balanced, healthy, and aware of her responsibilities is capable of being a "good" mother.

As we have seen, the curse which lies upon marriage is that too often the individuals are joined in their weakness rather than in their strength—each asking from the other instead of finding pleasure in giving. It is even more deceptive to dream of gaining through the child a plenitude, a warmth, a value, which one is unable to create for oneself; the child brings joy only to the woman who is capable of disinterestedly desiring the happiness of another, to one who without being wrapped up in self seeks to transcend her own existence. To be sure, the child is an enterprise to which one can validly devote oneself; but it represents a ready-made justification no more than any other enterprise does; and it must be desired for its own sake, not for hypothetical benefits. As Stekel well says:[2]

> Children . . . are neither playthings, nor tools for the fulfillment
> of parental needs or ungratified ambitions. Children are obligations;
> they should be brought up so as to become happy human beings.

There is nothing *natural* in such an obligation: nature can never dictate a moral choice; this implies an engagement, a promise to be carried out. . . .

And it is not true, even, that having a child is a privileged accomplishment for woman, primary in relation to all others; it is often said of a woman that she is coquettish, or amorous, or lesbian, or ambitious, "for lack of a child"; her sexual life, the aims, the values she pursues, would in this view be substituted for a child. In fact, the matter is originally uncertain, indeterminate: one can say as well that a woman wants a child for lack of love, for lack of occupation, for lack of opportunity to satisfy homosexual tendencies. A social and artificial morality is hidden beneath this pseudo-naturalism. That the child is the supreme aim of woman is a statement having precisely the value of an advertising slogan.

The second false preconception, directly implied by the first, is that the child is sure of being happy in its mother's arms. There is no such thing as an "unnatural mother," to be sure, since there is nothing natural about maternal love; but, precisely for that reason, there are bad mothers. And one of the major truths proclaimed by psychoanalysis is the danger to the child that may lie in parents who are themselves "normal." The complexes, obsessions, and neuroses of adults have their roots in the early family life of those adults; parents who are themselves in conflict, with their quarrels and their tragic scenes, are bad company for the child. Deeply scarred by their early home life, their approach to their own children is through complexes and frustrations; and this chain of misery lengthens indefinitely. . . .

. . . It would clearly be desirable for the good of the child if the mother were a complete, unmutilated person, a woman finding in her work and in her relation to society a self-realization that she would not seek to attain tyrannically through her offspring; and it would also be desirable for the child to be left to his parents infinitely less than at present, and for his studies and his diversions to be carried on among other children, under the direction of adults whose bonds with him would be impersonal and pure. . . .

We have seen that woman's inferiority originated in her being at first limited to repeating life, whereas man invented reasons for living more essential, in his eyes, than the not-willed routine of mere existence; to restrict woman to maternity would be to perpetuate this situation. She demands today to have a part in the mode of activity in which humanity tries continually to find justification through transcendence, through movement toward new goals and accomplishments; she cannot consent to bring forth life unless life has meaning; she cannot be a mother without endeavoring to play a role in the economic, political, and social life of the times. It is not the same thing to produce cannon fodder, slaves, victims, or, on the other hand, free men. In a properly organized society, where children would be largely taken in charge by the community and the mother cared for and helped, maternity would not be wholly incompatible with careers for women. On the contrary, the woman who works—farmer, chemist, or writer—is the one who undergoes pregnancy most easily because she is not absorbed in her own person; the woman who enjoys the richest individual life will have the most to give her children and will demand the least from them; she who acquires in effort and struggle a sense of true human values will be best able to bring them up properly. . . .

Notes

1. . . . [S]ome antifeminists are indignant in the name of nature and the Bible at any proposal to eliminate labor pains, which they regard as one of the sources of the maternal "instinct." Helene Deutsch seems somewhat drawn to this view, remarking that a mother who has not suffered from her labor pains does not feel the baby profoundly hers when it is placed in her arms. She agrees, however, that the same feelings of emptiness and estrangement are sometimes to be observed in women who have experienced the pangs of delivery; and she maintains throughout her book that maternal love is a sentiment, a conscious attitude, not an instinct, and that it is not necessarily connected with pregnancy. According to her, a woman may feel maternal love for an adopted child, for one her husband has had by a former wife, and so on. This contradiction evidently stems from the fact that she regards woman as doomed to masochism, her thesis compelling her to assign a high value to feminine suffering.

2. *Frigidity in Woman,* Vol. II, pp. 305, 306.

Genetic Puzzles and Stork Stories:
On the Meaning and Significance of
Having Children

Kenneth D. Alpern

A primary motivation for the development and use of reproduction-aiding techniques and services (RTs), such as artificial insemination, in vitro fertilization, and parenting through contract (surrogate motherhood), is the desire to have children.[1] This desire is regarded as natural, and having children, in the proper circumstances of personal maturity and stable relationship, is generally encouraged by both individuals and social practices. Having children is held to be a fundamental source of fulfillment for the parents, is an obvious good for the children, and is good for society, which benefits from well-raised new members. Thus, it would seem that considerations of prudence (personal well-being), of morality (proper regard for rights, interests, and character), and of good public policy all support having children and the desire to have children.

Most people assume that when the time comes, they will be able to have children without much difficulty. The problem, rather, is to avoid having children before the desired time. When obstacles, such as infertility, are encountered, couples are initially stunned and then embittered by the unfairness of impediments to this good, which they had assumed would be theirs and which they regularly observe others effortlessly enjoying. In order to overcome these obstacles, couples are willing to go to great lengths, enduring disruptive and invasive testing and therapy, such as drug treatment and surgery, often over many years and at the expense of thousands of dollars. Continued failure occasions great frustration and resentment. But for the fundamental good of having children, these actions and attitudes are generally regarded as natural and reasonable.

Many couples who experience continued failure at having children consider adoption but are deterred by long waits, expenses, or eligibility requirements (such as age).[2] Tens of thousands of couples whose problem is male infertility have for decades turned to artificial insemination with "donor" sperm, often without (seriously) looking into adoption. And increasingly, married couples (and single individuals and nontraditional couples) are turn-ing to more exotic RTs, including in vitro fertilization (in the thousands) and parenting through contract (over a thousand) in order to have children. Cer-tain of these new alternatives are particularly appealing, as they make it possible to have *one's own* children, that is, children to whom one or both parents are genetically related.

The RTs, then, hold out great hope for people who are in genuine, deep, and abiding distress. But these new options have also generated great contro-versy on moral, religious, public policy, and other grounds. Yet, even when the RTs are condemned, the basic motivation for turning to them—the desire to have (one's own) child—is almost always unquestioningly accepted and held to justify great personal and social costs to satisfy.

But should this desire be taken at face value, welcomed, supported, and indulged? At what costs, financial and otherwise, should its satisfaction be pursued? Exactly how important should the satisfaction of the desire to have (one's own) child be to the individuals immediately involved, to sympathetic third parties (e.g., family, friends, health care professionals), and to society in general? To answer such questions, we need a clearer understanding of exactly what it is that is being desired and why it should be so significant. The present essay seeks to work toward that clearer understanding.

It may seem that the meaning and significance of having children is so obvious that it does not need to be articulated or so fundamental that it cannot be set out in words. Yet, having a firm understanding of the meaning and significance of having children is essential to sound decisions, decent societies, and fulfilled lives. For example, is it primarily nurturing relationships with developing human beings that are desirable? If so, might not other options besides having children serve as well? What is the importance of the processes through which the child comes to be? Do the circumstances of conception, gestation, and parturition matter, or are they irrelevant as long as a child is the outcome? It is held best to have *one's own* child, but what does that mean: mere custody? nurturing the child? gestation? giving birth? having a genetic relationship to it? Why and to what extent are these different relationships significant? To what extent does having children through one or another RT satisfy or fail to satisfy properly understood desires and values, and how does development and use of these techniques affect our conceptions of ourselves and our well-being? Only with careful study of such issues can prudential, moral, and policy interests be understood and securely pursued.

The present essay does not presume to answer all of these questions. But it does attempt to initiate rational inquiry. In the first section, I consider a num-ber of challenges to the idea of rational inquiry into so fundamental a feature of human life. The second section surveys commonly offered reasons for having children. The third section points out certain conceptual features of desire and its satisfaction and applies these findings in a critique of the desire to have children. The fourth section probes the idea of a genetic relationship. Part of the title of this essay is taken from this inquiry into genetic relationships, not because this is the only focus of the essay, but because many people believe that in talk of genes is the firm and scientific basis for understanding what it is to have one's own child and why the genetic relation should be so significant to us. The fifth section offers a few concluding remarks. In the end, this essay may not have definitive answers to all the questions posed, but I do hope at least to make clear what the issues are, to help us to avoid certain confusions and mistakes, and to identify promising issues for further exploration.

Challenges to the Inquiry

A number of objections might be thought to undercut the inquiry from the start. First, it might be thought that the questions being asked are matters of personal decision and are not for others to answer. If a couple decides to use a certain RT and they feel satisfied with the outcome, then that shows that they got what they wanted. No one else can be in a better position to judge the value and the satisfaction to these individuals, and no one should intrude on their activities, at least not in the name of second-guessing these individuals' own desires, satisfaction, and well-being. Further, it might be objected that talk of reasons and critical examination of values are beside the point, because our biological makeup (genes, hormones, etc.) determines us to desire and to seek to have children. Having children is a basic biological drive or need, a "biological imperative," and this gives it an undeniable place in our lives. Finally, it might be claimed that there is in any case no point to worrying about conceptual clarification and justification, because in something as basic and dear as having children, people are going to do what they feel like doing, and reason and argument are not going to divert them.

Reply to the Challenges

It may be true that many people automatically follow their impulses and do not inquire very deeply into how best to serve even their own interests. And all of us to some degree fall back unreflectively on conventions and traditional values. But use of the RTs is sufficiently out of the ordinary and has occasioned enough controversy to cause most people to stop and reflect. We can do it, and we should. If we don't, it may be proper for others—friends, educators—to bring us to do so.

In connection with the first objection, one should not conflate the claim that deliberations about having children are personal and private with the claim that such deliberations cannot be guided by reason or by the insights of others. Perhaps we seek to insulate our personal deliberations because we think of reasons and morality in the context of an "authority" seeking to *force* us to do what the authority has decided is right and justified. But moral and rational discourse is not necessarily coercive. Though some sorts of coercion may sometimes be appropriate (as the need for criminal law attests), interpersonal moral reasoning can also be carried out in contexts of sympathy and *advice,* as when we seek counsel from a morally sensitive and reflective friend.

Mature, even minimally reflective, persons recognize their own fallibility and the value of others' insights, especially in matters as serious and emotional as bringing another human being into the world.

An adequate examination of the difficult notion of "biological imperatives" (biological drives and needs) is more than can be carried out in this essay. Such an inquiry would involve examining the nature of the relationships between (1) being biologically suited to reproduction, (2) feeling impelled toward reproductive activities and child rearing, (3) experiencing satisfaction in (various elements) of reproduction and child rearing, and (4) suffering distress or dysfunction if we do not have children. But even if we accept that something like biological imperatives are at work in the desire to have children, that would not establish the necessity or the proper place of having children in our lives. I offer the following brief observations in support of this claim.

First of all, whatever our notion of biological imperatives, they will vary in strength and content from person to person and may be functions of, and so modified by, contingencies of culture, personality, and sex.[3] Further, that biological forces are at work does not mean that we are powerless to restrain, redirect, or reshape them, or that we do so only at a loss to our well-being. Biology is not the only consideration or value that must be accommodated in living a good life.[4] Certainly, many people lead happy and fulfilled lives without having children.[5]

Concerning biological imperatives, we should also consider what their *objects* are and how the object of a drive is to be identified. At the very least, we should recognize that the connection between sexual intercourse and having children is something that has to be discovered by cultures and learned by each individual. An impulse to engage in sexual intercourse is not thereby a drive to have children. Even if biological drives are admitted, it is not clear whether the object of the drive in question should be identified as having children, nurturing children, going through pregnancy and parturition, merely engaging in sexual intercourse, or even just experiencing sexual gratification, which does not require engaging in intercourse. Thus, even to the extent that biology impels us and determines our good, it is not clear exactly what activities and experiences we are impelled toward or need.

One variation on the appeal to biological imperatives is the claim that built into humans through evolutionary processes is a drive to reproduce so as to perpetuate the species.[6] Perhaps all that needs to be said in response to this claim is to recall the observations just made about the objects of drives. Even if the outcome of a set of natural impulses is the continuation of the species, that does not mean that an individual is impelled toward anything more than activities (e.g., sexual intercourse) that have that outcome, nor does it mean that the individual's life is necessarily any worse for failing to contribute to that outcome. The actual perpetuation of the species may mean nothing at all to the individual. As a matter of pure biology, the continuation of the human species need matter no more to a human being than does the continuation of its species matter to a frog or to a petunia.

I am not denying that through biology and evolution we may have acquired certain behaviors, attitudes, and propensities that suit us well to having children or to finding satisfaction in having children. Rather, I have been trying to show that the implications of these facts for our motivations and our good are not obvious, and that a simple appeal to a drive to have children does not eliminate the need to inquire into the meaning and significance of the desire to have children.

Reasons for Desiring to Have Children

We may now turn to *reasons* for desiring to have or for valuing having children. My aim here is not only to bring to mind the different sorts of considerations that may be held to justify seeking to satisfy the desire, but also to help clarify exactly what it is about having children that is desired and valued—just as by setting out reasons for wanting a car (for status, for a sense of power, in order to get from place to place, for a sense of freedom), one acquires a better understanding of what the desire is for and of how it is best satisfied, as well as of its justification.

Reasons for desiring to have children are varied and complexly related. The following list, which no doubt is incomplete and overlapping, identifies many of the most important and commonly given reasons:[7]

- Having children is a cultural norm (it is the natural thing to do); it is expected by parents, peers, religions; it may even be felt to be a duty or fulfillment of God's command.
- Having children gives significance to marriage or to the personal relationship of two people; children symbolize, express, and actualize the union of the parents.
- Children are interesting, rewarding, challenging, and fulfilling; they provide opportunities for giving and for unconditional love. Having children can transform our ways of thinking and feeling. Children are persons with whom we can enter into specially intimate relationships of mutual knowledge, care, and dependence.
- Having children is a way of continuing oneself, one's line (family, bloodline, geneline), and one's species.
- Having children is participation in the processes of life and existence through intercourse, pregnancy, giving birth, and raising children.
- Children are a source of personal renewal, a way to recapture youth, innocence, and experiences and attitudes of wonder, discovery, etc.
- Having children is a way of expressing appreciation for one's own life.
- Having children is an activity of creation, participation in something beyond oneself; it gives a sense of power, competence, coming of age, and gender realization; it proves to oneself and to others one's independence and maturity.

- Children are sources of labor and of physical and emotional support, especially in old age.
- Having children contributes to the perpetuation and advancement of one's society, one's culture, one's ethnic group, etc.

Clearly, having children can be thought to serve, and to be constitutive of, a wide range of goods. And one's reasons for desiring to have children in part determine the content of that desire. For example, a person who seeks to have children primarily in order to love and nurture a child can be satisfied by quite different things than one who seeks to have children primarily for a sense of personal continuance. Each of the reasons in the above list can be further examined, dissected, and evaluated: Which are valid? Which are based on illusion? Which promote and which distort healthy and fulfilling human relationships? In what ways may these aims be achieved through the RTs, through adoption, or through different social arrangements? In what follows, rather than try to answer all these questions (which would require more space and insight than I presently have), I will first draw attention to a number of *general* features of desiring and follow out certain of their implications for the desire to have children. I will then turn to a more detailed inquiry into the meaning and significance of genetic relations, since this seems to many people to be the ultimate ground and explanation of the relation of parents and children.

Examinaton of the Desire to Have Children

It might be thought that a desire, such as the desire to have children, that is sincere and deeply felt should be accorded great weight in all types of decisions; that is, that it is in persons' interests that their desires be satisfied, that proper moral regard for persons demands respect for their desires, and that public policy should be formed to promote persons' interests as defined in part by their desires. But desires, even sincere and deeply felt desires, should not always be taken at face value. In this section, I draw attention to a number of general features of desire and of persons that may give reason to accord reduced weight to a desire in deliberations concerning a person's well-being.

A desire may be ascribed to a person, even oneself, on a number of different grounds, including what one says, what one feels attracted to and is motivated toward, what one does, what one feels good about having done and reflects with satisfaction upon, and what one identifies with and affirms. These different grounds, however, do not always coincide. In an attempt to resolve conflicts, appeal might be made to what one says or does *spontaneously*. Or, conversely, appeal might be made to what one feels, says, and does *upon reflection*. But neither of these appeals carries absolute authority. Appeal to spontaneity may reduce the chances for rationalization or self-deception, but a spontaneous response also can be simply the last thing one heard, something that was momentarily appealing, or merely an arbitrary pattern of response (such as a habit or mere convention). And though reflection may enable one to select a response with care, reflective responses are still vulnerable to the self-deception and rationalizations that spontaneity was supposed to help avoid. Thus, though each appeal can be instructive, neither is definitive of what one "really" desires. Indeed, I believe it is a mistake in this context to think in terms of what one "really" desires, as if there must be a "real desire" that one in fact has. We can describe what a person feels, what the person is motivated to do, what he or she spontaneously says and does, what the person judges on reflection, and so on. To ask further what the person *really* desires may then be pointless. The facts about the person have been described. There is no further entity (the putative "real desire") that remains to be defined, and it would provide no explanatory force. I will, nonetheless, speak in what follows of what persons (really) desire in contrast to the merely *apparent* contents of their desires. In doing so, however, I will be marking contrasts of a more limited sort than are marked by the use of the term "real" that I have rejected.

Now, how should we identify and weigh our own and others' desires? We do not have full awareness of ourselves, of what we desire, of what moves us, of what we value, or of what gives us satisfaction. Our self-conceptions develop gradually, incompletely, and in fragments that do not necessarily cohere. And what we do come to recognize of ourselves is always open to revision. Nonetheless, we do identify the content of desires, our own and those of others, and we arrive at reasonable estimates of the weight desires should be accorded. Sometimes we do this fairly consciously, as with children, judging what to make of their cries and their passionate declarations of need—Is the baby uncomfortable or just on a crying jag? Is the toy something the child really wants, or is she just parroting words that have been drummed into her head? We make such judgments regularly about ourselves and other adults as well. There may be no formula or method for making these judgments. But we recognize that it is necessary and proper to make such judgments and that it is possible to do so, if not with absolute certainty, even about ourselves, especially when we confront desires as complex as the desire to have (our own) children. In the following few paragraphs, I wish to draw attention to a number of considerations that should inform such judgments.

Weighing

The proper weight or importance of a desire can be misapprehended. The strength of one's feeling, for example, does not directly translate into a corresponding weight or value for the desire. A great many conditions can cause one to misjudge the weight that a particular desire should be accorded in thinking about a person's (one's own) life and well-being. For example, one might easily become obsessive about a desire if the thing desired is viewed not just as a matter of enjoyment and as external to one's self, but as central to one's conception of the good and as a matter of self-image and self-respect; if satisfaction of this desire has been taken for granted, thought to be natural, automatic, to be secured whenever sought; if failure to satisfy the desire is seen as dysfunctional and as a reason for embarrassment or shame; if what is desired is a matter of status or competition; if one constantly encounters other people enjoying, even flaunting,[8] their (seemingly effortless) success; if others are deeply interested in, press for, and pin their own hopes on one's success; if opportunities for success are limited by time constraints; if one's routine means for dealing with frustrations (money, avoidance, compensatory behavior) do not seem to work. Under conditions such as these, common to many infertile people, even legitimately important desires can be overly valued, and the person can be consumed by them. Though persons may be totally sincere and their emotional suffering undeniable, they may be less disposed toward self-reflection and less able to judge the proper place of this desire in even their own scheme of value, let alone in competition with the interests and rights of others. In such cases, prudence would seem to demand that one not automatically indulge the desire, but seek a critical perspective for evaluating it. Similarly, moral and policy considerations should not take the desire at face value. Merely to serve the desire, as intensely and sincerely as it may be felt, may not be the proper course for sympathetic individuals (relatives, friends, health care professionals, attorneys) or for a caring society.

Object

In addition to being overly valued, the object of a desire, just like the object of a drive, as discussed earlier, may be incorrectly identified. What is thought of as the object of persons' desires, even by the persons themselves, may better be understood as merely one way of satisfying a more generic object, or it may be a substitute or compensation for another object that it resembles or with which it is in some other way associated.[9] Thus, a desire to have children sometimes may be best understood within a larger context of desires for more generic objects, such as the desire for various types of human community, for a sense of participation in life and life processes, for contributions to others, or for creativity in general. If, for example, a person has been unable to develop certain forms of human relationship, as in a society that fragments families and provides scant opportunity for interaction between families and between generations, then having children may be seized upon as a substitute for these frustrated forms of interpersonal relationship. Or, again, if one feels lacking in power, in opportunity or ability to give to others, or in opportunities for meaningful productive activity, one may, consciously or unconsciously, seize upon having children as a replacement or compensation for these missing satisfactions. In such cases as these, it may be more correct to say that persons who identify their desire as the desire to have children more correctly desire, or would be better served by seeking, these other objects or by seeking to compensate for the failure to obtain these more generic objects in ways other than by having children. The list of reasons for desiring to have children given above (cf. the competing list below) suggests a number of other possible generic objects of desire.

Awareness of these more generic concerns (objects of desire) may suggest better alternatives for reacting to the expression of desire. Our society has fragmented and privatized family relationships and impoverished many other sorts of human affiliation. Few people would recognize intrinsic value in political activity, and even neighborhood community has been devitalized by frequent changes in residence, ease of transportation, and the elevated status of private pursuits. Opportunities for significant interaction with children have been reduced almost entirely to those within the nuclear family. Technology has distanced us from many life processes, including birth, death, and sickness, thus affording us less opportunity to be present, participate, serve, and be served. Given this impoverishment and privatization of forms of human affiliation and our removal from life processes, it is not surprising that we should seize more exclusively on having our own children as the most immediately available way to secure threatened values.[10] But the fact that having our own children becomes the most obvious way to secure or approximate what we ultimately desire or value does not mean that it is the best course for us as individuals or as a society. Indeed, the limited focus on having (our own) children may distort the values that we seek to preserve. Thus, it might be argued, it would be better for us to put less hope and fewer resources into esoteric ways of having children, and more into recovering and developing other ways of serving those values.

Autonomy, Authenticity, and Cooptation

So far it has been shown that the weight and object of expressed desires should sometimes be reassessed in light of the whole of a person's experiences and personality. Now I want to consider the claim that in certain cases expressed desires should not be taken at face value even if they are fully identified with by the person and integrated within the rest of the individual's personality. More specifically, I want to consider the claim that through socialization in early childhood we come to identify with values and desires that may be inauthentic and with which we should not be identified.

As a preliminary, take the case of a person who has been brainwashed, hypnotized, or otherwise "programmed" to desire, say, to eat asparagus. This person might well crave asparagus, be pained at being deprived of it, relish eating it, and reflect with satisfaction on having desired, eaten, and enjoyed it. But even though this person may be at peace in her own mind, it would be wrong to think that she is authentically expressed by this desire or that she is genuinely satisfied (though she may *feel* satisfied) by obtaining its object. It should be clear to anyone who is aware of the genesis of the desire that the person's identification with it is misconceived. Accordingly, it would be misguided of the person and of others to treat the desire as an authentic expression of the person and to take it at face value in deliberations concerning the person's well-being.

Now consider socialization. As in hypnosis, so too through socialization we acquire certain values and desires without choice or awareness. Indeed, in socialization we acquire deep values and ways of feeling that form an ultimate ground for what we later in life will, on reflection, accept and feel comfortable with. Our personalities are integrated around and in a sense defined by these early acquisitions. Yet, these values and ways of feeling, and the desires confirmed by them, may be arbitrary and potentially distorting, as they may be nothing more than products of the upbringing we happened to receive. The women's movement of the late 1960s used the term "cooptation" to characterize this sort of process, particularly in reference to women who were coopted by socialization into conventional gender roles. In this framework, then, the desire of a woman (or of a man, for that matter) to have a child, whatever the precise content of that desire, could be held to be more an expression of the norms of their society than an authentic expression of what they, themselves, are.

A problem for this position is giving a workable account of "what one is" and thereby giving sense to the claims of inauthenticity and distortion. For, unlike the case of hypnosis, in socialization, as imagined here, a person has no independent, pre-existing personality that his or her socialization could conflict with or fail to be integrated into. As the women's movement found, it was hard to convince people that women who were perfectly content in their socialized self-conceptions were somehow being untrue to themselves. So, what grounds could there be not to fully accept identification with one's socialized self? A thorough answer to this question would require much more space than can be given here (and would take us to the heart of relativism). But I hope a few brief remarks may make plausible the idea and relevance of cooptation through socialization.

I have little to say here about an appeal that might be made to the idea of autonomy. For that attempt to provide a ground from which to criticize a person's socialized identifications seems to me to rely on a dubious notion of unconditioned choice (by an "empty self" conceived as devoid of any acquired dispositions) and to render *all* socialization—even that which I would not take to be distorting—to be unacceptable.[11] Rather, I would appeal to the existence of certain *objective* human goods or human capacities essential for well-being.[12] On an objectivist view, socialized values and desires are cooptive if they conflict with these objective conditions.[13]

Objectivism is not without its problems,[14] but it may be supplemented by a sort of criticism that is at least intersubjective. For we have the capacity to become aware of and to reflect on the processes of socialization, and to do this informed by an understanding of a wide diversity of basic values. Our grasp need not be only intellectual or cognitive, but may include the type of understanding that comes through experience and imagination, as for example through travel, literature, and art. With recognition of how socialization works and with some appreciation of alternatives to the values to which we have been socialized, we can gain critical perspective on our own socialization and values, and so be able, at least to some extent, to accept, reject, and reform the results of that socialization and to form intersubjective conceptions of the good.[15] Desires, then, that conflict with these conceptions can be said to be inauthentic, distorting of persons, and should be regarded accordingly in deliberations about well-being.

In prudential reasoning we should, other things being equal, be circumspect about our unexamined desires, even when they are deep and abiding—and especially so in areas in which we have been alerted to serious bias by critiques of our culture regarding class, gender, age, species, and so on. Sympathetic others should not take uncritical desires at full value if there is reason to wonder whether the person would or should substantially reform those desires in light of critical examination, particularly when those desires are in competition with other desires of that person or of other persons. The same things might be said in regard to decisions of public policy, except that, at least in liberal political theory, persons have prima facie, though rebuttable, priority in defining their own interests. But that still does not mean that political processes must take all desires at face value. In the end, even our deepest personal and cultural values must be able to stand up to critical examination to have claim to full weight against other values and interests.

Reasons for Desiring to Have Children: A Competing List

Critics of contemporary society reflect with skepticism on many of the sorts of reasons listed in the second section for desiring to have children. Marxists, especially, claim to have discovered motives for having children that are less admirable, in that those motives lead to conceiving of and treating children as economic commodities in a capitalistic framework. One particularly succinct attack on the desire to have children in a capitalist society, by Robert Cooperstein,[16] charges that present attitudes toward having children are largely a form of enhancing one's economic and social capital. Among Cooperstein's charges are these: (1) Children are a vehicle of status and conspicuous consumption: the child's cuteness, spontaneity, and vitality are conferred upon the parents. (2) Children are used as compensatory substitutes: parents lacking value in their own lives seek to find value in the life of another. Having children is not then an overflowing of value but an attempt to gain value vicariously. (3) Children are a justification for self-abnegation, not so much in outpouring to another as in justification for self-denial borne of self-loathing, a justification for abandoning hope in oneself. (4) People have children merely to fit in. (5) Children are a source of consumable entertainment, like TV. (6) Children are a buttress to a weak and otherwise purposeless marital relationship and function as a shared possession. (7) Children are objects of love who cannot reject that love. (8) Children provide an excuse for greater accumulation of and absorption in possessions and power; they make possible a false sense of continued possession through inheritance, which distorts the activity of giving. (9) Children provide a vicarious and illusory sense of immortality.

In a similar vein, Germaine Greer[17] claims that in the West, rhetoric notwithstanding, children are not in fact valued for themselves, but in practice regarded as assets. This underlying valuation is in part shown, she maintains, by the fact that childbirth has been made a technological enterprise in economically advanced Western nations.

I do not offer this brief digression as a definitive critique of the desire to have children. I merely hope to bring to mind an alternative to the reigning sentiments. Having children may be a great and legitimate good, but it is a good that is easily misconceived and perverted.

Living Well without Having Children

In speaking of the value of having children, it should also be recognized that many people have lived fulfilled lives without having children and that many people are childless by choice. It may be charged, of course, that couples without children really want(ed) children or that, though they don't realize it, something essential to well-being is missing from their lives. But the fact is that a significant number of couples in fact do *not* want to have children,[18] and the charge that individuals and couples cannot be happy and fulfilled without having children seems to be more the expression of an ideology than a conclusion from sound evidence. It may be true, especially in our social conditions, that not having children cuts one off from certain significant goods, but it is also clear that having children does so as well. At bottom, it must be admitted that many individuals have found great fulfillment in the activities and relationships they are able to pursue free from the responsibilities of having children.

Couples who are childless by choice may be charged with selfishness. This may be an odd criticism in the context of trying to argue for the poverty of a life without children, since one way of taking the charge presupposes that living without children is in fact *more* personally rewarding. Otherwise, how could these couples be selfish?[19] Further, it should be noted that reasons for not having children needn't be narrowly self-serving, and may include thinking it unfair to a child to bring it into a world such as ours or thinking that one would not be a good parent. Indeed, one might return to the Marxist critique to charge that the selfishness is on the other side—that it is arrogant and narcissistic to seek to perpetuate or aggrandize oneself through the person of an unconsenting child.

Adoption

Many people faced with reproductive problems consider adoption. And adoption has resulted in extremely fulfilling relationships and lives for many couples and children. Quite a few of the reasons for desiring to have children can be satisfied through adoption.

But for most people, adoption is a second choice. Part of the reason for this is the unknowns of adoption—the child's parentage and its experiences prior to adoption. Another part is that with adopted children one cannot expect to find genetically based affinities of temperament, interest, or understanding, nor a genetically based physical resemblance to the parents who raise them.[20] Finally, an adopted child, it is generally felt, is just not, in the fullest sense, one's *own;* one is not a *real* parent of the child.

With the emergence of RTs, adoption is becoming for many, indeed, a third choice. For RTs such as artificial insemination, egg donorship, and parenting through contract make it possible for infertile people to avoid some or all of the supposed drawbacks of adoption. In particular, RTs hold out the possibility of having one's *own* child, being a *real* parent of the child (or at least of one partner standing in these relations), where this would otherwise not be possible. And having one's *own* child to love, raise, and care for is what most people most want.

This idea of "having one's own child" or "being a real parent," in a sense that contrasts with adoption, is thus a central concept in much thinking about having children and the use of RTs. We may assume that we understand what we mean by these terms, but as the next section seeks to show, we may not be so clear about either what we mean or why this relation to a child should be so significant to us.

Having One's Own Child: Genetic Puzzles and Stork Stories

We have been examining the desire to have children: What could warrant the desire? How should the desire be taken? We have recognized that there are good reasons for desiring to have children and that there are extremely strong attachments between parents and their children. But in some respects, we have been pretty much taking for granted that we understand what it means to have a child and to have one's own child.

As observed above, a number of different senses of "having (one's own) child" (and being a parent) would be readily acknowledged: having (legal) custody and responsibility for a child, being actively engaged in raising a child and in its life, having begotten a child, having carried a child in pregnancy and given birth to it, and so on. But primary in most people's thinking is the so-called biological relation. For practical purposes, the idea of the biological relation, and so of having one's own child, has been until recently quite unproblematic. A woman and man stand in the biological relation to a child if they have played their respective roles in the acts and processes of natural reproduction: intercourse, fertilization, gestation, parturition. With the advance of scientific knowledge, however, we have come to fix on the transmission of genes as the essence of these processes. Development and use of RTs has further brought us to recognize that the biological relation as we have conceived it is a composite of actions and processes that can be separated and certain of the separate parts either bypassed or performed in different ways and by different persons. As a result, we have become somewhat confused about how to use the term "biological relation" and whom to regard as a child's "real" parents. These confusions are exemplified in disputes over parentage in artificial insemination, embryo transfer, parenting through contract, and other RTs. In seeking to resolve our confusions, it seems to me that we have, under the impression of being scientific, come to regard the biological relation as consisting ultimately and most precisely in the "gene relation":[21] to have one's own child and to be a real parent, with all the significance we attach to these relations, is most fundamentally for the child to "have one's genes." And we feel that science can provide whatever explication we need of the concept of "gene relation" or "having one's genes."

But I am not so sure. My reservation is not about the truth of the science of genetics in this context. Rather, I am not so convinced that we know how to make best use of our knowledge of genetics when we consider the meaning and significance of having children. In the following "Genetic Puzzles and Stork Stories," I raise a number of questions and offer conjectures about how we might want to explicate our concepts and regard their significance. I must acknowledge from the start, however, that more questions are raised than answered. Indeed, there is no assurance that the concepts we are trying to explicate are ultimately coherent.

Genetic Puzzles and Stork Stories

How do we, how should we, understand our concepts of having one's own child, being a real parent, the gene relation, and a child's having one's genes? What significance do and should they have?[22]

1. Suppose that, walking down the street, you were to discover that a baby in a stroller happened by chance to have exactly the same genetic makeup as you. Would this make the child yours or you its parent? Would discovery of this identity of genes necessarily or naturally engender in you deep affection for the child and concern for its well-being? True, the baby might closely resemble you physically and psychologically. You might very well be fascinated (and frightened) at the prospect of observing and learning about the child. But merely happening to have the same pattern of genes surely is not enough to constitute having one's own child. Identical twins are not each other's child.

2. What is missing? Is it that one's child's genes do not only resemble one's own, but also are *derived* from them? Well, in what sense "derived"? Suppose that a mad geneticist had found a map of your genes and used that map as a model in creating your gene double in the stroller. The pattern of the child's genes now is both identical to and derived from yours. Does this make the child your own? Would this, should this, change the significance of the child to you?

There may be some temptation here to say yes. But exactly how is the child to be attached conceptually *to you*? If the name on the gene map were different—it turns out to have been your identical twin's name after all—then is the child now your twin's? If there is some controversy about the name at the top of the map, is the child's parentage in doubt? Are the true relations of this child to be worked out by deciding whose name was first listed, erased, corrected, or replaced at the head of the map? If not only your name, but also the names of six other people, several long dead, who happened to have had the same pattern of genes as you were listed, would all of you be the child's parents? Isn't this just not the sort of connection (derivation) we are looking for, even if yours is the only name on the map?

3. What if the mad geneticist, whatever the complications of the names on the map, *intended your* genes as the model? Would this make the connection with you less accidental? In working toward an answer, first recognize that mere intention, apart from any gene relation, does not make a child yours in the relevant sense:

(a) One day the stork flies over your house and drops a baby. Are you this child's parent? Is the child yours in the relevant sense? Did the stork get the right house? Is it your spouse's baby too? Even if a tag tied to the baby's toe indicates the intended recipients, being a recipient is not the same as being a parent. At bottom, is this case different from adopting a child who is intended *for* you?

(b) Add that the intentions involved are yours—you instigate and intend the process. You submit your order, and nine months later the stork makes a delivery. Your child? Well, you might be responsible for the child; you might willingly and happily accept it. But, again, is your relation to the child any different than if you had prearranged an adoption before conception?

(c) Now consider cases in which intentions are combined with a gene relation. The mad geneticist (call her MG), without your knowledge, creates a child by patterning its genes on yours—intending your genes, as distinguished from anyone else's genes that might be identical to yours, as the model. This child begins to seem like "another you." But is this the gene relation of parent and child? Why not regard MG's creation as your sibling or your "double" (a new category of relation[23])? This person's genes may be patterned on yours, but it seems that *one's child* derives from one through more than this external relation of intention and pattern. If MG used Cleopatra's gene pattern, why call the result *Cleopatra's* or Cleopatra's *child*? What sense could there be to distinguishing generations (children from grandchildren) in successive pattern-ings by MG?

(d) Finally, consider the case in which *you* instigate and intend MG's patterning of the child's genes on your (distinctive) genes. Your child? It may seem so. But the reasoning in the preceding scenarios should give pause. Why "your child" rather than "your sibling" or "your double"? The person may be due to you—you are responsible for its existence, its genes are patterned on yours, you may be accountable for its well-being—but it is still a different sort of deriving from you than we should regard as having one's own child. Perhaps the next scenario can help support this conclusion.

4. Add that you are MG—that you not only provide the pattern, insti-gate, and intend, but also that *you* perform the operations that bring the child into existence.[24] In this case you might be expected to take special interest in the child as a product of your art and skill. But this kind of making still doesn't seem to constitute having one's own child in the sense we are looking for. In the first cases, our initial temptation was not to say that it was the mad geneticist who is the real parent of your gene double. Nor are we tempted to say that Drs. Edwards and Steptoe are, except metaphorically, parents of Louise Brown.[25] This form of making children (construction, assembly, set-ting external processes in motion) does not seem to be what we have in mind

in having one's own children, and though one may take satisfaction in what one has produced by skill and art, this does not seem to be the significance of procreative relations.[26]

5. Can yet a closer connection be made? What if there were a *material* connection, if the genes came from your body? Then the baby could derive from you in matter as well as in form. Consider a number of variations[27]: (a) The raw materials making up the baby's genes come from materials taken from your body, broken down into their constitutive elements and reconstituted to form the genes of the double. (b) Does it matter what part of you the raw materials are taken from: sloughed-off skin cells, living tissue, chromosomes in the nuclei of non–sex cells or in sex cells? (c) Your genes were not broken down into elements and reconstituted but were taken and used whole. Why does this last variation in which the gene material maintains its physical integrity give greater pause? In the first case, one's body or genes go through a period of being "just stuff," with nothing that maintains their integrity as (part of) oneself. In either the first or the third scenario, the child is constituted by the same matter and the same form.[28] What seems to make a difference is that the form—the organizing principle that determines many of the characteristics of the child—is carried by certain material in a continuous and unified process that does not depend on an outside agency to reimpose order. A unity and continuity of form and material seems to be important in deeming the child one's own.

Further puzzles can be generated. But rather than multiply scenarios along this line of reasoning, we can with greater profit attend more closely to the facts of the genetics of reproduction.[29] First, we have been speaking of an *identity* of genes, but that is not what happens or is required in identifying one's own child in natural reproduction. The genes of a child, both in natural reproduction and to this time in RTs, are not identical to those of any one person but are, roughly, a combination of the genes of two people. More accurately, genes undergo significant modification, through crossing over in the formation of the parents' sex cells and recombination with the genes of the other parent in transmission of genes to the child. Consequently, a parent's sex cells will not be identical in their overall pattern of genes even to each other or to the corresponding parts of any other cells in the parent's body, let alone to the child's gene pattern. Further, the phenomenon of dominant and recessive genes (along with other factors) means that even though parent and child share individual genes, their expressed traits may be quite different. Let one (simplified) example, eye color, illustrate the complexities. Each person has a gene for eye color that is contributed by the person's mother and another gene for eye color that is contributed by the person's father. Suppose that for a particular individual the former codes for brown eyes, the latter for blue. Since the gene for brown eyes dominates the gene for blue, the person who has one gene of each type will express (have) the trait of brown eyes. Given these facts, we should not speak so simply of gene identity, but should take into account more complex relations of genes carried, genes expressed, and genes passed on.[30]

So, what exactly should we care about? In a sense, a child may be said to *have your genes* even though those genes are recessive and unexpressed in you and likewise in the child. In a strong sense, those recessive genes have nothing to do with what you or the child are like. So why care about this sense of shared genes? Should we then care about only shared genes that are *expressed?* Should genes be less important in our thinking and values? Should we be more concerned with actual traits, including those due more to "nurture" than to "nature," than with strings of genes?

I do not pose these as rhetorical questions; I am not convinced that gene relations are easily demoted. We still have a long way to go in clarifying and reforming our thinking. I have tried to start us on the way. In what remains of this section, I will briefly introduce one further line of thought that may supplement or contrast with the approach we have been considering so far.

Genetic Relations

In speaking of genes, we began with a purely formal relation between two static entities: the identity of the pattern of genes of two people. This approach turned out to be inadequate, and we found that, to the extent that gene relations can be made coherent, we need to appeal to dynamic relations of causation and temporal continuity of form and material. My reason for earlier reserving the term "*genetic* relation" was to be able to emphasize now that the meaning and significance of having (one's own) child essentially involves reference to the child's *genesis;* that is, reference not only to patterns of genes, but to the processes and activities through which a child comes to be. In the next few paragraphs I want to consider, briefly, one perspective on the relevance of these wider genetic relations for the meaning and significance of having a child.

In a sense that is sometimes overlooked, to have a child means to carry it in pregnancy and to give birth. It has been claimed by some writers that this sense should be seen as more important than any relation of genes to the meaning and significance of having (one's own) child. Thus, for example, Gena Corea asserts[31] that males are necessarily alienated from children and that they cannot recognize and experience them as fully their own, because the male role in reproduction is discontinuous with the child and is apprehended only intellectually; that is, intercourse is not experienced as continuous with the child's coming to be, and the male's connection to children must be discovered through deductions from observation of external events. In contrast, women experience a continuous relation to the child through pregnancy and giving birth. For women, the child is not an alien thing to which a connection must be forged through abstract reasoning, but is experienced and known as theirs (as "of them") by virtue of their reproductive activities. It is by going through these processes of generating the child that the most significant sort of identification with the child is formed, and mere gene relations are less significant in having one's own child than these genetic relations. In this light, the image of the stork can be seen to be a model only of the male experience of the processes of reproduction and to distort the relation in which women stand to the children they bear.

The attitude of most sperm donors in artificial insemination might support Corea's claims, at least at a psychological level. But if her claims are to be taken at this level, then they are jeopardized by the fact, recounted by Simone de Beauvoir,[32] that many women feel alienated from their pregnancies, as if they are being taken over by something external to themselves. And if, as has been argued,[33] bonding between mother and child is more significant after birth than during pregnancy, the necessary significance of the processes of genesis is further imperiled.

In a recent article,[34] Rosemarie Tong reasserts the primacy of pregnancy through the idea that gestation is a uniquely "lived commitment" to the child. Suggestive as the article is, we are unfortunately not told enough about any of the critical concepts and relations: what lived commitment is, how gestation is uniquely a lived commitment, or why having lived a commitment makes one "more of a parent" than anyone else. It remains unclear, for example, how a woman consumed by addiction to drugs and utterly uninterested in the welfare of her child could be said to have lived a commitment, though she is clearly the mother of her child. Or, to take another example mentioned earlier, Steptoe and Edwards were intimately involved with and intensely concerned for the offspring of their earliest successes with in vitro fertilization, but they are not literally parents of the offspring. And, finally, men who abandon women they impregnate surely are still parents of any resulting children and have obligations to the mothers and children in virtue of that fact.

It seems to me that Tong's arguments should be seen as targeting not what it is to *be* a parent, but what the grounds are for having a special claim to engage in parenting.[35] Indeed, Tong does speak in terms of rights to parenting, and it is a valuable contribution of her article that she moves us toward seeing many issues more in terms of what establishes rights to engage in the activity of parenting than in terms of what makes a person a parent or of who is "more" the parent. The most direct bearing of Tong's article on the argument I have been making, then, is that not only is the concept of what it is to be a parent and to have one's own child confused, it is in many contexts just not the relevant issue or not as relevant as is commonly thought.[36]

The genetic relation of a woman to her child, whether or not including a relation of gene patterns, may provide the *potential* for greater attachment and identification, but that potential need not be actualized. The *essential* significance of genetic relations may be somewhat in doubt, as is the essential significance of the relations of gene patterns. What we desire, what we should desire, and what we should best pursue as individuals, sympathetic third parties, and societies may be less dependent on "natural" relations than we seem normally to suppose. The science of genetics certainly does not provide full answers to the questions we have been asking, and the mere facts of the processes of genesis may not advance us much further.

Final Remarks

Having (one's own) children, in its many senses, is undeniably a fulfilling experience for most people. In the present state of our consciousness and culture, prudential, moral, and public policy decisions should all respect this important good. But the good of having (one's own) children should not be blindly indulged in any of these spheres of evaluation. We have seen how we are prone to misconceiving the nature and proper place of the desire for children, especially when we are confronted with obstacles to our will. And we have seen that exactly what it is we desire is not ultimately so clear.

Individuals can be more reflective. Well before coming face to face with the trauma of infertility, people can realize the value of a variety of creative interpersonal and intergenerational activities. We can form our lives to be less dependent on a single way of satisfying our desires for the generic goods of community, caring, and participation in the processes of life. Society, too, does better to support such broader conceptions of the good and to be less responsive to the unexamined will of individuals. Even taking the desire for children at face value, individuals as a whole may be better served by a society that focuses less on indulging the will of those suffering from infertility and more on removing conditions that cause infertility in the first place. Clearly, everyone, children and parents, would be better served by greater social support for adoption, in policy and in attitude.

In our children we seek to get beyond our finitude, beyond our limitations in power and in time. Having children is *one* way in which we seek to transcend ourselves. This may be a legitimate and healthy endeavor. But as individuals and as a society, we have impoverished both our conception of transcendence and our opportunities for it in creative, communal, intergenerational activities.[37] As we narrow our options, in conception and practice, and as we tighten our grip on the few remaining options we continue to recognize, we distort ourselves and the society that could support more humane attitudes and more fulfilled lives.

Appendix: Real Cases—Testicle and Ovary Transplantation

Several of the puzzles raised in fanciful ways in the fourth section have arisen in actual cases (or in close variations to those cases). Tim Twomey was born without testicles. In his thirties, he received a testicle transplant from his identical twin brother, and within several years fathered three children.[38] He is regarded as the real father of these children. However we think the term "real" should be used, what significance should be accorded to the relationship between Tim Twomey and these children? Would it be different if, say, his brother had served as a sperm donor for Tim and his wife, or if the brother had, by agreement, fathered a child for them through intercourse with Tim's wife? What differences in significance would there be if the brother were not an identical twin or if the testicle donor were totally unrelated?

Similarly, an ovary transplant between identical twins, and subsequent pregnancy, has been reported. How in this sort of case, and in imaginable variants, should the resulting relations between parents and children be understood and valued? What difference should it make if the ovary is just about to ovulate when it is transplanted? Who should be regarded as the mother—or rather, what should be the significance of the location of ovulation and conception? Should it matter whether fertilization takes place in the donor's body, in the recipient's body, or in a petri dish? What if only an egg were transferred between the identical twins? Does carrying the child through pregnancy make a difference? Further variations take only a moment's thought.

Notes

I would like to thank Ronald McLaren for very helpful comments on drafts of this essay.

1. Among other motives of interested parties, such as doctors, scientists, lawyers, and businesspeople, are the desire to help persons in distress, the pursuit of knowledge, the desire to exercise abilities to the fullest, and the desires for fame, profit, and power (control over nature and over people).

2. Among the affluent, who are the most avid users of RTs, attempts to have children tend to be postponed until later in life, when problems of infertility are greater. Then years may be spent in escalating attempts to overcome the problems before adoption and the more exotic RTs are seriously considered. By that time, the couple may be fairly old for adopting and, in the common case of white couples seeking healthy white babies, the wait may be as much as three to seven years for agency adoption, if that is even possible. Adoption of babies of color or nonhealthy or older children is considerably less difficult, as is international adoption (almost exclusively from economically less developed nations), though some of these nations are considering more restrictive policies.

3. For example, on the so-called maternal instinct and differences between women and men in their attachment to children, see Caroline Whitbeck, "The Maternal Instinct," *The Philosophical Forum* 6 (1974–1975), pp. 265–273; reprinted with afterword in Joyce Trebilcot, ed., *Mothering: Essays in Feminist Theory* (Totowa, NJ: Rowman & Allanheld, 1983), pp. 185–198.

4. A central argument of Simone de Beauvoir's classic *The Second Sex* (New York: Vintage Books, 1974; first published 1952) is that though women are physiologically constituted for the production of children, this fact does not determine what women can or should do with their lives, either morally or prudentially.

5. See, for example, Jean E. Veevers, *Childless by Choice* (Toronto: Butterworth, 1980).

6. This claim about biological drives is distinct from the claim that there is a moral obligation to reproduce or to continue the species—say, out of gratitude for one's own existence or from identification with others of one's kind.

7. See also the further reasons listed in the third section on p. 157.

8. The "Caution, Baby on Board" signs recently adorning many automobiles are clearly intended at least as much to advertise the possession of an object that confers status as to protect the child.

9. Space does not allow an examination here of the differences among substitution, replacement, compensation, and so on. For suggestive remarks, see Robert C. Solomon, "Is There Happiness After Death?" *Philosophy* 51 (1976), pp. 189–193. As brief illustrations of some of the distinctions, consider that a desire for a glass of milk may at times be just one way to satisfy the more generic desire to quench one's thirst; drinking orange juice or water might do just as well. A desire to go to loud parties may sometimes be better understood as a desire for friendly association that partygoing simulates. And a desire expressing itself in an eating binge may at times be best understood as compensation for having been wounded in love.

10. Our success even in this reduced area of activity should be seriously questioned, if figures are to be believed about the amount of time people spend away from home, watching television, and in meaningful interaction. A recent study by Fortino and Associates of New York City reported the average amount of time spent in meaningful conversation between spouses to be 4 minutes per day, and between parents and children to be 30 seconds. For a study of forms of community in America, see Robert Bellah et al., *Habits of the Heart* (New York: Harper & Row, 1985).

11. A view similar to the one I have in mind is articulated and criticized in Frithjof Bergmann, *On Being Free* (Notre Dame, IN: University of Notre Dame Press, 1977), especially chapters 1–3.

12. Aristotle's *Nicomachean Ethics* is perhaps the most celebrated account of an objective human good. Bernard Williams, *Ethics and the Limits of Philosophy* (Cambridge, MA: Harvard University Press, 1985), chapter 3, especially pages 40–44, suggests a modified objectivism in terms of human capacities. One need not accept the conclusions of either to appreciate the objectivist approach.

13. I speak of "conflict" for simplicity. A more detailed analysis would distinguish different sorts of conflict (e.g., the desire's undermining the conditions or replacing them with something inferior) and would be sensitive to other sorts of relations (e.g., the desire's being in tension with the conditions, failing to support them, or resisting integration into them). Different relations of desire and objective conditions would stipulate different levels of regard for the desire in deliberations about a person's well-being.

14. For example, how objective conditions can be established, whether they are general for humans as such or more specific (e.g., for females, for males), how much of well-being they specify, and why fidelity to what one objectively is should matter.

15. Which is not to say that all our endeavors, as individuals or as cultures, necessarily converge or resolve all problems. See, for example, Alasdair MacIntyre, *After Virtue* (Notre Dame, IN: University of Notre Dame Press, 1981).

16. *Notes on the Reproduction of Human Capital* (n.p., 1974), available from the main library of the University of California at Berkeley.

17. *Sex and Destiny* (New York: Harper & Row, 1984), especially chapter 1.

18. See, for example, Veevers, *Childless by Choice*. The attitude of such individuals is often expressed in the preferred term "child-*free*."

19. As pointed out to me by Ulf Nilsson, another way of lodging the criticism does hit the mark. A couple may be charged with selfishness not only because they maintain certain goods for themselves (e.g., money, travel), but because they fail to extend themselves into other goods (such as nurturing or community). A couple could be charged with selfishness in this latter sense without implying that their childless life was

more satisfying. Of course, as the rest of the paragraph in the text suggests, there may be good reasons for withholding from these other goods, and a couple childless for such reasons could be defended against the charge of selfishness.

20. On the other hand, it is still disputed just how much temperament, appearance, gestures, and so on are matters of nature (genes) and how much they are matters of nurture.

21. The more usual term is "genetic relation," but I prefer to speak of "gene relation" in order to mark a distinction that will be introduced below.

22. One way to approach the following cases is through Aristotle's famous "Doctrine of the Four Causes." In Aristotle's terms, a child's characteristics and the relation of child and parent can be analyzed in terms of the material that constitutes the child, the form (structure, organization) of the child, the causes (movements, events, actions) through which the child comes to be, and the purposes (of agents) or ends (of natural processes) that determine the child's coming to be (the so-called final cause). Aristotle's own exposition of the "causes" appears in his *Physics* (Book 2, chapters 3 and 7). The puzzles begin by addressing the significance of purely formal relations. Later puzzles consider the importance of one or more further relations of purpose, cause, material, or end.

Some of these puzzles push the notion of "having one's own children" fairly far. But, as the appendix at the end of this essay suggests, the fanciful puzzles may not be that far removed from actual events.

23. If we do adopt this new category of relation, why regard our "doubles" with parental affection and care?

24. Though I do not think it matters to the present cases, it should perhaps be pointed out that a person's causal role in this, as in any, causal process, may be greater or lesser, more active or more passive, from merely setting in motion a series of processes (as in popping coins into a soda machine), to choosing, directing, designing, and carrying out more and more of the process. No matter how minute one's involvement, though, one is always dependent at some level on natural causal connections (e.g., that certain substances have certain properties, that gravity works).

25. An Ontario judge's decision in an early artificial insemination case that the physician was the father of the child didn't stand long: *Orford v. Orford*, 49 Ont. L.R. 15, 58 D.L.R. 251 (1921). Among other things, the possibility of having a woman physician seemed to point to the absurdity of the decision.

26. Contrast Aristotle's views on the relation of production and reproduction in *Nicomachean Ethics*, Book 8, chapter 12 and Book 9, chapter 7. [These and other relevant passages are included above in this anthology.]

27. Given the conclusions of the preceding puzzle, it does not seem to me to matter who we imagine to be doing the constructing.

28. Compare the similar puzzles in Derek Parfit's examination of personal identity in connection with teletransportation in Part Three of his *Reasons and Persons* (Oxford: Oxford University Press, 1984).

29. This brief account will necessarily be oversimplified, but the key points can still be made validly.

30. We should also realize that the widest variation in genes between any two humans is on the order of only 0.1 to 0.01%.

31. *The Mother Machine* (New York: Harper & Row, 1985). [See excerpts below in this anthology.]

32. *The Second Sex*, chapter XVII: "Motherhood." [See excerpts above in this anthology.]

33. Whitbeck, "The Maternal Instinct."

34. "The Overdue Death of a Feminist Chameleon: Taking a Stand on Surrogacy Arrangements," *Journal of Social Philosophy,* 21 (1990), pp. 40–56. [Reprinted below in this anthology.]

35. That is, to have a claim to special access to the child, to nurture the child, to form reciprocal relations with it, and to have in general a wide range of opportunities, rights, and responsibilities regarding it.

36. More accurately, I think that as with my treatment of "real desire" above, so with the concept of "parent," once we identify the many and often conflicting criteria for applying the term, we should not attempt to resolve the conflicts in some arbitrary choice about how to use the term, but we should abandon the term and attend to the more concrete relations into which it has been splintered.

37. To offer just two examples, extended families and kibbutzim offer, as private families do not, rewarding relationships with children and involvement in life processes for adults who do not have "their own" children.

38. It should be mentioned that the operation was in no way frivolous and that Mr. Twomey's goal was not to have children. Before the operation, he suffered physical, emotional, and behavioral problems because of lack of testosterone production and had endured surgery and continuing drug treatment.

IV

MAKING AND SELLING BABIES: PRODUCTION AND COMMERCE

The readings in Part II introduced charges that reproductive technology degrades our lives by transforming intimate personal relationships into alienated commercial exchanges and procreation into production: babies are sold, pregnancy becomes a service comparable to prostitution, the loving union of husband and wife becomes a laboratory technique, and reproductive materials, embryos, and even children are turned into mere objects. (See the articles by Krimmel and Kass and the Vatican statement above.) Responses to these charges include arguments that participants in reproductive technology act voluntarily, that they get what they want (children whom they love, emotional and financial rewards), that we have already accepted and lived well with analogous changes in other parts of our lives, and that any detrimental effects do not affect the society at large. (See the articles by Robertson, Edwards, and Gorovitz, as well as those by Andrews and Keane.)[1] The readings in this part examine more deeply the significance of carrying out human reproduction within commercial and technological frameworks of meaning and value.[2] Though these readings do draw specific conclusions for practice, they have been chosen primarily because they address the underlying conceptual issues: What does it mean to commercialize or to objectify a person or activity? How do these things come about, and what precisely is objectionable about them?

The first article, "Market-Inalienability," selected from law professor Margaret Jane Radin's long and rewarding article of the same name, argues that proper conceptions of human personhood and human flourishing (what it is to live a good and rewarding life) cannot be secured if certain aspects of life are regarded as subject to economic activities and values. After a brief preface to the article, its three sections offer, respectively, an account of the role of rhetoric in determining what a thing is, a theoretical justification for limiting commodification, and applications of the theory to prostitution, baby selling, and parenting through contract.[3] Overall, Radin's article can be seen as setting out key elements of a theory of commodification—of what it is to be a commodity, how economic relations make something into a commodity, the significance of regarding something as a commodity, and the justification for limiting commodification.

One defense of economic activity is that at most it affects only those who are engaged in the activities themselves: reproductive technology affects only the individuals voluntarily engaged in them. Radin's account of rhetoric is essential to responding to this defense. She contends that not only do economic *activities* (being monetarily priced, bought and sold, etc.) have a role in determining what a thing is and can do, but so too do the ways these things are *thought* about and *spoken* about. If this is true, then it can be argued that the effects of economic activities and values extend beyond the few individuals actually involved in the economic transaction. Taking one of Radin's examples, if a child can be traded for a Chevy, if such transactions are recognized and allowed in society, then not only is the particular child affected, but children in general may be conceived of more in terms of market values— thereby, it is claimed, distorting and limiting their potential for personhood and self-realization. If this argument is correct, then even limited commercialization of reproduction in private transactions can be a legitimate concern for social and legal regulation.

In the next article, Protestant theologian Oliver O'Donovan examines one aspect of bringing human procreation within human control. Drawing on theological insights, O'Donovan sketches an account of what distinguishes procreation from production (making), how reproductive technology threatens to transform procreation into production, and why that transformation, both of activities and of our ways of conceiving of them, should be resisted. The heart of O'Donovan's argument is that procreation transmits being and thereby makes the parents one with the resulting child, while production, in contrast, is an act of will and control that, though it may result in a valuable product, does not embody one's self. If all activities are conceived as production, we may expand the realm of our will, but we lose the fullness of our being; we diminish our selves.

The distinctions and relations O'Donovan seeks to draw, if they can be made, are of the utmost importance. If production—that is, activities of the will involving control, design (forming, foreseeing, selecting, and directing processes and outcomes), and power (action, efficient causation)—secures only one kind of value and is just one kind of creativity, namely, the realization of our will in objects external to us, while procreation involves a unique transmission of our being, then we have strong reason to resist techniques that threaten to reduce procreation to production. The most difficult task for O'Donovan's view, as a rationally articulated position, is to render intelligible what it means for being to be transmitted and how procreation, unlike production, can accomplish that end. If we must rely on faith for such understanding, then the account and its conclusions will be unconvincing to nonbelievers and will be of dubious authority in policy decisions.

O'Donovan's position may be compared with claims made in a number of other selections. Aristotle, for example, appears to accept production as a model for procreation; de Beauvoir appears to regret the apparent passivity of women in the biological processes of procreation; and Tong argues that gestation is an active process. O'Donovan, in contrast, contends that there is value in the passivity of humans in procreation and in procreation's remaining outside the realm of human will and control. To some extent, O'Donovan's conclusion, though not his theological arguments for it, resembles the position of feminist Gena Corea (see below), who holds that technological intrusion into the biological processes of reproduction destroys the continuity of experience crucial to the mother's identification with her offspring.[4]

Notes

1. For a more extensive defense of commercialization, see Elisabeth M. Landes and Richard Posner, "The Economics of the Baby Shortage," *Journal of Legal Studies* 7 (1978), pp. 323–348 and Gary Becker, *A Treatise on the Family* (Cambridge, MA: Harvard University Press, 1981); for criticism, see J. Robert S. Prichard, "A Market for Babies?" *University of Toronto Law Journal* 34 (1984), pp. 341–357, and Elizabeth S. Anderson, "Is Women's Labor a Commodity?," *Philosophy and Public Affairs* 19 (1990), pp. 71–92, as well as the complete text of the original article by Margaret Jane Radin excerpted in this part, "Market-Inalienability," *Harvard Law Review* 100 (1987), pp. 1849–1937.

2. To conceive of human reproduction within an economic framework of value is to think of it in terms of ownership, markets, supply and demand, pricing, marketing, sale, and other economic activities. To conceive of it within a technological framework of value is to think of it in terms of such things as power, control, efficiency, quality, and outcome.

3. Parts of the original article not included in this anthology offer a more complete and qualified analysis, including extensive criticism of competing conceptions of commodification.

4. For further discussion, see Alison M. Jaggar and William L. McBride, " 'Reproduction' as Male Ideology," *Hypatia—Woman's Studies International Forum* 8 (1985), pp. 185–196, where it is argued that there is "no adequate rationale for insisting on a theoretical distinction between the production of things and the production of people."

Market-Inalienability

Margaret Jane Radin

Editor's Note and Summary

The selection from Professor Radin's article begins after the following brief summary of key points and terminology from parts of the article not included below.

Among Professor Radin's aims in the complete article are to clarify what it is for something to be a commodity and to present reasons for refusing to treat something as a commodity (i.e., for refusing to commodify it). The heart of her argument is the claim that a proper conception of human personhood and flourishing cannot be secured if certain aspects of life are regarded as in principle subject to being priced, bought, and sold.

Terminology

A thing is "market-inalienable," as Radin uses the term, if it "is not to be sold, which in our economic system means it is not to be traded in the market." A nonsalable item may still be transferred in other ways, such as by gift. Indeed, sales may be precluded in part to encourage gifts, as is the case with human organs or, in some countries, human blood. The term "commodification," most broadly construed, includes not only actual buying and selling of something (commodification in the narrow sense), but also regarding the thing in terms of market rhetoric, "the practice of thinking about interactions as if they were sale transactions," and applying market methodology to it. Commodification thus includes owning, pricing, selling, and evaluating interactions in terms of monetary cost-benefit analysis or regarding these activities as appropriate. Professor Radin also distinguishes two types of property: personal and fungible. Property is personal "when it has become identified with a person, with her self-constitution and self-development in the context of her environment. Personal property cannot be taken away and replaced with money or other things without harm to the person." "Property is fungible when there is no such personal attachment. Thus, fungible objects are commodified: trading them is like trading money."

From *Harvard Law Review* 100 (1987), pp. 1849–1937. Abridged. Copyright © 1987 by the Harvard Law Review Association. Reprinted by permission of the publisher and author.

Positions and Arguments

Universal commodifiers hold "that anything some people are willing to sell and others are willing to buy in principle can and should be the subject of free market [laissez-faire] exchange" and that everything people need or desire is to be conceived of as a commodity. Thus, "everything that is desired or valued is an object that can be possessed, that can be thought of as equivalent to a sum of money, and that can be alienated. The person is conceived of and spoken of as the possessor and trader of these goods, and hence all human interactions are sales." Though universal commodification is a caricature, certain economic analysts, such as Richard Posner, come close. Among the attractions of universal commodification are claimed to be the freedom it allows individuals to trade and its absence of paternalism.

In criticism of universal commodification, universal non-commodifiers hold that commodification brings about an inferior form of life. Karl Marx, in particular, argues that economic alienation (separating something from oneself as a piece of property) expresses and creates human alienation (estrangement from one's self). A problem for universal noncommodification, indeed for any theory that seeks to change the status quo, is the transition problem: how, with justice, can society be transformed from its current degree of commodification to the more desirable degree of commodification?

Market pluralisms are a range of intermediate positions holding that a limited realm of commodification ought to be allowed to coexist with one or more nonmarket realms. The burden of market pluralists is to justify distinctions between things that should and things that shouldn't be commodified. As a market pluralist, Radin sketches an attempt to solve this problem.

Though Radin rejects universal noncommodification, she takes several of its key insights as grounds for limiting universal commodification. These insights include recognition of the importance of rhetoric—our discourse, how we think and talk about a thing—to what the thing is for us; and recognition of the ways in which commodification, both in practice and in rhetoric, forms the sort of life we can lead. Radin recognizes the attractions of universal commodification, among which are the apparent freedom and absence of paternalism it allows to each individual in choosing whether or not to buy or sell a thing. Against this, Radin contends that if we reject the notion that freedom means negative liberty, that is, doing whatever one prefers to do as long as it doesn't harm others, and "adopt a positive view of liberty that includes proper self-development as necessary for freedom, then inalienabilities needed to foster that development will be seen as freedom-enhancing, rather than as impositions of unwanted restraint on our desires to transact in markets."

I. Rhetoric and Reality

"The word is not the thing," we were taught, when I was growing up. Rhetoric is not reality; discourse is not the world. Why should it matter if someone conceptualizes the entire human universe as one giant bundle of scarce goods subject to free alienation by contract, especially if reasoning in market rhetoric can reach the same result that some other kind of normative reasoning reaches on other grounds? . . .

. . . Recall that Posner conceives of rape in terms of a marriage and sex market. Posner concludes that "the prevention of rape is essential to protect the marriage market . . . and more generally to secure property rights in women's persons." . . .[1] Bodily integrity is an owned object with a price.

What is wrong with this rhetoric? [A] risk-of-error argument . . . is one answer. Unsophisticated practitioners of cost-benefit analysis might tend to undervalue the "costs" of rape to the victims. But this answer does not exhaust the problem. Rather, for all but the deepest enthusiast, market rhetoric seems intuitively out of place here, so inappropriate that it is either silly or somehow insulting to the value being discussed.

One basis for this intuition is that market rhetoric conceives of bodily integrity as a fungible object.[2] A fungible object is replaceable with money or other objects; in fact, possessing a fungible object is the same as possessing money. A fungible object can pass in and out of the person's possession without effect on the person as long as its market equivalent is given in exchange. To speak of personal attributes as fungible objects—alienable "goods"—is intuitively wrong. Thinking of rape in market rhetoric implicitly conceives of as fungible something that we know to be personal, in fact conceives of as fungible property something we know to be too personal even to be personal property.[3] Bodily integrity is an attribute and not an object. We feel discomfort or even insult, and we fear degradation or even loss of the value involved, when bodily integrity is conceived of as a fungible object.

Systematically conceiving of personal attributes as fungible objects is threatening to personhood, because it detaches from the person that which is integral to the person. Such a conception makes actual loss of the attribute easier to countenance. For someone who conceives bodily integrity as "detached," the same person will remain even if bodily integrity is lost; but if bodily integrity cannot be detached, the person cannot remain the same after loss.[4] Moreover, if my bodily integrity is an integral personal attribute, not a detachable object, then hypothetically valuing my bodily integrity in money is not far removed from valuing *me* in money. For all but the universal commodifier, that is inappropriate treatment of a person.

. . . The difference between conceiving of bodily integrity as a detached, monetizable object and finding that it is "in fact" detached is not great, because there is no bright line separating words and facts. The modern philosophical turn toward coherence or antifoundationalist theories[5] means that we cannot be sanguine about radically different normative discourses reaching the "same" result. Even if everybody agrees that rape should be punished criminally, the normative discourse that conceives of bodily integrity as detached and monetizable does not reach the "same" result as the normative discourse that conceives of bodily integrity as an integral personal attribute. If we accept the gist of the coherence or antifoundationalist theories, facts are not "out there" waiting to be described by a discourse. Facts are theory-dependent and value-dependent. Theories are formed in words. Fact- and value-commitments are present in the language we use to reason and describe, and they shape our reasoning and description, and the shape (for us) of reality itself.

These concerns are relevant to the conceptualization of rape as theft of a property right. A particular conception of human flourishing is advanced by this pervasive use of market rhetoric. To think in terms of costs to the victim and her sympathizers versus benefits to the rapist is implicitly to assume that raping "benefits" rapists. Only an inferior conception of human flourishing would regard rape as benefiting the rapist. . . .

[Thus,] one way to see how universal market rhetoric does violence to our conception of human flourishing is to consider its view of personhood. In our understanding of personhood we are committed to an ideal of individual uniqueness that does not cohere with the idea that each person's attributes are fungible, that they have a monetary equivalent, and that they can be traded off against those of other people. Universal market rhetoric transforms our world of concrete persons, whose uniqueness and individuality is expressed in specific personal attributes, into a world of disembodied, fungible, attribute-less entities possessing a wealth of alienable, severable "objects." This rhetoric reduces the conception of a person to an abstract, fungible unit with no individuating characteristics.

Another way to see how universal market rhetoric does violence to our conception of human flourishing is to consider its view of freedom. Market rhetoric invites us to see the person as a self-interested maximizer in all respects. Freedom or autonomy, therefore, is seen as individual control over how to maximize one's overall gains. In the extreme, the ideal of freedom is achieved through buying and selling commodified objects in order to maximize monetizable wealth. . . . Marx argued with respect to those who produce and sell commodities that this is not freedom but fetishism; what and how much is salable is not autonomously determined. Whether or not we agree with him, it is not satisfactory to think that marketing whatever one wishes defines freedom. Nor is it satisfactory to think that a theoretical license to acquire all objects one may desire defines freedom.

Market rhetoric, if adopted by everyone, and in many contexts, would indeed transform the texture of the human world. This rhetoric leads us to view politics as just rent seeking, reproductive capacity as just a scarce good for which there is high demand, and the repugnance of slavery as just a cost. To accept these views is to accept the conception of human flourishing they imply, one that is inferior to the conception we can accept as properly ours. An inferior conception of human flourishing disables us from conceptualizing the world rightly. Market rhetoric, the rhetoric of alienability of all "goods," is also the rhetoric of alienation of ourselves from what we can be as persons.

To reject the slogan, "The word is not the thing," is not to deny that there is a difference between thought and action. To say "I wish you were dead" is not to kill you. Rather, rejecting the slogan is a way of understanding that the terms in which human life is conceived matter to human life. Understanding this, we must reject universal commodification, because to see the rhetoric of the market—the rhetoric of fungibility, alienability, and cost-benefit analysis—as the sole rhetoric of human affairs is to foster an inferior conception of human flourishing. . . .

II. Toward Evolutionary Pluralism

I now wish to develop a pluralist view that differs in significant respects from liberal pluralism and negative liberty. My central hypothesis is that market-inalienability is grounded in noncommodification of things important to personhood. In an ideal world markets would not necessarily be abolished, but market-inalienability would protect all things important to personhood. But we do not live in an ideal world. In the nonideal world we do live in, market-inalienability must be judged against a background of unequal power. In that world it may sometimes be better to commodify incompletely than not to commodify at all. Market-inalienability may be ideally justified in light of an appropriate conception of human flourishing, and yet sometimes be unjustifiable because of our nonideal circumstances.

Because of the ideological heritage of the subject-object dichotomy, we tend to view things internal to the person as inalienable and things external as freely alienable. A better view of personhood, one that does not conceive of the self as pure subjectivity standing wholly separate from an environment of pure objectivity, should enable us to discard both the notion that inalienabilities relate only to things wholly subjective or internal and the notion that inalienabilities are paternalistic.

1. Rethinking Personhood: Freedom, Identity, Contextuality

In searching for such a better view, it is useful to single out three main, overlapping aspects of personhood: freedom, identity, and contextuality. The freedom aspect of personhood focuses on will, or the power to choose for oneself. In order to be autonomous individuals, we must at least be able to act for ourselves through free will in relation to the environment of things and other people. The identity aspect of personhood focuses on the integrity and continuity of the self required for individuation. In order to have a unique individual identity, we must have selves that are integrated and continuous over time. The contextuality aspect of personhood focuses on the necessity of self-constitution in relation to the environment of things and other people. In order to be differentiated human persons, unique individuals, we must have relationships with the social and natural world.

A better view of personhood—a conception of human flourishing that is superior to the one implied by universal commodification—should present more satisfactory views of personhood in each of these three aspects. I am not seeking here to elaborate a complete view of personhood. Rather, I focus primarily on a certain view of contextuality and its consequences: the view that connections between the person and her environment are integral to personhood. I also suggest that to the extent we have already accepted certain views of freedom, identity, and contextuality, we are committed to a view of personhood that rejects universal commodification.

Universal commodification conceives of freedom as negative liberty, indeed as negative liberty in a narrow sense, construing freedom as the ability to trade everything in free markets. In this view, freedom is the ability to use the will to manipulate objects in order to yield the greatest monetizable value. Although negative liberty has had difficulty with the hypothetical problem of free choice to enslave oneself, even negative liberty can reject the general notion of commodification of persons: the person cannot be an entity exercising free will for itself if it is a manipulable object of monetizable value for others.

A more positive meaning of freedom starts to emerge if one accepts the contextuality aspect of personhood. Contextuality means that physical and social contexts are integral to personal individuation, to self-development. Even under the narrowest conception of negative liberty, we would have to bring about the social environment that makes trade possible in order to become the person whose freedom consists in unfettered trades of commodified objects. Under a broader negative view that conceives of freedom as the ability to make oneself what one will, contextuality implies that self-development in accordance with one's own will requires one to will certain interactions with the physical and social context because context can be integral to self-development. The relationship between personhood and context requires a positive commitment to act so as to create and maintain particular contexts of environment and community. Recognition of the need for such a commitment turns toward a positive view of freedom, in which the self-development of the individual is linked to pursuit of proper social development, and in which proper self-development, as a requirement of personhood, could in principle sometimes take precedence over one's momentary desires or preferences.

Universal commodification undermines personal identity by conceiving of personal attributes, relationships, and philosophical and moral commitments as monetizable and alienable from self. A better view of personhood should understand many kinds of particulars—one's politics, work, religion, family, love, sexuality, friendships, altruism, experiences, wisdom, moral commitments, character, and personal attributes—as integral to the self. To understand any of these as monetizable or completely detachable from the person—to think, for example, that the value of one person's moral commitments is commensurate or fungible with those of another, or that the "same" person remains when her moral commitments are subtracted—is to do violence to our deepest understanding of what it is to be human.

To affirm that work, politics, or character is integral to the person is not to say that persons cease to be persons when they dissociate themselves from their jobs, political engagements, or personal attributes. Indeed, the ability to dissociate oneself from one's particular context seems integral to personhood. But if we must recognize the importance of the ability to detach oneself, we must recognize as well that interaction with physical and social contexts is also integral to personhood. One's surroundings—both people and things—can become part of who one is, of the self. From our understanding that attributes and things can be integral to personhood, which stems mainly from our understanding of identity and contextuality, and from our rejection of the idea of commodification of the person, which stems mainly from our understanding of freedom, it follows that those attributes and things identified with the person cannot be treated as completely commodified. Hence, market-inalienability may attach to things that are personal.

2. Protecting Personhood: Noncommodification of Personal Rights, Attributes, and Things

In my discussion of possible sources of dissatisfaction with thinking of rape in market terms, I suggested that we should not view personal things as fungible commodities. We are now in a better position to understand how conceiving of personal things as commodities does violence to personhood, and to explore the problem of knowing what things are personal.

To conceive of something personal as fungible assumes that the person and the attribute, right, or thing, are separate. This view imposes the subject-object dichotomy to create two kinds of alienation. If the discourse of fungibility is partially made one's own, it creates disorientation of the self that experiences the distortion of its own personhood. For example, workers who internalize market rhetoric conceive of their own labor as a commodity separate from themselves as persons; they dissociate their daily life from their own self-conception. To the extent the discourse is not internalized, it creates alienation between those who use the discourse and those whose personhood they wrong in doing so. For example, workers who do not conceive of their labor as a commodity are alienated from others who do, because, in the workers' view, people who conceive of their labor as a commodity fail to see them as whole persons.

To conceive of something personal as fungible also assumes that persons cannot freely give of themselves to others. At best they can bestow commodities. At worst—in universal commodification—the gift is conceived of as a bargain. Conceiving of gifts as bargains not only conceives of what is personal as fungible, it also endorses the picture of persons as profit-maximizers. A better view of personhood should conceive of gifts not as disguised sales, but rather as expressions of the interrelationships between the self and others. To relinquish something to someone else by gift is to give of yourself. Such a gift takes place within a personal relationship with the recipient, or else it creates one. Commodification stresses separateness both between ourselves and our things and between ourselves and other people. To postulate personal interrelationship and communion requires us to postulate people who can yield personal things to other people and not have them instantly become fungible. Seen this way, gifts diminish separateness. . . .

Not everything with which someone may subjectively identify herself should be treated legally or morally as personal.[6] Otherwise the category of personal things might collapse into "consumer surplus": anything to which someone attached high subjective value would be personal. The question whether something is personal has a normative aspect: whether identifying oneself with something —constituting oneself in connection with that thing— is justifiable. What makes identifying oneself with something justifiable, in turn, is an appropriate connection to our conception of human flourishing. More specifically, such relationships are justified if they can form part of an appropriate understanding of freedom, identity, and contextuality. A proper understanding of contextuality, for example, must recognize that, although personhood is fostered by relations with people and things, it is possible to be involved too much, or in the wrong way, or with the wrong things.

There is no algorithm or abstract formula to tell us which items are (justifiably) personal. A moral judgment is required in each case. To identify something as personal, it is not enough to observe that many people seem to identify with some particular kind of thing, because we may judge such identification to be bad for people. An example of a justifiable kind of relationship is people's involvement with their homes. This relationship permits self-constitution within a stable environment. An example of an unjustifiable kind of relationship is the involvement of the robber baron with an empire of "property for power." The latter is unjustified because it ties into a conception of the person we can recognize as inferior: the person as self-interested maximizer of manipulative power.

If some people wish to sell something that is identifiably personal, why not let them? In a market society, whatever some people wish to buy and others wish to sell is deemed alienable. Under these circumstances, we must formulate an affirmative case for market-inalienability, so that no one may choose to make fungible—commodify—a personal attribute, right, or thing. I shall now propose and evaluate three possible methods of justifying market-inalienability based on personhood: a prophylactic argument, assimilation to prohibition, and a domino theory. . . .

[Editor's summary:

a. The Prophylactic Argument.
In some cases, commodifying a personal attribute may fairly reliably indicate that one was coerced, such as selling oneself into slavery or selling one's sexual services. In such cases, banning such sale may be society's most reliable strategy for protecting individual freedom and personhood. A problem with this view, however, is that if poverty is perceived as a form of coercion, then banning sales coerced by poverty would deny impoverished people access to goods that may be even more central to their personhood.[7]

b. Prohibition.
The prohibition argument is that commodification is bad in itself or is bad
because a thing commodified is never the "same" as the thing noncommodified.
This view, however, would lead to universal noncommodification and the im-
plausible view that the commodification of nuts and bolts is as damaging as the
commodification of love, friendship, and sexuality.]

c. The Domino Theory.
The domino theory envisions a slippery slope leading to market domination.
The domino theory assumes that for some things, the noncommodifed version
is morally preferable; it also assumes that the commodified and noncommodified versions of some interactions cannot coexist. To commodify
some things is simply to preclude their noncommodified analogues from existing. Under this theory, the existence of some commodified sexual interactions
will contaminate or infiltrate everyone's sexuality so that all sexual relationships will become commodified. If it is morally required that noncommodified
sex be possible, market-inalienability of sexuality would be justified. This
result can be conceived of as the opposite of a prohibition: there is assumed to
exist some moral requirement that a certain "good" be socially available. The
domino theory thus supplies an answer (as the prohibition theory does not) to
the liberal question why people should not be permitted to choose both market and nonmarket interactions: the noncommodified version is morally preferable when we cannot have both. . . .

The argument that market-inalienabilities are necessary to encourage altruism relies upon the domino theory. . . . But why do we need to forbid sales to
preserve opportunities for altruism for those who wish to give? In a gifts-only
regime, a donor's gift remains nonmonetized, whereas if both gifts and sales
are permitted, the gift has a market value. This market value undermines our
altruism and discourages us from giving, the argument runs, because our gift
is now equivalent merely to giving fifty dollars (or whatever is the market
price of a pint of blood) to a stranger, rather than life or health.

The "domino" part of this argument—that once something is commodified for some it is willy-nilly commodified for everyone—posits that once
market value enters our discourse, market rhetoric will take over and characterize every interaction in terms of market value. If this is true, some special
things . . . must be completely noncommodified if altruism is to be possible.
But the feared domino effect of market rhetoric need not be true. To suppose
that it must necessarily be true seems to concede to universal commodification
the assumption that thinking in money terms comes "naturally" to us.[8] Most
people would probably think the assumption false in light of their common
experience. For example, many people value their homes or their work in a
nonmonetary way, even though those things also have market value.

Rather than merely assuming that money is at the core of every transaction in "goods," thereby making commodification inevitable and phasing out
the noncommodified version of the "same" thing (or the nonmarket aspects of

sale transactions), we should evaluate the domino theory on a case-by-case basis. We should assess how important it is to us that any particular contested thing remain available in a noncommodified form and try to estimate how likely it is that allowing market transactions for those things would engender a domino effect and make the nonmarket version impossible. This might involve judging how close to universal commodification our consciousness really is, and how this consciousness would affect the particular thing in question.

The possible avenues for justifying market-inalienability must be reevaluated in light of our nonideal world. One ideal world would countenance no commodification; another would insist that all harms to personhood are unjust; still another would permit no relationships of oppression or disempowerment. But we are situated in a nonideal world of ignorance, greed, and violence; of poverty, racism, and sexism. In spite of our ideals, justice under nonideal circumstances, pragmatic justice, consists in choosing the best alternative now available to us. In doing so we may have to tolerate some things that would count as harms in our ideal world. Whatever harms to our ideals we decide we must now tolerate in the name of justice may push our ideals that much farther away. How are we to decide, now, what is the best transition toward our ideals, knowing that our choices now will help to reconstitute those ideals?

In light of the desperation of poverty, a prophylactic market-inalienability may amount merely to an added burden on would-be sellers; under some circumstances we may judge it, nevertheless, to be our best available alternative. We might think that both nonmarket and market interactions can exist in some situations without a domino effect leading to a more commodified order, or we might think it is appropriate to risk a domino effect in light of the harm that otherwise would result to would-be sellers. We might find prohibition of sales not morally warranted, on balance, in some situations, unless there is a serious risk of domino effect. These will be pragmatic judgments.

Nonideal evaluation of market-inalienability faces a characteristic double bind. Often commodification is put forward as a solution to powerlessness or oppression, as in the suggestion that women be permitted to sell sexual and reproductive services. But is women's personhood injured by allowing or by disallowing commodification of sex and reproduction? The argument that commodification empowers women is that recognition of these alienable entitlements will enable a needy group—poor women—to improve their relatively powerless, oppressed condition, an improvement that would be beneficial to personhood. If the law denies women the opportunity to be comfortable sex workers and baby producers instead of subsistence domestics, assemblers, clerks, and waitresses—or pariahs (welfare recipients) and criminals (prostitutes)—it keeps them out of the economic mainstream and hence the mainstream of American life.

The rejoinder is that, on the contrary, commodification will harm personhood by powerfully symbolizing, legitimating, and enforcing class division and gender oppression. It will create the two forms of alienation that correlate with commodification of personal things. Women will partly internalize the notion that their persons and their attributes are separate, thus creating the pain of a divided self. To the extent that this self-conception is not internalized, women will be alienated from the dominant order that, by allowing commodification, sees them in this light. Moreover, commodification will exacerbate, not ameliorate, oppression and powerlessness, because of the social disapproval connected with marketing one's body.[9]

But the surrejoinder is that noncommodification of women's capabilities under current circumstances represents not a brave new world of human flourishing, but rather a perpetuation of the old order that submerges women in oppressive status relationships, in which personal identity as market-traders is the prerogative of males. We cannot make progress toward the non-commodification that might exist under ideal condition of equality and freedom by trying to maintain noncommodification now under historically determined conditions of inequality and bondage.

These conflicting arguments illuminate the problem with the prophylactic argument for market-inalienability. If we now permit commodification, we may exacerbate the oppression of women—the suppliers. If we now disallow commodification—without what I have called the welfare-rights corollary, or large-scale redistribution of social wealth and power—we force women to remain in circumstances that they themselves believe are worse than becoming sexual commodity-suppliers. Thus, the alternatives seem subsumed by a need for social progress, yet we must choose some regime now in order to make progress. The dilemma of transition is the double bind.

The double bind has two main consequences. First, if we cannot respect personhood either by permitting sales or by banning sales, justice requires that we consider changing the circumstances that create the dilemma. We must consider wealth and power redistribution. Second, we still must choose a regime for the meantime, the transition, in nonideal circumstances. To resolve the double bind, we have to investigate particular problems separately; decisions must be made (and remade) for each thing that some people desire to sell.

If we have reason to believe with respect to a particular thing that the domino theory might hold—commodification for some means commodification for all—we would have reason to choose market-inalienability. But the double bind means that if we choose market-inalienability, we might deprive a class of poor and oppressed people of the opportunity to have more money with which to buy adequate food, shelter, and health care in the market, and hence deprive them of a better chance to lead a humane life. Those who gain from the market-inalienability, on the other hand, might be primarily people whose wealth and power make them comfortable enough to be concerned about the inroads on the general quality of life that commodification would make. Yet, taking a slightly longer view, commodification threatens the personhood of everyone, not just those who can now afford to concern themselves about it. Whether this elitism in market-inalienability should make us risk the dangers of commodification will depend upon the dangers of each case.

One way to mediate the dilemma presented by the double bind is through what I shall call incomplete commodification. Under nonideal circumstances the question whether market-inalienability can be justified is more complicated than a binary decision between complete commodification and complete noncommodification. Rather, we should understand there to be a continuum reflecting degrees of commodification that will be appropriate in a given context. An incomplete commodification—a partial market-inalienability—can sometimes substitute for a complete noncommodification that might accord with our ideals but cause too much harm in our nonideal world.

Before considering examples, it may be helpful to distinguish two aspects of incomplete commodification: participant and social. The participant aspect draws attention to the meaning of an interaction for those who engage in it. For many interactions in which money changes hands, market rhetoric cannot capture this significance. In other words, market and non market aspects of an interaction coexist: although money changes hands, the interaction also has important nonmonetizable personal and social significance. The social aspect of incomplete commodification draws attention instead to the way society as a whole recognizes that things have nonmonetizable participant significance by regulating (curtailing) the free market. . . .

III. Evolutionary Pluralism Applied: Problems of Sexuality and Reproductive Capacity

I now offer thoughts on how the analysis that I recommend might be brought to bear on a set of controversial market-inalienabilities. It is not my purpose to try to provide the detailed, practical evaluation that is needed, but only to sketch its general contours. The example I shall pursue is the contested commodification of aspects of sexuality and reproductive capacity: the issues of prostitution, baby-selling, and surrogacy. I conclude that market-inalienability is justified for baby-selling and also—provisionally—for surrogacy, but that prostitution should be governed by a regime of incomplete commodification.

1. Prostitution
[Editor's summary:

In the application of her theory to prostitution, Professor Radin argues that though an ideal of personhood would seem to include equal, nonmonetized sexual sharing, the criminalization of commodified sexual activities such as prostitution in our present social circumstances tends to undermine the personhood of poor and powerless women who feel forced to engage in prostitution in order to survive. Yet to allow all forms of free market activity in relation to sex—such as public advertising on billboards and TV, agencies to recruit and train—would foster a rhetoric that would harmfully reshape our conceptions of sexuality and personhood. Radin's suggested solution is incomplete commodification of sexual activity: prostitution should be decriminalized so as to protect poor women from the degradation and danger of the black market and of occupations that appear even less desirable to them than prostitution, but other organized marketing of sexual services such as brokerage (pimping), recruitment, and, probably, advertising should be prohibited.]

2. Baby-Selling

A different analysis is warranted for baby-selling. Like relationships of sexual sharing, parent-child relationships are closely connected with personhood, particularly with personal identity and contextuality. Moreover, poor women caught in the double bind raise the issue of freedom: they may wish to sell a baby on the black market, as they may wish to sell sexual services, perhaps to try to provide adequately for other children or family members. But the double bind is not the only problem of freedom implicated in baby-selling. Under a market regime, prostitutes may be choosing to sell their sexuality, but babies are not choosing for themselves that under current nonideal circumstances they are better off as commodities. If we permit babies to be sold, we commodify not only the mother's (and father's) baby-making capacities—which might be analogous to commodifying sexuality—but we also conceive of the baby itself in market rhetoric. When the baby becomes a commodity, all of its personal attributes—sex, eye color, predicted IQ, predicted height, and the like—become commodified as well. This is to conceive of potentially all personal attributes in market rhetoric, not merely those of sexuality. Moreover, to conceive of infants in market rhetoric is likewise to conceive of the people they will become in market rhetoric, and to create in those people a commodified self-conception.

Hence, the domino theory has a deep intuitive appeal when we think about the sale of babies. An idealist might suggest, however, that the fact that we do not now value babies in money suggests that we would not do so even if babies were sold. Perhaps babies could be incompletely commodified, valued by the participants to the interaction in a nonmarket way, even though money changed hands. Although this is theoretically possible, it seems too risky in our nonideal world.[10] If a capitalist baby industry were to come into being, with all of its accompanying paraphernalia, how could any of us, even those who did not produce infants for sale, avoid subconsciously measuring the dollar value of our children? How could our children avoid being preoccupied with measuring their own dollar value? This makes our discourse about ourselves (when we are children) and about our children (when we are parents) like our discourse about cars. Seeing commodification of babies as an inevitable and grave injury to personhood appears rather easy. In the worst case, market rhetoric could create a commodified self-conception in everyone, as the result of commodifying every attribute that differentiates us and that other people value in us, and could destroy personhood as we know it.

I suspect that an intuitive grasp of the injury to personhood involved in commodification of human beings is the reason many people lump baby-selling together with slavery. But this intuition can be misleading. Selling a baby, whose personal development requires caretaking, to people who want to act as the caretakers is not the same thing as selling a baby or an adult to people who want to act only as users of her capacities. Moreover, if the reason for our aversion to baby-selling is that we believe it is like slavery, then it is unclear why we do not prohibit baby-giving (release of a child for adoption) on the ground that enslavement is not permitted even without consideration. We might say that respect for persons prohibits slavery but may require adoption in cases in which only adoptive parents will treat the child as a person, or in the manner appropriate to becoming a person. But this answer is still somewhat unsatisfactory. It does not tell us whether parents who are financially and psychologically capable of raising a child in a manner we deem proper nevertheless may give up the child for adoption, for what we could consider less than compelling reasons. If parents are morally entitled to give up a child even if the child could have (in some sense) been raised properly by them[11] our aversion to slavery does not explain why infants are subject only to market-inalienability. There must be another reason why baby-giving is unobjectionable.

The reason, I think, is that we do not fear relinquishment of children unless it is accompanied by market rhetoric. The objection to market rhetoric may be part of a moral prohibition on market treatment of any babies, regardless of whether nonmonetized treatment of other children would remain possible. To the extent that we condemn baby-selling even in the absence of any domino effect, we are saying that this "good" simply should not exist. Conceiving of any child in market rhetoric wrongs personhood. In addition, we fear, based on our assessment of current social norms, that the market value of babies would be decided in ways injurious to their personhood and to the personhood of those who buy and sell on this basis, exacerbating class, race, and gender divisions. To the extent the objection to baby-selling is not (or is not only) to the very idea of this "good" (marketed children), it stems from a fear that the nonmarket version of human beings themselves will become impossible. Conceiving of children in market rhetoric would foster an inferior conception of human flourishing, one that commodifies every personal attribute that might be valued by people in other people. In spite of the double bind, our aversion to commodification of babies has a basis strong enough to recommend that market-inalienability be maintained.

3. Surrogate-Mothering

The question of surrogate mothering seems more difficult. I shall consider the surrogacy situation in which a couple desiring a child consists of a fertile male and an infertile female. They find a fertile female to become impregnated with the sperm of the would-be father, to carry the fetus to term, to give birth to the child, and to relinquish it to them for adoption. This interaction may be paid, in which case surrogacy becomes a good sold on the market, or unpaid, in which case it remains a gift.

Those who view paid surrogacy as tantamount to permitting the sale of babies point out that a surrogate is paid for the same reasons that an ordinary adoption is commissioned: to conceive, carry, and deliver a baby. Moreover, even if an ordinary adoption is not commissioned, there seems to be no substantive difference between paying a woman for carrying a child she then delivers to the employers, who have found her through a brokerage mechanism, and paying her for an already "produced" child whose buyer is found through a brokerage mechanism (perhaps called an "adoption agency") after she has paid her own costs of "production." Both are adoptions for which consideration is paid. Others view paid surrogacy as better analogized to prostitution (sale of sexual services) than to baby-selling. They would say that the commmodity being sold in the surrogacy interaction is not the baby itself, but rather "womb services."

The different conceptions of the good being sold in paid surrogacy can be related to the primary difference between this interaction and (other) baby-selling: the genetic father is more closely involved in the surrogacy interaction than in a standard adoption. The disagreement about how we might conceive of the "good" reflects a deeper ambiguity about the degree of commodification of mothers and children. If we think that ordinarily a mother paid to relinquish a baby for adoption is selling a baby, but that if she is a surrogate, she is merely selling gestational services, it seems we are assuming that the baby cannot be considered the surrogate's property, so as to become alienable by her, but that her gestational services can be considered property and therefore become alienable. If this conception reflects a decision that the baby cannot be property at all—cannot be objectified—then the decision reflects a lesser level of commodification in rhetoric. But this interpretation is implausible because of our willingness to refer to the ordinary paid adoption as baby-selling. A more plausible interpretation of conceiving of the "good" as gestational services is that this conception reflects an understanding that the baby is already someone else's property—the father's. This characterization of the interaction can be understood as both complete commodification in rhetoric and an expression of gender hierarchy. The would-be father is "producing" a baby of his "own,"[12] but in order to do so he must purchase these "services" as a necessary input. Surrogacy raises the issue of commodification and gender politics in how we understand even the description of the problem. An oppressive understanding of the interaction is the more plausible one: women—their reproductive capacities, attributes, and genes—are fungible in carrying on the male genetic line.

Whether one analogizes paid surrogacy to [the] sale of sexual services or to baby-selling, the underlying concerns are the same. First, there is the possibility of even further oppression of poor or ignorant women, which must be weighed against a possible step toward their liberation through economic gain from a new alienable entitlement—the double bind. Second, there is the possibility that paid surrogacy should be completely prohibited because it expresses an inferior conception of human flourishing. Third, there is the possibility of a domino effect of commodification in rhetoric that leaves us all inferior human beings.

Paid surrogacy involves a potential double bind. The availability of surrogacy option could create hard choices for poor women. In the worst case, rich women, even those who are not infertile, might employ poor women to bear children for them. It might be degrading for the surrogate to commodify her gestational services or her baby, but she may find this preferable to her other choices in life. But although surrogates have not tended to be rich women, nor middle-class career women, neither have they (so far) seemed to be the poorest women, the ones most caught in the double bind.

Whether surrogacy is paid or unpaid, there may be a transition problem: an ironic self-deception. Acting in ways that current gender ideology characterizes as empowering might actually be disempowering. Surrogates may feel they are fulfilling their womanhood by producing a baby for someone else, although they may actually be reinforcing oppressive gender roles. Even if surrogate mothering is subjectively experienced as altruism, the surrogate's self-conception as nurturer, caretaker, and service-giver might be viewed as a kind of gender role-oppression. It is also possible to view would-be fathers as (perhaps unknowing) oppressors of their own partners. Infertile mothers, believing it to be their duty to raise their partners' genetic children, could be caught in the same kind of false consciousness and relative powerlessness as surrogates who feel called upon to produce children for others. Some women might have conflicts with their partners that they cannot acknowledge, either about raising children under these circumstances instead of adopting unrelated children, or about having children at all. These considerations suggest that to avoid reinforcing gender ideology, both paid and unpaid surrogacy must be prohibited.

Another reason we might choose prohibition of all surrogacy, paid or unpaid, is that allowing surrogacy in our nonideal world would injure the chances of proper personal development for children awaiting adoption. Unlike a mother relinquishing a baby for adoption, the surrogate mother bears a baby only in response to the demand of the would-be parents: their demand is the reason for its being born. There is a danger that unwanted children might remain parentless even if only unpaid surrogacy is allowed, because those seeking children will turn less frequently to adoption. Would-be fathers may strongly prefer adopted children bearing their own genetic codes to adopted children genetically strange to them; perhaps women prefer adopted children bearing their partners' genetic codes. Thus, prohibition of all surrogacy might be grounded on concern for unwanted children and their chances in life.

Perhaps a more visionary reason to consider prohibiting all surrogacy is that the demand for it expresses a limited view of parent-child bonding; in a better view of personal contextuality, bonding should be reconceived. Although allowing surrogacy might be thought to foster ideals of interrelationships between men and their children, it is unclear why we should assume that the ideal of bonding depends especially on genetic connection. Many people who adopt children feel no less bonded to their children than responsible genetic parents;[13] they understand that relational bonds are created in shared life more than in genetic codes.[14] We might make better progress toward ideals of interpersonal sharing—toward a better view of contextual personhood—by breaking down the notion that children are fathers'—or parents'—genetic property.

In spite of these concerns, attempting to prohibit surrogacy now seems too utopian, because it ignores a transition problem. At present, people seem to believe that they need genetic offspring in order to fulfill themselves; at present, some surrogates believe their actions to be altruistic. To try to create an ideal world all at once would do violence to things people make central to themselves. This problem suggests that surrogacy should not be altogether prohibited.

Concerns about commodification of women and children, however, might counsel permitting only unpaid surrogacy (market-inalienability). Market-inalienability might be grounded in a judgment that commodification of women's reproductive capacity is harmful for the identity aspect of their personhood and in a judgment that the closeness of paid surrogacy to baby-selling harms our self-conception too deeply. There is certainly the danger that women's attributes, such as height, eye color, race, intelligence, and athletic ability, will be monetized. Surrogates with "better" qualities will command higher prices in virtue of those qualities. This monetization commodifies women more broadly then merely with respect to their sexual services or reproductive capacity. Hence, if we wish to avoid the dangers of commodification and, at the same time, recognize that there are some situations in which a surrogate can be understood to be proceeding out of love or altruism and not out of economic necessity or desire for monetary gain, we could prohibit sales but allow surrogates to give their services. We might allow them to accept payment of their reasonable out-of-pocket expenses—a form of market-inalienability similar to that governing ordinary adoption in some jurisdictions.

Fear of a domino effect might also counsel market-inalienability. At the moment, it does not seem that women's reproductive capabilities are as commodified as their sexuality. Of course, we cannot tell whether this means that reproductive capabilities are more resistant to commodification or whether the trend toward commodification is still at an early stage. Reproductive capacity, however, is not the only thing in danger of commodification. We must also consider the commodification of children. The risk is serious indeed, because, if there is a significant domino effect, commodification of some children means commodification of everyone. Yet, as long as fathers do have an unmonetized attachment to their genes (and as long as their partners tend to share it), even though the attachment may be nonideal, we need not see children born in a paid surrogacy arrangement—and they need not see themselves—as fully commodified. Hence, there may be less reason to fear the domino effect with paid surrogacy than with baby-selling. The most credible fear of a domino effect—one that paid surrogacy does share with commissioned adoption—is that all women's personal attributes will be commodified. The pricing of surrogates' services will not immediately transform the rhetoric in which women conceive of themselves and in which they are conceived, but that is its tendency. This fear, even though remote, seems grave enough to take steps to ensure that paid surrogacy does not become the kind of institution that could permeate our discourse.

Thus, for several reasons market-inalienability seems an attractive solution. But, in choosing this regime, we would have to recognize the danger that the double bind might force simulations of altruism by those who would find living on an expense allowance preferable to their current circumstances. Furthermore, the fact that they are not being paid "full" price exacerbates the double bind and is not really helpful in preventing a domino effect. We would also have to recognize that there would probably not be enough altruistic surrogates available to alleviate the frustration and suffering of those who desire children genetically related to fathers,[15] if this desire is widespread.

The other possible choice is to create an incomplete commodification similar to the one suggested for sale of sexual services. The problem of surrogacy is more difficult, however, primarily because the interaction produces a new person whose interests must be respected. In such an incomplete commodification, performance of surrogacy agreements by willing parties should be permitted, but women who change their minds should not be forced to perform. The surrogate who changes her mind before birth can choose abortion; at birth, she can decide to keep the baby. Neither should those who hire a surrogate and then change their minds be forced to keep and raise a child they do not want. But if a baby is brought into the world and nobody wants her, the surrogate who intended to relinquish the child should not be forced to keep and raise her. Instead, those who, out of a desire for genetically related offspring, initiated the interaction should bear the responsibility for providing for the child's future in a manner that can respect the child's personhood and not create the impression that children are commodities that can be abandoned as well as alienated.[16]

We should be aware that the case for incomplete commodification is much more uneasy for surrogacy than for prostitution. The potential for commodification of women is deeper, because, as with commissioned adoption, we risk conceiving of all of women's personal attributes in market rhetoric, and because paid surrogacy within the current gender structure may symbolize that women are fungible baby-makers for men whose seed must be carrried on. Moreover, as with commissioned adoption, the interaction brings forth a new person who did not choose commodification and whose potential personal identity and contextuality must be respected even if the parties to the interaction fail to do so.

Because the double bind has similar force whether a woman wishes to be a paid surrogate or simply to create a baby for sale on demand, the magnitude of the difference between paid surrogacy and commissioned adoption is largely dependent on the weight we give to the father's genetic link to the baby. If we place enough weight on this distinction, then incomplete commodification for surrogacy, but not for baby-selling, will be justified. But we should be aware, if we choose incomplete commodification for surrogacy, that this choice might seriously weaken the general market-inalienability of babies, which prohibits commissioned adoptions. If paid surrogacy is permitted, it will become a substitute for commissioned adoption.

If, on balance, incomplete commodification rather than market-inalienability comes to seem right for now, it will appear so for these reasons:

because we judge the double bind to suggest that we should not completely foreclose women's choice of paid surrogacy, even though we foreclose commissioned adoptions; because we judge that people's (including women's) strong commitment to maintaining men's genetic lineage will ward off commodification and the domino effect, distinguishing paid surrogacy adequately from commissioned adoptions; and because we judge that the commitment cannot be overridden without harm to central aspects of people's self-conception. If we instead choose market-inalienability, it will be because we judge the double bind to suggest that poor women will be further disempowered if paid surrogacy becomes a middle-class option, and because we judge that people's commitment to men's genetic lineage is an artifact of gender ideology that can neither save us from commodification nor result in less harm to personhood than its reinforcement would now create. In my view, a form of market-inalienability similar to our regime for ordinary adoption is the better nonideal solution. . . .

IV. Conclusion

. . . Market-inalienability ultimately rests on our best conception of human flourishing, which must evolve as we continue to learn and debate. Likewise, market-inalienabilities must evolve as we continue to learn and debate; there is no magic formula that will delineate them with utter certainty, or once and for all. In our debate, there is no such thing as two radically different normative discourses reaching the "same" result. The terms of our debate will matter to who we are.

Notes

1. Posner, Economic Analysis of Law, 202 (3rd. ed., 1986).
2. In Radin, *Property and Personhood*. 34 Stan L. Rev. 957 (1982), I suggest that property may be divided into fungible and personal categories for purposes of moral evaluation. Property is personal in a philosophical sense when it has become identified with a person, with her self-constitution and self-development in the context of her environment. Personal property cannot be taken away and replaced with money or other things without harm to the person—to her identity and existence. In a sense, personal property becomes a personal attribute. On the other hand, property is fungible when there is no such personal attachment. *See* id. at 959–61, 978–79, 986–88.
3. The distinction between fungible and personal property is intended to distinguish between, on the one hand, things that are really "objects" in the sense of being "outside" the person, indifferent to personal constitution and continuity, and on the other hand, things that have become at least partly "inside" the person, involved with one's continuing personhood. The traditional subject-object dichotomy makes the notion of personal property hard to grasp, and, in the present context, poses a danger. To analogize bodily integrity to personal property may simply reintroduce the suggestion inherent in market rhetoric that I am trying to argue against: the suggestion that

bodily integrity is somehow an owned object separate from personhood, rather than an inseparable attribute of personhood.

4. This should not be understood to argue that someone who is raped is changed into a completely different person. To assert either that she is altogether the "same" afterwards or that she is completely "different" afterwords would trivialize her experience: we must have a way of conceptualizing our understanding both that she is different afterwards, so that we recognize that she has been changed by the experience, and simultaneously that she is the same afterwards, or else there would be no "she" that we can recognize to have had the experience and been changed by it. Just as personal attributes should not be seen as separate from an abstract self, neither should our experience be seen as separate from ourselves.

5. Antifoundationalism denies that rationality or truth consists of linear deductions from an unquestioned foundational reality or truth. Coherence theories stress holistic interdependence of an entire body of beliefs and commitments; they judge truth or rightness by fit, not by correspondence with an external foundational standard. . . .

6. Those who subjectively identify with things not properly personal might be said to be alienated, improper object-relations keep them from being integrated persons according to the conception of human flourishing we accept.

7. The puzzle about whether poverty can constitute coercion is a philosophical red herring that conceals a deeper problem. Insofar as preventing sales seems harmful or disempowering to poor people who otherwise would sell personal things, it is so even if we think of the choice to sell as not coerced. Because allowing sales, even if we think of them as freely chosen, also seems harmful or disempowering, we are caught in a double bind, a painful dilemma of transition.

8. The assumption is a concession to universal commodification if it means that thinking in money terms comes naturally to people *sub specie aeternitatis*. But noncommodifiers might assume that thinking in money terms comes naturally to people who live in a commodified social order. This assumption expresses the link between rhetoric and the world, discussed above. My argument is that it should be evaluated more particularly, not that it should be ignored.

9. If marketing one's body is an available option, then those who fail to commodify themselves to feed their families might be thought blameworthy as well. *See* Shapiro, "Regulation as Language: Communicating Values by Reducing the Contingencies of Choice," forthcoming.

10. Perhaps we should separately evaluate the risk in the cases of selling "unwanted" babies and selling babies commissioned for adoption or otherwise "produced" for sale. The risk of complete commodification may be greater if we officially sanction bringing babies into the world for purposes of sale than if we sanction accepting money once they are already born. It seems such a distinction would be quite difficult to enforce, however, because nothing prevents the would-be seller from declaring any child to be "unwanted." Thus, permitting the sale of babies is perhaps tantamount to permitting the production of them for sale.

11. But perhaps we should prophylactically decline to trust any parents who wished to give a child away for "frivolous" reasons adequately to raise a child if forced to keep her.

12. *See,* e.g., *To Serve "the Best Interest of the Child,"* N.Y. Times, Apr. 1, 1987, § B, at 2, col. 2 (The trial judge in the Baby M case said, "At birth, the father does not purchase the child. It is his own biological genetically related child. He cannot purchase what is already his."). Indeed, the very label we now give the birth mother reflects the father's ownership: she is a "surrogate" for "his" wife in her role of bearing "his" child.

13. There has been very little study, however, of the emotional aftermath of adoption. *See* C. Foote, R. Levy and F. Sander, *Cases and Materials on Family Law,* 404–24 (3rd ed. 1985). As we can recognize from the widespread incidence of child abuse and neglect, not all genetic parents are bonded to their children in any ideal sense.

14. True, there is usually a deep bond between a baby and the woman who carries her, but it seems to me that this bond too is created by shared life, the physical and emotional interdependence of mother and child, more than by the identity of the genetic material. It will be difficult to study this question unless childbearing by embryo transfer, in which a woman can carry a fetus that is not genetically related to her, becomes widespread.

15. In light of the apparent strength of people's desires for fathers' genetic offspring, the ban on profit would also be difficult to enforce. As with adoption, we would see a black market develop in surrogacy.

16. The special dangers of commodification in the surrogacy situation should serve to distinguish it from the way we treat children generally. Perhaps a regulatory scheme should require bonding, insurance policies, or annuities for the child in case of death of the adoptive parents or reneging by them. *See* Note, *Developing a Concept of the Modern "Family": A Proposed Uniform Surrogate Parenthood Act* 73 Geo. L. J. 1283 (1985), 1304. *But* cf. Hollinger, (arguing that financial requirements for surrogate parents are unwarranted because the state does not require that "children generated by coital means be similarly protected"). Perhaps a better scheme (because less oriented to market solutions) could require that alternative adoptive parents at least be sought in advance. *From Coitus to Commerce: Legal and Social Consequences of Noncoital Reproduction,* 18 U. Mich J. L. Ref. 865, 911 n. 174 (1985)

Begotten or Made?

Oliver O'Donovan

Being and Making

. . . As I looked through evidence submitted by Christian bodies to the Warnock Committee,[1] and compared it with writings from other Christian sources in the last quarter-century, it seemed to me that a consistent concern emerged. It was expressed as clearly by those who accepted these new techniques as by those who rejected them. It was common to Roman Catholics, Protestants, and Jews. It arose from a caution about the impact of technology (which is, above all, the impact of certain ways of *thinking*) on our self-understanding as human beings. It found common expression in a distinction that constantly recurred: between the use of technique to assist human procreation and the transformation of human procreation into a technical operation. It was a concern about the capacity of technology to change, not merely the conditions of our human existence, but its essential characteristics. . . .

When the fathers of the Council of Nicaea declared, in words familiar to every Christian who recites their creed, that the only Son of God the Father was "begotten, not made," they intended to make a simple point. The Son was "of one being with the Father." He was God, just as God the Father was God. And to emphasize the point they used an analogy, based upon our twofold human experience of forming things other than ourselves. That which we beget is *like* ourselves. (I shall use the word "beget," as the ancients did, to speak of the whole human activity of procreation, and not in the modern way, meaning especially the male side of the activity.) Our offspring are human beings, who share with us one common human nature, one common human experience and one common human destiny. We do not determine what our offspring is, except by ourselves being that very thing which our offspring is to become. Just so, the fathers said, the eternal Son of God who was not made, was of the Father's *being,* not his *will.* But that which we make is *unlike* ourselves. Whether it is made of matter, like a wooden table, or of words like a lecture, or of sounds like a symphony, or of colors and shapes like a picture, or of images like an idea, it is the product of our own free determination. We

From *Begotten or Made?* Oxford: Oxford University Press, 1984. Abridged. © Oliver O'Donovan, 1984. Used by permission of Oxford University Press.

have stamped the decisions of our will upon the material which the world has offered us, to form it in this way and not in that. What we "make," then, is alien from our humanity. In that it has a human maker, it has come to existence as a human project, its being at the disposal of mankind. It is not fit to take its place alongside mankind in fellowship, for it has no place beside him on which to stand: man's will is the law of its being. That which we beget can be, and should be, our companion; but the product of our art—whatever immeasurable satisfaction and enjoyment there may be both in making it and in cherishing it—can never have the independence to be that "other I," equal to us and differentiated from us, which we acknowledge in those who are begotten of human seed.

In making this contrast with reference to the eternal Son of God the Nicene fathers used an analogy. Like all analogies, it has its limitations. We cannot speak of "begetting" in the divine being without making it clear what aspects of the analogy are not applicable to the life of godhead. At the same time, we cannot say that any human beings are "begotten, not made" in the same absolute sense that we can say it of the Son of God. For all human beings begotten of other human beings are, at the same time, "made" by God. Of no human being can it be said that he is simply "not made," that he is at nobody's disposal, that no higher will acts as the law of his being. God's will is such a law for every human being, and every human being is at the disposal of God. Human beings, begotten of human seed, are also made; even Jesus Christ, considered simply as a human being is a "creature" of God. Nevertheless, the ground of the analogy holds. A being who is the "maker" of any other being is alienated from that which he has made, transcending it by his will and acting as the law of its being. To speak of "begetting" is to speak of quite another possibility than this: the possibility that one may form another being who will share one's own nature, and with whom one will enjoy a fellowship based on radical equality.

In this essay we have to speak of "begetting"—not the eternal begetting of the godhead, but the temporal begetting of one creature by another. We have to consider the position of this human "begetting" in a culture which has been overwhelmed by "making"—that is to say, in a technological culture. And here we must stress a point that is often made by those who have taught us how to think about our technological culture—we may mention George Grant's *Technology and Empire*[2] and Jacques Ellul's *The Technological Society*[3]—that what marks this culture out most importantly, is not anything that it does, but what it thinks. It is not "technological" because its instruments of making are extraordinarily sophisticated (though that is evidently the case), but because it thinks of everything it does as a form of instrumental making. Politics (which should surely be the most noninstrumental of activities) is talked of as "making a better world"; love is "building a successful relationship". There is no place for simply *doing*. The fate of a society which sees, wherever it looks, nothing but the products of the human will is that it fails, when it does see some aspect of human activity which is not a matter of construction, to recognize the significance of what it sees and to think about it appropriately. This blindness in the realm of thought is the heart of what it is to be a technological culture.

Nevertheless, though thought comes first, there are implications in the realm of practice too. Such a society is incapable of acknowledging the inappropriateness of technical intervention in certain types of activity. When every activity is understood as making, then every situation in which we act is seen as a raw material, waiting to have something made out of it. If there is no category in thought for an action which is not artifactual, then there is no restraint in action which can preserve phenomena which are not artificial. This imperils not only, or even primarily, the "environment" (as we patronizingly describe the world of things which are not human); it imperils what it is to be human, for it deprives human existence itself of certain spontaneities of being and doing, spontaneities which depend upon the reality of a world which we have not made or imagined, but which simply confronts us to evoke our love, fear, and worship. Human life, then, becomes mechanized because we cannot comprehend what it means that some human activity is "natural." Politics becomes controlled by media of mass communication, love by analytical or counselling techniques. And begetting children becomes subject to the medical and surgical interventions. . . .

We are asking about our human "begetting," that is to say, our capacity to give existence to another human being, not by making him the end of a project of our will, but by imparting to him our own being, so that he is formed by what we are and not by what we intend. And we are asking what must become of our begetting in a revolutionary climate of thought in which "making" is the conceptual matrix by which we understand all human activity. . . .

The great intellectual challenge that faces our age in view of these innovations is not to understand *that* this or that may or may not be done, but to understand *what* it is that would be done, if it were to be done. And it would be mere intellectual evasiveness to pretend that the human mode of reproduction was a contingency that chanced upon our human race, and might as well not have done.

To this given connection in our nature between male-female relationship and procreation it is possible to respond in only two ways. We may welcome it, or we may resent it. Christian teaching has encouraged us to welcome it. Christian thinkers have said, in the first place, that the connection is good for the *man-woman relationship,* which is protected from debasement and loss of mutuality by the fact that it is fruitful for procreation. When erotic relationships between the sexes are conceived merely as relationships—with no further implications, no "end" within the purposes of nature—then they lack the significance which they need if they are to be undertaken responsibly. They become simply a profound form of play, undertaken for the joy of the thing alone, and depending upon the mutual satisfaction which each partner affords the other for their continuing justification. The honoring of each partner by the other must be founded on the honor which the relationship itself claims, by serving a fundamental good of the human race. Saint Peter's counsel to Christian husbands (1 Pet.3:7) has often been understood (rightly or wrongly) in this sense: "Bestow honor on the woman, as you are joint heirs of the gift of life." Paradoxically, this mutual honoring for the dignity of the procreative task can sometimes be seen most clearly in the midst of that mutual dishonoring which accompanies marital breakdown. When partners engage in a bitter struggle with each other over the custody of children, what does it mean but that even while they cannot bring themselves to live with each other, neither can they live without the image of the other gazing out at them through the child's eyes?

Christian teachers have said, in the second place, that the true character of *procreation* is secured by its belonging to the man-woman relationship. The status of the child as "begotten, not made" is assured by the fact that she is not the primary object of attention in that embrace which gave her her being. In that embrace the primary object of attention to each partner is the other. The I-Thou predominates. The She (or He) which will spring from the I-Thou is always present as possibility, but never as project pure and simple. And precisely for that reason she cannot be demeaned to the status of artifact, a product of the will.

From these two complementary perspectives (the former more Catholic and the second more Protestant) Christian thinkers in the West have argued that the procreative and relational aspects of marriage strengthen one another, and that each is threatened by the loss of the other. This is a knot tied by God, which men should not untie. It is clear that any attempt to convert begetting into making constitutes a loosening of that knot, a severing of the relational from the procreative and the procreative from the relational. And for this to happen it is not necessary for anyone to deny the value of either procreation or sexual relationship. It is enough to think, as many moderns do seem to think, that each would flourish better if relieved of the burden of marching *pari passu* with the other. . . .

Contingency and Artifice: *In Vitro* Fertilization

Granted that *in vitro* fertilization intends to treat pathology and not contingency, does it not have the effect of abolishing the contingency at the same time as it compensates for the pathology? If this is so, there will be a strong ground of objection to it (one which will not apply in the same way to some other means of compensating for infertility, such as artificial insemination). For the element of chance is one of the factors that most distinguishes the act of begetting from the act of technique. In allowing something to randomness, we confess that, though we might, from a purely technical point of view, direct events, it is beyond our competence to direct them well. We commit ourselves to divine providence because we have reached the point at which we know we must stop making, and simply be. To say "randomness," of course, is not to say "providence." Randomness is the inscrutable face which providence turns to us when we cannot trace its ways or guess its purpose. To accept that face is to accept that we cannot plan for the best as God plans for the best, and that we cannot read his plans before the day he declares them. There are, to be sure, ways in which we reduce the degree of unpredictability indirectly, by choosing the time of intercourse carefully, for example, to fit in with natural rhythms of fertility. Yet for all that we may encourage conception to take place, its occurrence is not the direct object of our technique. We do not, in natural begetting, bring sperm and ovum together, and, as it were, forcibly introduce them to each other. Thus we distinguish the act of begetting from those other acts in which we attempt to control the outcome directly, mastering with our hands or with their implements the material resistance which stands between the will and its proposed artifact.

But it is not the case that conception by *in vitro* fertilization abolishes contingency. It is true that it does so at one point: the actual fertilization of the ovum by the sperm is made the direct object of technique. There is therefore more difference between *in vitro* and *in vivo* than the mere difference of location that those phrases may suggest: there is a new, technical relationship to an event which has hitherto been subject only to indirect influences. But what is lost to contingency at the point of *fertilization* is not lost, but may even be enhanced, at the point of *implantation*. Implantation is still unpredictable and unmanipulable, an event which can only be encouraged, and not yet directly managed.

As one might expect, this very factor, which in our view goes some way to saving the humanity of the whole undertaking, is regarded by its practitioners as a technical imperfection to be overcome as soon as suitable means can be found. Since the early days of the practice it has been customary to reduce the element of unpredictability by replacing not one, but two or even three embryos in the womb, to increase the chance that one of them will implant. It is at least arguable that this does no further injury to the others than that which they might suffer in the course of nature anyway, for the fate of every new conceptus is doubtful. But it does reduce the doubtfulness which must attach to every *act* of embryo-replacement. It is easy to see why, from the administrative point of view, it is desirable to minimize the contingencies and maximize the rate of success at first attempt. Time, patience and resources are all consumed in repeated attempts which could be avoided. Yet this observation, while making the practice of multiple replacement intelligible, does so in a way that rather strengthens than mitigates the force of the case against it; for it is precisely the integration of human fertilization into the general demands of an administrative system that more than anything else confirms its status as an act of "making" rather than of "begetting." We pointed out in [the first section] that the primary characteristic of a technological society is not the things it may *do* with the aid of machines, but the way it *thinks* of everything it does as a kind of mechanical production. Once begetting is acknowledged to be under the laws of time and motion efficiency, then its absorption into the world of productive technique is complete. The laws of operation cease to be the laws of natural procreation, aided discreetly by technical assistance; they become the laws of production, which swallow up all that is natural into their own world of artifice. That is why I think there is a great deal of symbolic importance in resisting multiple replacement of embryos. We should expect the practitioners to act inefficiently at this point, just as we expect researchers to act inefficiently when they are dealing with human subjects. Inefficiency is the worship they pay to the *humanum,* the human person and personal relationships, objects which cannot be subject to the laws which govern productive efficiency. . . .

Union and Procreation

In my earlier discussions[4] of transsexual surgery and gamete-donation I attempted to show that the issue of the making or begetting of children is correlated to another issue, the unity or separation of the procreative and relational goods of marriage. I argued that when procreation is not bound to the relational union established by the sexual bond, it becomes a chosen "project" of the couple rather than a natural development of their common life. Sexual relationship, correspondingly, loses the seriousness which belongs to it because of our common need for a generation of children, and degenerates into merely a form of play. The document submitted to the Warnock Commission by the Catholic Bishops' Joint Committee on Bioethical Issues has made this point the basis of its objections to *in vitro* fertilization, and has argued the case with great eloquence.[5]

If in the course of natural procreation, the Committee maintains, the parents' hope for a child is fulfilled, then "the child will be a gift embodying the parents' acts of personal . . . involvement with each other. Procreation will thus have been an extension of the parents' whole common life" (para. 21). But the same cannot be said of the child born as a result of *in vitro* fertilization, who will tend to be assigned "to the same status as other objects of acquisition. The technical skills and decisions of the child's makers will have produced, they hope, a good product, a desirable acquisition" (para. 27). Although good parents "will strive to assign the child his or her true status . . . they will be laboring against the real structure of the decisive choices and against the deep symbolism of all that was done to bring their child into being." The "structure of the decisive choices": that is what makes the decisive difference in the view of the Catholic Bishops' Committee.

> In procreation by sexual intercourse *one and the same act of choice* made by each spouse governs *both* the experienced and expressive sexual union *and* the procreation of the child. There is one intentional act. . . . But in IVF there are irreducibly separate acts of choice, all indispensible, and all the independent acts of different people. . . . Thus the IVF child comes into existence, not as a gift supervening on an act expressive of marital union . . . but rather in the manner of a product of a making (and indeed, typically, as the end-product of a process managed and carried out by persons other than his parents) [para. 24].

Within this argument we may notice two features. One is the principle that I have maintained, that procreation is safeguarded from degeneration by springing from a sexual relationship in which the child is not the immediate object of attention. The other is the further stipulation that these twin goods of marriage must be held together in *one intentional act* of sexual intercourse. The complaint against IVF is that there are "separate acts of choice," that the unity of the procreative and the relational goods is not maintained in each single act. Now, it might seem that this further stipulation is merely a necessary clarification of what was implied in my principle. For the unity of procreative and relational goods will certainly be an empty thing if there is not some concrete expression of it. Anyone can agree, after all, that marriage should have both a relational good and a procreative one—and then pursue the two so distinctly that they become quite unrelated projects. And what other concrete point of unity can there be than the act of sexual intercourse, of its nature both procreative and relational? . . .

[I]n the Catholics' argument against IVF, we have an instance of "strict act-analysis" [which holds that "each and every marriage act" must express the two goods equally]. They argue that the offensiveness of IVF and AIH resides in the "irreducibly separate acts of choice . . . the independent acts of different people," by which the IVF procedure is carried through. To which we may reply that there are *distinct* acts of choice, which involve persons other than the couple, in any form of aided conception, including those forms of which the document approves. Whether they are *independent* acts of choice is precisely the question which requires moral insight. If they are indeed independent (and not subordinate to the couple's quest for fruitfulness in their sexual embrace) then they are certainly offensive. But that point cannot be settled simply by asserting that they are distinct. The question remains: is there a moral unity which holds together what happens at the hospital with what happens at home in bed? Can these procedures be understood appropriately as the couple's search for help within their sexual union (the total life-union of their bodies, that is, not a single sexual act)? And I have to confess that I do not see why not. News reports tell us that some IVF practitioners advise their Roman Catholic patients to have sexual intercourse following embryo-replacement, in order to respect the teachings of their church. It would seem to me that such advice might well be given to all patients, in order to help them form a correct view of what is, or should be, meant by the technique: not the making of a baby apart from the sexual embrace, but the aiding of the sexual embrace to achieve its proper goal of fruitfulness. . . .

The Child

I confess that I do not know how to think of an IVF child except (in some unclear but inescapable sense) as the *creature* of the doctors who assisted at her conception—which means, also, of the society to which the doctor belongs and for whom he acts.

If anyone finds this conception grotesque and self-evidently wrong, I congratulate him on his good habits of thought—but with a warning. Good habits of thought teach us to find the notion of one human being as the creature of another odd and repulsive; but habit alone will not protect a culture against the "paradigm shift" in its perceptions which will occur when too much in what it observes and does is more obviously thought of in a new way. If our habits of thought continue to instruct us that the IVF child is radically equal to the doctors who produced her, then that is good—for the time being. But if we do not live and act in accordance with such conceptions, and if society welcomes more and more institutions and practices which implicitly deny them, then they will soon appear to be merely sentimental, the tatters and shreds which remind us of how we used once to clothe the world with intelligibility.

For myself, I do not *believe* that the doctor has become the child's creator. I do not believe it, though, as I have admitted, I do not know how to reconcile my unbelief with the obvious significance of *in vitro* fertilization. I can only confess, as a matter of Christian faith, that I believe in another and unique Creator who will not relinquish to others his place as the maker and preserver of mankind. To those who wish to make this confession with me let me put this closing question: should we not expect that a humanity which is so made will vindicate its maker, and his creatures, against every false claim to lordship?

Notes

1. [Report of the British Committee of Inquiry into Human Fertilisation and Embryology, now published in book form: Mary Warnock, *A Question of Life: The Warnock Report on Human Fertilisation & Embryology*, (Oxford: Basil Blackwell, 1985).]

2. (Anansi: Toronto, 1969).

3. Tr. J. Wilkinson (Jonathan Cape: London, 1965).

4. [Not included in this selection—Editor.]

5. *In Vitro Fertilization: Morality and Public Policy* (Catholic Information Services, 1983).

V

REPRODUCTIVE TECHNOLOGY AND WOMEN: OPPORTUNITY OR OPPRESSION?

What is the significance of reproductive technology for women? From early in the women's movement, it had been argued that women's biology and existing social arrangements have burdened women with bearing and rearing children, thereby robbing them of opportunities to become fully aware of and able to exercise their capacities as human beings. Technological developments, such as contraception and abortion, which increased women's control over reproductive processes, were welcomed by most in the women's movement, and at first, innovations in reproductive technology were similarly hailed as having the potential to free women from "the tyranny of their biology." Continuing to express this enthusiasm, lawyer Lori Andrews, in the first article in this part, catalogues the ways in which reproductive technology maintains and expands the choices and control individual women have with respect to their own bodies. She attempts to demonstrate that parenting through contract in particular gives women greater freedom while not harming women (either the individuals involved in the practice or women in general), children, or society.

Many in the women's movement do not share Andrews's enthusiasm. One of the most provocative critics is feminist writer Gena Corea. Corea argues that whereas men are, by the facts of biology, alienated from the processes of procreation and life, women concretely experience continuity with their children and the processes through which those children are born. Men, through abstract, intellectual thought, can come to conceive of children as their own, but this process, claims Corea, cannot ultimately overcome men's alienation. Corea traces a history in which women and their reproductive functions were originally revered, but then were progressively denigrated and appropriated by men in their attempt to overcome their alienation. Reproductive technology is, Corea concludes, a completing step in men's attempt to appropriate women's reproductive processes, reducing women's involvement in procreation to the same state of external, intellectual alienation as that in which men are claimed to have originally stood.[1] On the nature and significance of women's experiences in reproduction, see also the articles by de Beauvoir and Tong.

A critical problem for the women's movement, especially in regard to social policy, is reconciling the feminist position that individual women should have freedom of choice in reproductive matters with the recognition that those choices can be informed by and reinforce values that are antithetical to women's fulfillment. It is hard to deny the obvious joy and satisfaction experienced by women who have, after years of frustration, succeeded in having children through the aid of reproductive technology. Even if somehow women's and men's conceptions of women themselves, children, and childbearing are changed, can't the trade-off be worth it? Or might it be argued that it is not the techniques themselves that are damaging to women, but rather the consciousness with which they are regarded? In that case, feminist critics should not oppose the techniques themselves, but instead should aim to change our cultural and individual consciousness so that we are properly receptive to them. Any attempt to take up this line of thought should attend to the positions developed by Radin and O'Donovan in Part IV of this anthology.[2]

Being able to choose the sex of one's offspring has long been a dream not only in our culture, but in many others as well. Generally, the preference has been to have male children. Thus, the growing possibility that reliable methods of sex preselection will be found has worried people who are concerned with the interests and rights of women. In the final article in this part, philosopher Mary Anne Warren addressed the question of the morality of sex preselection. She considers both whether the practice is intrinsically sexist and whether it can be shown with any degree of certainty to have harmful consequences. She concludes that neither charge can be sustained and consequently that the practice cannot be judged to be immoral. In evaluating Warren's article, attention should be given to Radin's argument, especially as it concerns tensions between individual rationality (what may be prudent for a particular individual) and the conceptions of self that thinking and acting according to individual rationality may exemplify and promote.

Notes

1. For a literary expression of similar ideas, see Margaret Atwood, *The Handmaid's Tale* (New York: Ballantine Books, 1985). For further reflection on the nature and significance of women's experiences in reproduction, see also the articles by de Beauvoir and Tong in this anthology. Tong's article could well have been included in this section, but it is placed in the section on law because of its practical focus on the legal status of parenting through contract.

2. The tensions here between nature and control and between individual freedom and promoting degrading self-conceptions arise in other connections as well, such as in some women's willing (and profitable) participation in the production of pornographic representations of themselves or in modifications of their bodies through, for example, breast augmentation or dieting.

Surrogate Motherhood: The Challenge for Feminists

Lori B. Andrews

Surrogate motherhood presents an enormous challenge for feminists. During the course of the *Baby M* trial, the New Jersey chapter of the National Organization of Women met and could not reach consensus on the issue. "The feelings ranged the gamut," the head of the chapter, Linda Bowker, told the *New York Times*. "We did feel that it should not be made illegal, because we don't want to turn women into criminals. But other than that, what you may feel about the Baby M case may not be what you feel about another.

"We do believe that women ought to control their own bodies, and we don't want to play big brother or big sister and tell them what to do," Ms. Bowker continued. "But on the other hand, we don't want to see the day when women are turned into breeding machines."[1]

Other feminist groups have likewise been split on the issue, but a vocal group of feminists came to the support of Mary Beth Whitehead with demonstrations[2] and an amicus brief[3]; they are now seeking laws that would ban surrogate motherhood altogether. However, the rationales that they and others are using to justify this governmental intrusion into reproductive choice may come back to haunt feminists in other areas of procreative policy and family law.

As science fiction has taught us, the types of technologies available shape the nature of a society. Equally important as the technologies—and having much farther-reaching implications—are the policies that a society devises and implements to deal with technology. In Margaret Atwood's *The Handmaid's Tale,* a book often cited as showing the dangers of the technology of surrogacy, it was actually policy changes—the criminalization of abortion and the banning of women from the paid labor force—that created the preconditions for a dehumanizing and harmful version of surrogacy.

From *Law, Medicine and Health Care* 16 (1988), pp. 72–80. Copyright American Society of Law and Medicine, Inc. Reprinted by permission.

The Feminist Legacy

In the past two decades, feminist policy arguments have refashioned legal policies on reproduction and the family. A cornerstone of this development has been the idea that women have a right to reproductive choice—to be able to contracept, abort, or get pregnant. They have the right to control their bodies during pregnancy, such as by refusing Cesarean sections. They have a right to create non-traditional family structures such as lesbian households or single-parent families facilitated by artificial insemination by donor. According to feminist arguments, these rights should not be overridden by possible symbolic harms or speculative risks to potential children.

Another hallmark of feminism has been that biology should not be destiny. The equal treatment of the sexes requires that decisions about men and women be made on other than biological grounds. Women police officers can be as good as men, despite their lesser strength on average. Women's larger role in bearing children does not mean they should have the larger responsibility in rearing children. And biological fathers, as well as nonbiological mothers or fathers, can be as good parents as biological mothers.

The legal doctrine upon which feminists have pinned much of their policy has been the constitutional protection of autonomy in decisions to bear and rear one's biological children.[4] Once this protection of the biologically related family was acknowledged, feminists and others could argue for the protection of non-traditional, non-biological families on the grounds that they provide many of the same emotional, physical, and financial benefits that biological families do.[5]

In many ways, the very existence of surrogacy is a predictable outgrowth of the feminist movement. Feminist gains allowed women to pursue educational and career opportunities once reserved for men, such as Betsy Stern's position as a doctor and medical school professor. But this also meant that more women were postponing childbearing and suffering the natural decline in fertility that occurs with age. Women who exercised their right to contraception, such as by using the Dalkon Shield, sometimes found that their fertility was permanently compromised. Some women found that the chance for a child had slipped by them entirely and decided to turn to a surrogate mother.

Feminism also made it more likely for other women to feel comfortable being surrogates. Feminism taught that not all women relate to all pregnancies in the same way. A woman could choose not to be a rearing mother at all. She could choose to lead a child-free life by not getting pregnant. If she got pregnant, she could choose to abort. Reproduction was a condition of her body over which she, and no one else, should have control. For some women, those developments added up to the freedom to be a surrogate.

In the surrogacy context, feminist principles have provided the basis for a broadly held position that contracts and legislation should not restrict the surrogate's control over her body during pregnancy (such as by a requirement that the surrogate undergo amniocentesis or abort a fetus with a genetic defect). The argument against enforcing such contractual provisions resounds with the notion of gender equality, since it is in keeping with common law principles that protect the bodily integrity of both men and women, as well as with basic contract principles rejecting specific performance of personal-services provisions.[6] It is also in keeping with constitutional principles giving the pregnant woman, rather than the male progenitor, the right to make abortion decisions. In this area, feminist lobbying tactics have met with considerable success. Although early bills on surrogacy contained provisions that would have constrained surrogates' behavior during pregnancy, most bills regulating surrogacy that have been proposed in recent years specifically state that the surrogate shall have control over medical decisions during the pregnancy.[7] Even the trial court decision in the Baby M case, which enforced the surrogacy contract's termination of parental rights, voided the section that took from the surrogate the right to abort.[8]

Now a growing feminist contingent is moving beyond the issue of bodily control during pregnancy and is seeking to ban surrogacy altogether. But the rationales for such a ban are often the very rationales that feminists have fought against in the contexts of abortion, contraception, non-traditional families, and employment. The adoption of these rationales as the reason to regulate surrogacy could severely undercut the gains previously made in these other areas. These rationales fall into three general categories: the symbolic harm to society of allowing paid surrogacy, the potential risks to the woman of allowing paid surrogacy, and the potential risks to the potential child of allowing paid surrogacy.

The Symbolic Harm to Society

For some feminists, the argument against surrogacy is a simple one: it demeans us all as a society to sell babies. And put that way, the argument is persuasive, at least on its face. But as a justification for policy, the argument is reminiscent of the argument that feminists roundly reject in the abortion context: that it demeans us as a society to kill babies.

Both arguments, equally heartfelt, need closer scrutiny if they are to serve as a basis for policy. In the abortion context, pro-choice people criticize the terms, saying we are not talking about "babies" when the abortion is done on an embryo or fetus still within the woman's womb. In the surrogacy context, a similar assault can be made on the term "sale." The baby is not being transferred for money to a stranger who can then treat the child like a commodity, doing anything he or she wants with the child. The money is being paid to enable a man to procreate his biological child; this hardly seems to fit the characterization of a sale. Am I buying a child when I pay a physician to be my surrogate fallopian tubes through in vitro fertilization (when, without her aid, I would remain childless)? Am I buying a child when I pay a physician to perform a needed Cesarean section, without which my child would never be born alive?

At most, in the surrogacy context, I am buying not a child but the pre-conception termination of the mother's parental rights. For decades, the pre-conception sale of a father's parental rights has been allowed with artificial insemination by donor. This practice, currrently facilitated by statutes in at least thirty states, has received strong feminist support. In fact, when, on occasion, such sperm donors have later felt a bond to the child and wanted to be considered legal fathers, feminist groups have litigated to hold them to their pre-conception contract.[9]

Rather than focusing on the symbolic aspects of a sale, the policy discussion should instead analyze the advisability of pre-conception terminations for both women and men. For example, biological parenting may be so important to both the parent and the child that either parent should be able to assert these rights after birth (or even later in the child's life). This would provide sperm donors in artificial insemination with a chance to have a relationship with the child.

Symbolic arguments and pejorative language seem to make up the bulk of the policy arguments and media commentary against surrogacy. Surrogate motherhood has been described by its opponents not only as the buying and selling of children but as reproductive prostitution,[10] reproductive slavery,[11] the renting of a womb,[12] incubatory servitude,[13] the factory method of childbearing,[14] and cutting up women into genitalia.[15] The women who are surrogates are labeled paid breeders,[16] biological entrepreneurs,[17] breeder women,[18] reproductive meat,[19] interchangeable parts in the birth machinery,[20] manufacturing plants,[21] human incubators,[22] incubators for men's sperm,[23] a commodity in the reproductive marketplace,[24] and prostitutes.[25] Their husbands are seen, alternatively, as pimps[26] or cuckolds.[27] The children conceived pursuant to a surrogacy agreement have been called chattel[28] or merchandise to be expected in perfect condition.[29]

Feminists opposing surrogacy have also relied heavily on a visual element in the debate over Baby M. They have been understandably upset at the vision of a baby being wrenched from its nursing mother or being slipped out a back window in a flight from governmental authorities. But relying on the visceral and visual, a long-standing tactic of the right-to-life groups, is not the way to make policy. Conceding the value of symbolic arguments for the procreative choice of surrogacy makes it hard to reject them for other procreative choices.

One of the greatest feminist contributions to policy debates on reproduction and the family has been the rejection of arguments relying on tradition and symbolism and an insistence on an understanding of the nature and effects of an actual practice in determining how it should be regulated. For example, the idea that it is necessary for children to grow up in two-parent, heterosexual families has been contested by empirical evidence that such traditional structures are not necessary for children to flourish.[30] This type of analysis should not be overlooked in favor of symbolism in discussions of surrogacy.

The Potential Harm to Women

A second line of argument opposes surrogacy because of the potential psychological and physical risks that it presents for women. Many aspects of this argument, however, seem ill founded and potentially demeaning to women. They focus on protecting women against their own decisions because those decisions might later cause them regret, be unduly influenced by others, or be forced by financial motivations.

Reproductive choices are tough choices, and any decision about reproduction—such as abortion, sterilization, sperm donation, or surrogacy—might later be regretted. The potential for later regrets, however, is usually not thought to be a valid reason to ban the right to choose the procedure in the first place.

With surrogacy, the potential for regret is thought by some to be enormously high. This is because it is argued (in biology-is-destiny terms) that it is unnatural for a mother to give up a child. It is assumed that because birth mothers in traditional adoption situations often regret relinquishing their children, surrogate mothers will feel the same way. But surrogate mothers are making their decisions about relinquishment under much different circumstances. The biological mother in the traditional adoption situation is already pregnant as part of a personal relationship of her own. In many, many instances, she would like to keep the child but cannot because the relationship is not supportive or she cannot afford to raise the child. She generally feels that the relinquishment was forced upon her (for example, by her parents, a counselor, or her lover).[31]

The biological mother in the surrogacy situation seeks out the opportunity to carry a child that would not exist were it not for the couple's desire to create a child as a part of their relationship. She makes her decision in advance of pregnancy for internal, not externally enforced reasons. While 75 percent of the biological mothers who give a child up for adoption later change their minds,[32] only around 1 percent of the surrogates have similar changes of heart.

Entering into a surrogacy arrangement does present potential psychological risks to women. But arguing for a ban on surrogacy seems to concede that the *government,* rather than the individual woman, should determine what risks a woman should be allowed to face. This conflicts with the general legal policy allowing competent individuals to engage in potentially risky behavior so long as they have given their voluntary, informed consent.

Perhaps recognizing the dangers of giving the government widespread powers to "protect" women, some feminists do acknowledge the validity of a general consent to assume risks. They argue, however, that the consent model is not appropriate to surrogacy since the surrogate's consent is neither informed nor voluntary.

It strikes me as odd to assume that the surrogate's consent is not informed.

The surrogacy contracts contain lengthy riders detailing the myriad risks of pregnancy, so potential surrogates are much better informed on that topic than are most women who get pregnant in a more traditional fashion. In addition, with volumes of publicity given to the plight of Mary Beth White-head, all potential surrogates are now aware of the possibility that they may later regret their decisions. So, at that level, the decision is informed. Yet a strong element of the feminist argument against surrogacy is that women cannot give an informed consent until they have had the experience of giving birth. Robert Arenstein, an attorney for Mary Beth Whitehead, argued in congressional testimony that a "pre-birth or at-birth termination, is a termination without informed consent. I use the words informed consent to mean full understanding of the personal psychological consequences at the time of sur-render of the child."[33] The feminist amicus brief in *Baby M* made a similar argument.[34]

The New Jersey Supreme Court picked up this characterization of in-formed consent, writing that "quite clearly any decision prior to the baby's birth is, in the most important sense, uninformed."[35] But such an approach is at odds with the legal doctrine of informed consent. Nowhere is it expected that one must have the experience first before one can make an informed judgment about whether to agree to the experience. Such a requirement would preclude people from ever giving informed consent to sterilizations, abortions, sex change operations, heart surgery, and so forth. The legal doc-trine of informed consent presupposes that people will predict in advance of the experience whether a particular course will be beneficial to them.

A variation of the informed consent argument is that while most compe-tent adults can make such predictions, hormonal changes during pregnancy may cause a woman to change her mind. Virtually a whole amicus brief in the *Baby M* appeal was devoted to arguing that a woman's hormonal changes during pregnancy make it impossible for her to predict in advance the conse-quences of her relinquishment.[36] Along those lines, adoption worker Elaine Rosenfeld argues that

> [t]he consent that the birth mother gives prior to conception is not the consent of . . . a woman who has gone through the chemical, biological, endocrinological changes that have taken place during pregnancy and birth, and no matter how well prepared or well inten-tioned she is in her decision prior to conception, it is impossible for her to predict how she will feel after she gives birth.[37]

In contrast, psychologist Joan Einwohner, who works with a surrogate mother program, points out that

> women are fully capable of entering into agreements in this area and of fulfilling the obligations of a contract. Women's hormonal changes have been utilized too frequently over the centuries to enable male dominated society to make decisions for them. The Victorian era allowed women no legal rights to enter into contracts. The Victorian

era relegated them to the status of dependent children. Victorian ideas are given renewed life in the conviction of some people that women are so overwhelmed by their feelings at the time of birth that they must be protected from themselves.[38]

Surrogate Carol Pavek is similarly uncomfortable with hormonal arguments. She posits that if she is allowed the excuse of hormones to change her mind (thus harming the expectant couple and subjecting the child to the trauma of litigation), what's to stop men from using their hormones as an excuse for rape or other harms? In any case, feminists should be wary of a hormone-based argument, just as they have been wary of the hormone-related criminal defense of premenstrual syndrome.

The consent given by surrogates is also challenged as not being voluntary. Feminist Gena Corea, for example, in writing about another reproduction arrangement, in vitro fertilization, asks, "What is the real meaning of a woman's 'consent' . . . in a society in which men as a social group control not just the choices open to women but also women's *motivation* to choose?"[39]

Such an argument is a dangerous one for feminists to make. It would seem to be a step backward for women to argue that they are incapable of making decisions. That, after all, was the rationale for so many legal principles oppressing women for so long, such as the rationale behind the laws not allowing women to hold property. Clearly, any person's choices are motivated by a range of influences—economic, social, religious.

At a recent conference of law professors, it was suggested that surrogacy was wrong because women's boyfriends might talk them into being surrogates and because women might be surrogates for financial reasons. But women's boyfriends might talk them into having abortions or women might have abortions for financial reasons; nevertheless, feminists do not consider those to be adequate reasons to ban abortions. The fact that a woman's decision could be influenced by the individual men in her life or by male-dominated society does not by itself provide an adequate reason to ban surrogacy.

Various feminists have made the argument that the financial inducement to a surrogate vitiates the voluntariness of her consent. Many feminists have said that women are exploited by surrogacy.[40] They point out that in our society's social and economic conditions, some women—such as those on welfare or in dire financial need—will turn to surrogacy out of necessity rather than true choice. In my view, this is a harsh reality that must be guarded against by vigilant efforts to assure that women have equal access to the labor market and that there are sufficient social services so that poor women with children do not feel they must enter into a surrogacy arrangement in order to obtain money to provide care for their existing children.

However, the vast majority of women who have been surrogates do not allege that they have been tricked into surrogacy, nor have they done it because they needed to obtain a basic of life such as food or health care. Mary Beth Whitehead wanted to pay for her children's education. Kim Cotton wanted money to redecorate her house.[41] Another surrogate wanted money to buy a car. These do not seem to be cases of economic exploitation; there is no consensus, for example, that private education, interior decoration, and an automobile are basic needs, nor that society has an obligation to provide those items. Moreover, some surrogate mother programs specifically reject women who are below a certain income level to avoid the possibility of exploitation.

There is a sexist undertone to an argument that Mary Beth Whitehead was exploited by the paid surrogacy agreement into which she entered to get money for her children's education. If Mary Beth's husband, Rick, had taken a second job to pay for the children's education (or even to pay for their mortgage), he would not have been viewed as exploited. He would have been lauded as a responsible parent.

It undercuts the legitimacy of women's role in the workforce to assume that they are being exploited if they plan to use their money for serious purchases. It seems to harken back to a notion that women work (and should work) only for pin money (a stereotype that is the basis for justifying the firing of women in times of economic crisis). It is also disturbing that in most instances, when society suggests that a certain activity should be done for altruism, rather than money, it is generally a woman's activity.

Some people suggest that since there is a ban on payment for organs, there should be a ban on payment to a surrogate.[42] But the payment for organs is different from the payment to a surrogate, when viewed from either the side of the couple or the side of the surrogate. As the New Jersey Supreme Court has stated, surrogacy (unlike organ donation) implicates a fundamental constitutional right—the right to privacy in making procreative decisions.[43] The court erroneously assumed that the constitutional right did not extend to commercial applications. This is in conflict with the holdings of other right-to-privacy cases regarding reproductive decisions. In *Carey v. Population Services,* for example, it was acknowledged that constitutional protection of the use of contraceptives extended to their commercial availability.[44] The Court noted that "in practice, a prohibition against all sales, since more easily and less offensively enforced, might have an even more devastating effect on the freedom to choose contraception" than a ban on their use.[45]

Certainly, feminists would feel their right to an abortion was vitiated if a law were passed prohibiting payment to doctors performing abortions; such a law would erect a major barrier to access to the procedure. Similarly, a ban on payment to surrogates would inhibit the exercise of the right to produce a child with a surrogate. For such reasons, it could easily be argued that the couple's right to pay a surrogate is constitutionally protected (unlike the right to pay a kidney donor).

From the surrogate's standpoint, the situation is different as well. An organ is not meant to be removed from the body; it endangers the life of the donor to live without the organ. In contrast, babies are conceived to leave the body and the life of the surrogate is not endangered by living without the child.[46]

At various legislative hearings, women's groups have virtually begged that women be protected against themselves, against their own decisions. Adria

Hillman testified against a New York surrogacy bill on behalf of the New York State Coalition on Women's Legislative Issues. One would think that a women's group would criticize the bill as unduly intruding into women's decisions—it requires a double-check by a court on a contract made by a woman (the surrogate mother) to assure that she gave voluntary, informed consent and does not require oversight of contracts made by men. But the testimony was just the opposite. The bill was criticized as empowering the court to assess whether a surrogacy agreement protects the health and welfare of the potential child, without specifying that the judge should look into the agreement's potential effect on the natural mother.[47] What next? Will women have to go before a court when they are considering having an affair—to have a judge discern whether they will be psychologically harmed by, or later regret, the relationship?

Washington Post writer Jane Leavy has written:

> I have read volumes in defense of Mary Beth, her courage in taking on a lonely battle against the upper classes, the exploited wife of a sanitation man versus the wife of a biochemist, a woman with a 9th grade education versus a pediatrician. It all strikes me as a bit patronizing. Since when do we assume that a 29-year-old mother is incapable of making an adult decision and accepting the conse- quences of it?[48]

Surrogate mother Donna Regan similarly testified in New York that her will was not overborne in the surrogacy context: "No one came to ask me to be a surrogate mother. I went to them and asked them to allow me to be a surrogate mother.[49]

"I find it extremely insulting that there are people saying that, as a woman, I cannot make an informed choice about a pregnancy that I carry," she contin- ued, pointing out that she, like everyone, "makes other difficult choices in her life."[50]

Potential Harm to Potential Children

The third line of argument opposes surrogacy because of the potential harm it represents to potential children. Feminists have had a long-standing concern for the welfare of children. But much feminist policy in the area has been based on the idea that mothers (and family) are more appropriate decision- makers about the best interests of children than the government. Feminists have also fought against using traditions, stereotypes, and societal tolerance or intolerance as a driving force for determining what is in a child's best interest. In that respect, it is understandable that feminists rallied to the aid of Mary Beth Whitehead in order to expose and oppose the faulty grounds on which custody was being determined.[51]

However, the opposition to stereotypes being used to determine custody in a best-interests analysis is not a valid argument against surrogacy itself (which is premised not on stereotypes about the child's best interest being used to determine custody, but on a preconception agreement being used to determine custody). And when the larger issue of the advisability of surrogacy itself comes up, feminists risk falling into the trap of using arguments about potential harm to the child that have as faulty a basis as those they oppose in other areas of family law.

For example, one line of argument against surrogacy is that it is like adoption and adoption harms children. However, such an argument is not sufficiently borne out in fact. There is evidence that adopted children do as well as non-adopted children in terms of adjustment and achievement.[52] A family of two biological parents is not necessary to assure the child's well-being.

Surrogacy has also been analogized to baby-selling. Baby-selling is prohibited in our society, in part because children need a secure family life and should not have to worry that they will be sold and wrenched from their existing family. Surrogacy is distinguishable from baby-selling since the resulting child is never in a state of insecurity. From the moment of birth, he or she is under the care of the biological father and his wife, who cannot sell the child. There is thus no psychological stress to that child or to *any other existing child* that he or she may someday be sold. Moreover, no matter how much money is paid through the surrogacy arrangement, the child, upon birth, cannot be treated like a commodity—a car or a television set. Laws against child abuse and neglect come into play.

Paying a biological mother to give her child up for traditional adoption is criticized since the child may go to an "undeserving" stranger, whose mere ability to pay does not signify sufficient merit for rearing a child. In paid surrogacy, by contrast, the child is turned over to the biological father. This biological bond has traditionally been considered to be a sufficient indicator of parental merit.

Another argument about potential harm to the resulting children is that parents will expect more of a surrogate child because of the $10,000 they have spent on her creation. But many couples spend more than that on infertility treatments without evidence that they expect more of the child. A Cesarean section costs twice as much as natural childbirth, yet the parents don't expect twice as much of the children. Certainly, the $10,000 is a modest amount compared to what parents will spend on their child over her lifespan.

Surrogacy has also been opposed because of its potential effect on the surrogate's other children. Traditionally, except in cases of clear abuse, parents have been held to be the best decision-makers about their children's best interests. Applying this to surrogacy, the surrogate (and not society) would be the best judge of whether on not her participation in a surrogacy program will harm her children. Not only are parents thought best able to judge their child's needs, but parents can profoundly influence the effects of surrogacy on the child. Children take their cues about things from the people around them. There is no reason to believe that the other children of the surrogate will necessarily feel threatened by their mother's contractual pregnancy. If the children are told from the beginning that this is the contracting couple's child—not a part of their own family—they will realize that they themselves are not in danger of being relinquished.

Surrogate Donna Regan told her child that "the reason we did this was because they [the contracting couple] wanted a child to love as much as we love him." Regan contrasted her case to the Whitehead case: "In the Mary Beth Whitehead case, the child did not see this as something her mother was doing for someone else, so, of course, the attitude that she got from that was that something was being taken away rather than something being given."[53]

It seems ironic for feminists to embrace the argument that certain activities might inherently lead their children to fear abandonment, and that consequently such activities should be banned. Feminists have fought hard to gain access for women to amniocentesis and late-stage abortions of fetuses with a genetic defect[54]—even in light of similarly anecdotal evidence that when the woman aborts, her *other* children will feel that, they too, might be "sent to heaven" by their mother.[55] Indeed, it could be argued that therapeutic abortion is more devastating to the remaining children than is surrogacy. After all, the brother or sister who is aborted was intended to be part of the family; moreover, he or she is dead, not just living with other people. I personally do not feel that the potential effect of either therapeutic abortion or surrogacy on the pregnant woman's other children is a sufficient reason to ban the procedures, particularly in light of the fact that parents can mediate how their children perceive and handle the experiences.

The reactions of outsiders to surrogacy may, however, be beyond the control of parents and may upset the children. But is this a sufficient reason to ban surrogacy? William Pierce seems to think so. He says that the children of surrogates "are being made fun of. Their lives are going to be ruined."[56] It would seem odd to let societal intolerance guide what relationships are permissible. Along those lines, a judge in a lesbian custody case replied to the argument that children could be harmed by stigma by stating:

> It is just as reasonable to expect that they will emerge better equipped to search out their own standards of right and wrong, better able to perceive that the majority is not always correct in its moral judgments, and better able to understand the importance of conforming their beliefs to the requirements of reasons and tested knowledge, not the constraints of currently popular sentiment or prejudice.[57]

Feminism Revisited

Feminists are taking great pride that they have mobilized public debate against surrogacy. But the precedent they are setting in their alliance with politicians like Henry Hyde and groups like the Catholic church is one whose policy is "protect women, even against their own decisions" and "protect children at all costs" (presumably, in latter applications, even against the needs and desires of women). This is certainly the thrust of the New Jersey Supreme Court decision against surrogacy, which cites as support for its holding the notorious *In re A. C.* case. In that case a woman's decision to refuse a Cesarean section was overridden based on an unsubstantiated possibility of benefit to her future child.[58]

In fact, the tenor of the New Jersey Supreme Court decision is reminiscent of earlier decisions "protecting" women that have been roundly criticized by feminists. The U.S. Supreme Court in 1872 felt it was necessary to prevent Myra Bradwell and all other women from practicing law—in order to protect women and their children. And when courts upheld sexist employment laws that kept women out of employment that men were allowed to take, they used language that might have come right out of the New Jersey Supreme Court's decision in the Baby M case. A woman's

> physical structure and a proper discharge of her maternal functions— having in view not merely her health, but the well-being of the race— justify legislation to protect her from the greed as well as the passion of man. The limitations which this statute place upon her contractual powers, upon her right to agree with her employer as to the time she shall labor, are not imposed solely for her benefit, but also largely for the benefit of all.[59]

The New Jersey Supreme Court rightly pointed out that not everything should be for sale in our society. But the examples given by the court, such as occupational safety and health laws prohibiting workers from voluntarily accepting money to work in an unsafe job, apply to both men and women. In addition, an unsafe job presents risks that we would not want people to undertake, whether or not they received pay. In contrast, a policy against paid surrogacy prevents women from taking risks (pregnancy and relinquishment) that they are allowed to take for free. It applies disparately—men are still allowed to relinquish their parental rights in advance of conception and to receive money for their role in providing the missing male factor for procreation.

Some feminists are comfortable with advocating disparate treatment on the grounds that gestation is such a unique experience that it has no male counterpart at law and so deserves a unique legal status.[60] The special nature of gestation, according to this argument, gives rise to special rights—such as the right for the surrogate to change her mind and assert her legal parenthood after the child is born.

The other side of the gestational coin, which has not been sufficiently addressed by these feminists, is that with special rights come special responsibilities. If gestation can be viewed as unique in surrogacy, then it can be viewed as unique in other areas. Pregnant women could be held to have responsibilities that other members of society do not have—such as the responsibility to have a Cesarean section against their wishes in order to protect the health of a child (since only pregnant women are in the unique position of being able to influence the health of the child).

Some feminists have criticized surrogacy as turning participating women, albeit with their consent, into reproductive vessels. I see the danger of the anti-surrogacy arguments as potentially turning *all* women into reproductive vessels, without their consent, by providing government oversight for women's decisions and creating a disparate legal category for gestation. Moreover, by breathing life into arguments that feminists have put to rest in other contexts, the currrent rationales opposing surrogacy could undermine a larger feminist agenda.

Notes

1. Iver Peterson, "Baby M Custody Trial Splits Ranks of Feminists over Issue of Exploitation," *New York Times,* Feb. 24, 1987 (quoting Linda Bowker).

2. Bob Port, "Feminists Come to the Aid of Whitehead's Case," *St. Petersburg Times,* Feb. 23, 1987, 1A.

3. Brief filed on behalf of Amici Curiae, the Foundation on Economic Trends et at., In the matter of Baby M, New Jersey Supreme Court, Docket No. FM-25314-86E (hereafter cited as "Brief"). (The feminists joining in the brief included Betty Friedan, Gloria Steinem, Gena Corea, Barbara Katz Rothman, Lois Gould, Michelle Harrison, Kathleen Lahey, Phyllis Chesler, and Letty Cottin Pogrebin.)

4. See, e.g., Roe v. Wade, 410 U.S. 113 (1973); Griswold v. Connecticut, 381 U.S. 479 (1965); Meyer v. Nebraska, 262 U.S. 390 (1923); Pierce v. Society of Sisters, 268 U.S. 510 (1928).

5. See, e.g., Karst, "The Freedom of Intimate Association," *Yale Law Journal,* 89 (1980): 624.

6. Prior to conception and during pregnancy, the surrogate mother contract is a personal service contract. However, after the child's birth, no further services on the part of the surrogate are needed. Thus, enforcing a provision providing for the father's custody of the child is not the enforcement of a personal services contract. It is like the enforcement of a court order on custody or the application of a paternity statute.

7. Lori Andrews, "The Aftermath of Baby M: Proposed State Laws on Surrogate Motherhood," *Hastings Center Report,* 17 (Oct./Nov. 1987): 31–40, at 37.

8. In re Baby M, 217 N.J. Super, 313, 525 A.2d 1128, 1159 (1987).

9. Jhordan C. v. Mary K., 179 Cal. App. 3d 386, 224 Cal. Rptr. 530 (1986).

10. *Surrogate Parenthood and New Reproductive Technologies, A Joint Public Hearing, before the N.Y. State Assembly, N.Y. State Senate, Judiciary Committees* (Oct. 16, 1986) (statement of Bob Arenstein at 103–4, 125); *In The Matter of a Hearing on Surrogate Parenting before the N.Y. Standing Committee on Child Care* (May 8, 1987) [statement of Adria Hillman at 174, statement of Mary Ann Dibari at 212 ("the prostitution of motherhood")].

11. *Surrogacy Arrangement Act of 1987: Hearing on H.R. 2433, before the Subcomm. on Transportation, Tourism, and Hazardous Materials,* 100th Cong., 1st Sess. (Oct. 15, 1987) (statement of Gena Corea at 3, 5); Robert Gould, N.Y. Testimony (May 8, 1987), supra note 10, at 233 (slavery).

12. Arthur Morrell, U.S. Testimony (Oct. 15, 1987), supra note 11, at 1.

13. William Pierce, U.S. Testimony (Oct. 15, 1987), supra note 11, at 2, citing Harvard Law Professor Lawrence Tribe.

14. Brief, supra note 3, at 19.

15. Port, supra note 2, at 7A, quoting Phyllis Chesler.

16. Gena Corea, U.S. Testimony (Oct. 15, 1987), supra note 11, at 3; Hillman, N.Y. Testimony (May 8, 1987), supra note 10, at 174.

17. Ellen Goodman, "Checking the Baby M Contract," *Boston Globe,* March 24, 1987, 15.

18. Gena Corea, U.S. Testimony (Oct. 15, 1987), supra note 11, at 5; Hillman, N.Y. Testimony (May 8, 1987) supra note 10, at 174.

19. Gena Corea, U.S. Testimony (Oct. 15, 1987), supra note 11, at 5.

20. Id.

21. Id.: 2.

22. Elizabeth Kane, U.S. Testimony (Oct. 15, 1987), supra note 11, at 1.

23. Kay Longcope, "Standing up for Mary Beth," *Boston Globe,* March 5, 1987, 81, 83 (quoting Janice Raymond).

24. Brief, supra note 3, at 14.

25. Robert Gould, N.Y. Testimony (May 8, 1987), supra note 10, at 232.

26. Judianne Densen-Gerber, N.Y. Testimony (May 8, 1987), supra note 10, at 253; Robert Gould, N.Y. Testimony (May 8, 1987), supra note 10, at 232.

27. Robert Gould, N.Y. Testimony (May 8, 1987), supra note 10, at 232.

28. Henry Hyde, U.S. Testimony (Oct. 15, 1987), supra note 11, at 1 ("Commercial surrogacy arrangements, by rendering children into chattel, are in my opinion, immoral."); DiBari, N.Y. Testimony (May 8, 1987), supra note 10, at 212.

29. John Ray, U.S. Testimony (Oct. 15, 1987), supra note 11, at 7.

30. See, e.g., Maureen McGuire and Nancy J. Alexander, "Artificial Insemination of Single Women," *Fertility and Sterility,* 43 (Feb. 1985): 182–84; Raschke and Raschke, "Family Conflict and Children's Self-Concept: A Comparison of Intact and Single Parent Families," *Journal of Marriage and the Family,* 41 (1979): 367; Weiss, "Growing up a Little Faster," *Journal of Social Issues,* 35 (1979): 97.

31. See, e.g., Rynearson, "Relinquishment and Its Maternal Complications: A Preliminary Study," *American Journal of Psychiatry,* 139 (1982): 338; Deykin, Campbell, Patti, "The Postadoption Experience of Surrendering Parents," *American Journal of Orthopsychiatry,* 54 (1984): 271.

32. Betsy Aigen, N.Y. Testimony (May 8, 1987), supra note 10, at 18.

33. Robert Arenstein, U.S. Testimony (Oct. 15, 1987), supra note 11, at 9.

34. Brief, supra note 3, at 30–31.

35. In re Baby M, 109 N.J. 396; 537 A.2d 1227, 1248 (1988).

36. See Brief filed on behalf of Amicus Curiae the Gruter Institute, In the Matter of Baby M, New Jersey Supreme Court, Docket No. FM-25314-86E.

37. *Hearing in re Surrogate Parenting: Hearing on S.B. 1429, before Senators Goodhue, Dunne, Misters Balboni, Abramson, and Amgott* (April 10, 1987) (statement of Elaine Rosenfeld at 187). A similar argument made by Adria Hillman, N.Y. Testimony (May 8, 1987), supra note 10, at 175.

38. Joan Einwohner, N.Y. Testimony (April 10, 1987), supra note 37, at 110–11.

39. Gena Corea, *The Mother Machine* (New York: Harper & Row, 1985), 3.

40. Brief, supra note 3, at 10, 13; Judy Breidbart, N.Y. Testimony (May 8, 1987), supra note 10, at 168.

41. K. Cotton and D. Winn, *Baby Cotton: For Love and Money* (1985).

42. Karen Peters, N.Y. Testimony (May 8, 1987), supra note 10, at 121.

43. In re Baby M, 109 N.J. 396; 537 A.2d 1227, 1253 (1988).

44. Carey v. Population Services Int'l., 431 U.S. 678 (1977).

45. Carey v. Population Services, Int'l., 431 U.S. 678, 688 (1976) (citation omitted).

46. Betsy Aigen, N.Y. Testimony (May 8, 1987), supra note 10, at 11–12.

47. Adria Hillman, N.Y. Testimony (May 8, 1987), supra note 10, at 177–78.

48. Jane Leavy, "It Doesn't Take Labor Pains to Make a Real Mom," *Washington Post,* April 4, 1987.

49. Donna Regan, N.Y. Testimony (May 8, 1987), supra note 10, at 157.

50. Id.

51. Michelle Harrison, "Social Construction of Mary Beth Whitehead," *Gender and Society,* 1 (Sept. 1987): 300–11.

52. Teasdale and Owens, "Influence of Paternal Social Class on Intelligence Level in Male Adoptees and Non-Adoptees," *British Journal of Educational Psychology,* 56 (1986): 3.

53. Donna Regan, N.Y. Testimony (May 8 1987), supra note 10, at 156.

54. See, e.g., the briefs filed by feminist organizations in Thornburgh v. American College of Obstetricians, 476 U.S. 747 (1986).

55. See, e.g., J. Fletcher, *Coping with Genetic Disorders: A Guide for Counseling* (San Francisco: Harper & Row, 1982).

56. William Pierce, N.Y. Testimony (May 8, 1987), supra note 10, at 86. It should be pointed out that kids hassle other kids for a wide range of reasons. A child might equally be made fun of for being the recipient of a kidney transplant or being the child of a garbage man.

57. M.P. v. S.P., 169 N.J. Super, 425, 438, 404 A.2d 1256, 1263 (Super. Ct. App. Div. 1979).

58. In re Baby M, 109 N.J. 396; 537 A.2d 1227, 1254 n. 13 (1988), citing In re A. C., 533 A.2d 611 (D.C. App. 1987).

59. Muller v. Oregon, 208 U.S. 412, 422 (1907).

60. See Brief, supra note 3, at 11.

The Mother Machine

Gena Corea

Reproductive Continuity: *Capturing the "Magic" of Maternity*

I want to . . . go back to the beginning, to the time, centuries ago, when woman was the sole creator of the child. I go back in order to understand how the male's role in procreation—at first perceived to be none at all—affected his consciousness.[1]

In Neolithic society, man knew nothing of his part in procreation and made no connection between sexual intercourse and the birth of a baby nine months later. A woman's body, he saw, ripened with child as a tree ripened with fruit. Clearly a spirit impregnated a woman, perhaps entering her body through the wind, a star, a bird, the rain, or the moon.

Humankind revered woman's awe-inspiring power to bring forth life and to nourish life with the milk of her body. For thousands of years, they worshiped a female deity, the Great Goddess, in the image of this human mother. The Goddess was worshiped for a period five times as long as recorded history, far longer than any other deities. (We will return to the Goddess later to record her violent overthrow).

Man's belief that he played little or no part in procreation affected him deeply, as we see in the overwhelming evidence of birth or parturition envy noted by psychiatrists, sociologists, historians, anthropologists and mothers observing small sons. Early man, primitive man, and Christian man have all had various methods of trying to make woman's procreative power their own. He has mutilated his genitals in an attempt to render him capable of giving birth. Or simulated labor and delivery (couvade). Or worn women's clothing. Or conducted initiation ceremonies in which the male sponsors of boys give birth to men. Psychiatrist Bruno Bettelheim has written at length about some of these methods.

First, self-mutilation. The Galloi, priests of the goddess Cybele, voluntarily castrated themselves, and ran through the streets holding their genitals in their hands. At a certain point, each priest would throw his genitals into a

From *The Mother Machine*, Chapters 15 & 16. New York: Harper & Row, 1985, pp. 283–317. Abridged. Copyright © 1985 by Gena Corea. Reprinted by permission of HarperCollins Publishers.

woman's house and the woman would give him female clothing, a type of clothing he would wear for the rest of his life. This custom, prevalent in Rome from the second century B.C. through the fourth century A.D., shows that men were willing "to become 'female' in order to share woman's superior powers" (Bettelheim, 1968, p. 93).

In less drastic surgery, men often gave women the products of the mutilation—blood or foreskin. Bettelheim suggests that what men expected in return for this offering was "a share in women's great and secret power of procreation, a gift that only women can bestow because only women possess it."

Male expectations in performing subincision appear to be similar. Subincision is an initiation ceremony practiced among many primitive tribes, including the central Aborigine tribes of Australia. The ceremony involves the slitting of the penis in an apparent attempt to make the male genitals into female ones. The subincision hole is called a "vagina" or a "penis womb." The subincision wound, called a "vulva," is repeatedly opened so that it bleeds again, mimicking menstruation. The people themselves compare the blood from the wound to menses. In New Guinea, where the men also practice subincision, a man bleeding from his penis must observe the same taboos a menstruating woman must.

One commentator has concluded that "through subincision the young man is supposed to be changed into a woman. . . . The initiation ceremonies change boys into women, or, rather, man-woman" (Bryk, quoted in Bettelheim, 1968, p. 106).

Couvade, often explained as a custom practiced to distract evil spirits so that they do not harm the baby, is another male attempt to take over the function of women. Under the extreme form of this custom, the pregnant woman works until a few hours before the birth, then goes into the forest with some women and bears the child. Within a few hours, she must return to work. Her husband, however, lies on a hammock, sometimes simulating labor and childbirth. While the women nurse and care for him, he fasts or eats a weak gruel. His confinement may last for days or even weeks. The full couvade has been observed on all continents in both ancient and recent time. According to the *Encyclopedia Britannica,* it has been reported as recently as the early twentieth century in the Basque country and in Brazil.

Through this custom, men detract from the woman's importance and pretend to give birth themselves. But, Bettelheim comments, they copy only the insignificant externals of the birth experience, and not the essentials, which they cannot duplicate. "Such an apeing of superficials only emphasizes the more how much the real, essential powers are envied," he wrote.

Transvestism is also an attempt to acquire woman's power. It prevailed in the majority of ancient priesthoods. Sometimes, as among the Naven tribe of New Guinea, transvestism plays a part in an initiation ceremony for boys. A boy's male sponsor dresses up in widow's clothing, makes himself look pregnant, is referred to as "mother," and wanders among the people crying out in a high, falsetto voice for his child, the boy initiate.

Initiation ceremonies are rebirth rituals in which the male sponsors of boys give birth to men. Their purpose seems to be to assert that men, too, can bear life. Men frankly act out childbirth in some of the ceremonies. In the Liberian Poro society, the crocodile spirit, a representative of the male group, swallows up the boy initiates and remains pregnant with them for up to four years. (During this time the boys are living in the bush.) When the boys—now young men—return home, they must pretend to be newborns. Such initiation rituals are sometimes accompanied by the myth that they were stolen from women and sometimes that women were killed to get them.

Christian priests rebirth children even today through the power of their God, a phenomenon about which Una Stannard, author of *Mrs. Man,* has written. The early Christians believed one was not truly born until after baptism. Women merely birthed human beings into mortal, fleshly life while men birthed humans into eternal, immortal life through their own amniotic fluid, the baptismal waters. A Catholic rite for the consecration of the baptismal font actually refers to the font as a "stainless womb." In a letter written in 256 A.D., Cyprian wrote: "The birth of Christians is in baptism. He, Christ, generated us from our mother— the [baptismal] water" (Stannard, 1977). As Stannard points out, the Church, embodiment of the Father god, had taken over the procreation power of women and become *Mater Ecclesia.* She quotes Tertullian, who said the Church was "the true mother of the living . . . the second Adam," and Paul in Galatians in the New Testament who asserted that the Church was "the mother of us all."

Men not only birth; they suckle. It is Christ's word, not woman's milk, which truly nourishes man. Clement, for example, compared seeking Christ to suckling: "For to those babes that suck the Word, the Father's breasts of love supply the milk" (Stannard, 1977, p. 294).

Evidence of a male desire to possess woman's procreative power has been found not only by anthropologists working among primitive peoples and feminists observing Christian practices, but also by psychologists treating adolescent boys. For example, in a paper on the desire of boys to bear children, Edith Jacobson mentioned that among her male patients she had had "occasion to observe . . . an intense and persistent envy of female reproductive ability—an envy which is often disguised by a seemingly normal masculinity" (quoted in Bettelheim, 1968). She protested that pertinent studies on male birth envy had been conspicuously neglected by psychiatrists. Commenting on this protest, psychiatrist Dr. Wolfgang Lederer wrote: "Indeed, of our fear and envy of women, we, the psychoanalytic-papers-writing-men, have managed to maintain a dignified fraternal silence" (Lederer, 1968, p. 153).

That the desire to bear babies is not confined to psychiatric patients is suggested by an acknowledgment in the children's book *The Boy Who Wanted a Baby.* Author Wendy Lichtman thanks "the men and boys who were vulnerable and brave in telling me their feelings of longing for that which is not possible" (Lichtman, 1982).

So in the beginning, woman was the sole creator of the child. But at some unknown time, some unknown people discovered paternity, the connection between intercourse and a child's birth. Man then realized that by lying with a woman, he impregnated her and fathered the child she bore. He understood that he was physically linked with the child, that it was flesh of his flesh. He came to see the child as a continuation of himself. In order to understand how the discovery of paternity relates to the new reproductive technologies, we must step back a moment and look at a theory proposed by Mary O'Brien, a sociologist at the Ontario Institute for Studies in Education and a former midwife. In *The Politics of Reproduction,* O'Brien points out the following: Impressive bodies of philosophical thought have examined certain human biological necessities—the need to eat, to express sexuality, and to die—and have shown how these needs have shaped human understanding (or consciousness) and our relationship to the world. Marx transformed our need to eat into a theoretical system in which productive labor remakes our consciousness. The existentialists did the same for death, and Freud, showing how libido shapes our consciousness, for sexuality. But there is another biological necessity that male philosophers have ignored: birth. There is no philosophy of birth comparable to those concerned with labor, sexuality, and death.

Yet birth, too, shapes our human understanding. O'Brien notes that the reproductive experience for men and women differs, so men and women have a different reproductive consciousness. For woman, reproduction is a continuous experience. She participates in intercourse. The fertilized egg grows within her body during the nine months of pregnancy. She births the child in an act of labor, sometimes nourishes the child with her milk, and raises the child.

For man, reproduction is a discontinuous experience. He ejaculates his sperm into the woman and then goes about his business. Nine months later, a woman bears a child that is his as well as hers. But he has a hard time imagining that child as his. To make a connection between copulation and the birth of a child much later requires an intellectual act. Paternity, then, is an abstract idea—conceptualizing a cause and effect relationship between copulation and childbirth—while maternity is an experience, O'Brien points out.

Man's sperm is alienated (that is, separated) from him in the sex act and this alienation negates him as a parent. He has no certainty that the child born nine months later is *his* child. Woman's seed, unified with the man's and developed into a baby within her body, is also alienated from her at birth. But she undergoes a process that reconciles her to this separation. Her labor in childbirth confirms for her the certainty that this child is *her* child, and gives her a relationship to the child similar to that which a worker has toward a product. After her labor, she need take no further action to annul her separation from the human race.

When his seed is alienated, man is separated from the continuity of the human species, from a sense of unity with natural process. He does not actually experience a link between generations. While woman has a sense of her connection with the next generation in the labor through which she births that generation, man is isolated within the dimensions of his own lifespan. He has not labored to produce the child, except in the relatively trivial expenditure of energy in sexual intercourse.

Alienation is the separation of a human being from the world and from the experience of the world; it is a negation of self. O'Brien points out, as the philosopher Hegel did before her, that human consciousness resists alienation and negation of the self.

Man's nullity as a parent appears to be unbearable to him. To make that nullity bearable, to neutralize his separation from his seed and from genetic continuity, man had to do something. What he has done is appropriate the child.[2] Defying the uncertainty of paternity, he works in cooperation with other men to assert a proprietorial right to a child, one that nature has not provided for him. His assertion of a right to the child must be supported by ideologies of male supremacy and by a host of social structures. The legal ownership of children and man's need to legitimate on the basis of biological fatherhood can be seen as attempts on the part of the male to reclaim the child, to overcome the discontinuous nature of his reproductive experience. The idea that women contribute only "matter" to babies while men contribute spirit—an idea that, as we will later see, prevailed for centuries—is also an attempt by men to resist the alienation of their seed and reclaim the child.

We see man's appropriation of the child in the laws throughout the world, which, until less than a century ago, gave fathers sole guardianship of children. The father had an absolute right to take the children away from his wife during marriage and, upon his death, could bequeath that guardianship to another male rather than to their mother. Fathers were routinely granted custody of children upon divorce. It was not until 1886 in England that, under certain rare circumstances, a woman could get custody of her children. All but five states in America in the 1890s gave fathers sole legal guardianship of children.

To assure paternity, man had to control the sexual activities of his woman, allowing no other man to impregnate her. Then he could pass his name, power and property down through his sons. In this way (although O'Brien does not state this), he could achieve continuity over time. The creation of the private realm helped men to control their women. Men separated social life into private and public realms in order to ensure themselves exclusive rights to a particular woman, rights buttressed by the woman's physical separation from other men. With marriage and the patriarchal family, two of the institutions men developed to solve the problem of male separation from reproduction, wives who committed "adultery" (a new crime) were severely punished and children born out of wedlock were declared "illegitimate."[3]

It seems to me that whether O'Brien's theory is fully right or not is unimportant. What *is* important is that she has opened up the issue to discussion. She has pointed out how the effect of reproduction on consciousness has been rendered invisible in patriarchal society. She has demonstrated the need for a philosophy of birth, a philosophy that remains to be worked out.[4]

O'Brien has pointed out that because of the discontinuous nature of man's reproductive experience, he lacks a sense of genetic continuity. Reproductive technologies can give him that continuity over time through these means:

Sperm banks and artificial insemination, which will allow a man to engender children even after he is dead. If fact, the man who originated the concept of frozen sperm banks in 1866, Mantegazza, suggested that a man, while dying on a battlefield, could still beget a legal heir through his frozen sperm at home. More than a century later, Dr. Jerome K. Sherman, American pioneer in techniques for freezing human sperm, observed that by storing his sperm, "man can induce conception in absence of testes, in old age, and long after his death" (Sherman, 1973).

Sex determination. By ensuring the birth of a son, a man assures himself a form of immortality. He sees himself reborn in his son.

The creation of an exact replica of man, his clone. One commentator has noted that "having oneself cloned is yet another effort to assure some form of personal continuity; it is simply more direct than having normal offspring, a child formed by sexual union and incorporating a variety of genetic strains [that is, a mother's as well as a father's]. A human clone would be totally identical to its donor-father, and could step directly into his shoes, as it were, carry on and perfect whatever he had begun, be his heir in the most immediate and literal sense of the term" (Ebon, 1978, pp. 2–3).

Reproductive technologies do more than give males a sense of continuity over time. They are transforming the experience of motherhood and placing it under the control of men. Woman's claim to maternity is being loosened, man's claim to paternity strengthened. Moreover, these techniques are creating for women the same kind of discontinuous reproductive experience men now have. "That is one of the absolutely crucial things about them," comments Jalna Hanmer, a sociologist at England's University of Bradford who has studied the technologies. The woman begins to feel that the baby is not hers, Hanmer observes. The more complex the technologies become, the more a woman must use her intellect to figure out in what way she contributed to the child's birth. Through her egg? Through her womb? Through her labor? As paternity always has been, maternity is becoming an act of intellect—for example, making a causal connection between the extraction of an egg and the birth of a child to another woman nine months later. Meanwhile, those men who extract eggs, culture them, transfer embryos, surgically birth babies, or control the dials on the artificial womb will have a more continuous reproductive experience than men have ever before had.

How will woman's claim to maternity be loosened? As one pioneer in reproductive technology explained to me, in the future there will be three kinds of mothers:

The genetic mother who "donates" or sells her eggs
The surrogate or natal mother who carries the baby
The social mother who raises the child

Under this system of dismembered motherhood, none of these three women will have a compelling claim to her child. Nor does Dr. Joseph Fletcher think she ought to. Fletcher is a medical ethicist associated with the University of Virginia School of Medicine. He believes that a woman whose egg is used to produce a baby should have no claim of any kind on the child born of that egg. Parental relationships need to be "reconceptualized," he writes. "They cannot anymore be based on blood or wombs or even genes. . . . The mere fact of conceiving a child or donating the elements of its conception or gestating it does not establish anybody as a father or mother." Parenthood, he maintains, will have to be understood morally rather than biologically.

As Fletcher notes, with uterine and ovarian transplants, with egg and embryo transfers, "Maternity now is in question too, as paternity used to be."

The modern reproductive technologist championed by men like Fletcher is, in his quest, a brother to the alchemist who looked for one universal medicine, "some powerful substance that would enable men to control matter and live forever" (Cummings, 1966). The alchemist sought nothing less than "the magic of maternity" conferred upon men. This is the conclusion of scholars Sally G. Allen and Joanne Hubbs, who studied a treatise by a prominent seventeenth century alchemist. They found that it describes man's aggressive arrogation of woman's procreation power. The great alchemist Paracelsus answered "yes" to the question: "Whether it was possible for art and nature that a man should be born outside a woman's body and a natural mother's." The culmination of the alchemical process is frequently depicted through the image of the birth of a male child, who, Paracelsus wrote: "By art received life, through art . . . received a body, flesh, bones and blood and through art . . . was born" (Allen and Hubbs, 1980, p. 211).

Reproductive technologists now aim to bring forth life through "art" rather than nature and enable a man to be not only the father but also the mother of his child.

Transsexual surgery may someday help transform men into mothers. This surgery is, in the majority of cases, now performed on men in order to construct artificial females. Men cut off the penises and testicles of other men, surgically construct a "vagina" and inject hormones into their patients. Fletcher comments on this surgery and then continues: "Furthermore, transplant or replacement medicine foresees the day, after the automatic rejection of alien tissues is overcome, when a uterus can be implanted in a human male's body—his abdomen has spaces—and gestation started by artificial fertilization and egg transfer." By decreasing the activity of the testes, physicians could also "stimulate milk from the man's rudimentary breasts—men too have mammary glands. If surgery could not construct a cervical canal the delivery could be effected by a cesarean section and the male or transsexualized mother could nurse his own baby. . . .

"As it is at present," he continued, "women have four reproductive functions: to menstruate, ovulate, gestate, and lactate—while men only impregnate. But . . . surgery may soon be trading these functions back and forth; they have already begun doing it with both surgery and hormones."

In this way, reproductive technologists, like the alchemists, would be conferring "the magic of maternity" on men. . . .

While much experimentation remains to be done before men can indeed bear babies (if they ever really can), the fact that some researchers in reproductive technology are already predicting the advent of male mothers is noteworthy. . . .

Fletcher points out that in the biblical creation story, there is no mother at all. In Genesis, God the Father was the first mother. God formed Adam artificially from the dust. Then Adam became the second mother, birthing Eve while the male God acted as obstetrician. Only on the third round did we get a female mother with Eve birthing Cain and Abel. Fletcher writes: "Women have continued to be the mothers ever since, until now when reproduction once more takes the form of artifice as it did in the Garden of Eden— including motherless children and male mothers." We have come full circle, he writes. The new biology is restoring the modes of birth in effect before the Fall (Fletcher, 1974).

The Father God's birthing of Adam and later of Jesus, his "only-begotten" son (a phrase which does not mean "this *one,* or *only* son" but rather "alone-begotten" by the Father without a mate), are expressions of what bioethicist Dr. Janice Raymond terms a basic patriarchal myth: Single parenthood by the father. The reproductive technologies are an acting out of that myth. Fathers can be, or appear to be, the sole parent through: surrogate motherhood; destruction of the female genetic component of the egg and injection into the egg of two sperm; cloning; and gestation in an artifical womb. One embryologist wonders how women will react "to being deprived of their role in reproduction not just as provider of the egg and a nine-month incubator, but also of anything to do with the process at all, from start to finish? A single male, alone on another planet, could theoretically reproduce a whole population from a piece of his own skin, given efficient incubators and a cloning technique!" (Francoeur, 1970, p. 158)

If or when technology makes it possible for men to create life and give birth in their laboratories, women need not maintain their procreative capacity. Indeed, commentator Edward Grossman has written that women who use artificial wombs might choose to be sterilized.

In an article entitled "The Obsolescent Mother: A Scenario," Grossman explains approvingly how technology may destroy the awesomeness of woman's childbearing process, a spectacle "with its final event as if something were coming to inexorable term," which "still has about it a sense of prehistory, savage and elemental." This spectacle strikes both the savage and the civilized mind as awesome, he writes. Childbirth, together with the other "striking biological events" in a woman's body, may lead some to conclude that anatomy is destiny. But men are changing that. Their medicine and technology are transforming woman into a male-like being. Her cyclical, periodic nature is obliterated with hormones (such as those found in the Pill) to give her the linear biology of a man.

Still, she continues to give birth. "So long as we reproduce ourselves, we also reproduce the spectacle of a woman withdrawing into herself, becoming huge, and in blood and tumult bringing forth the succeeding generation. This is the stuff myths are made of. . . . Technology, which has gone part of the way toward destroying it [the myth], may yet destroy the rest" (Grossman, 1971).

To describe what we are now witnessing, "revolution" is too small a word. . . .[5]

Reproductive Control: *The War against the Womb*

Men employ the "old reproductive technologies in their obstetrics and gynecology specialty and, in this way, hold a monopoly on childbirth, contraceptive, abortion, and sterilization services. So they are able to exercise a primitive control over reproduction. But soon the "new" reproductive technologies will enable them to actually take over the life-giving powers of women. "Thank you for my baby," Lesley Brown said to her obstetrician Patrick Steptoe who, with Robert Edwards, was "lab-parent" to the world's first test-tube baby.

In papers reporting research on these technologies, men frequently state that they are taking control over woman's ovulation and imply that by doing so they are creating a more efficient method of reproduction. . . .

When reproductive engineers manipulate the bodies of female animals today, they are clear, blunt and unapologetic about why they are doing it. They want to turn the females into machines for producing "superior" animals or into incubators for the embryos of more "valuable" females. They want, as one entrepreneur told me, to "manufacture embryos at a reduced cost.". . .

When reproductive engineers manipulate the bodies of human females—those beings, who, like animals, are a part of nature men must control—their language changes. Today they say they are manipulating women's bodies out of compassion; to bring new hope to the infertile; to prevent birth defects; to increase women's options, expand their freedom. Obscuring the impact of reproductive engineering on women as a class, they exphasize the "rights" of individual women to use these technologies.

The decision to change the language used when discussing the application of animal breeding techniques to women may in some cases be quite conscious. Reviewing the medical and legal literature on AID, Dr. Bernard Rubin noted that such phrases as "therapeutic donor insemination" and "semi-adoption" had been coined "to get away from the comparisons with animal husbandry" (Rubin, 1965).

Although *today,* the language men employ in speaking of the use of reproductive technology on women differs from that employed in speaking of its use on animals, it may not always be so. Women may find that the connection men have made for centuries between women and animals still lives on in patriarchal minds just as it lives on in men's laws and practices. Women and animals remain parts of nature to be controlled and subjugated. . . .

Now men are far beyond the stage at which they expressed their envy of woman's procreative power through couvade, transvestism, subincision. They are beyond merely giving spiritual birth in their baptismal-font wombs, beyond giving physical birth with their electronic fetal monitors, their forceps, their knives.

Now they have laboratories.

Notes

1. [In the introduction to her book *The Mother Machine,* from which this selection comes, Gena Corea writes: ". . . I often refer to the developers and supporters of reproductive technology as 'men.' In doing so, I recognize the following: The overwhelming majority of reproductive engineers are male. The overwhelming majority of persons on whose bodies these men experiment are female. The technology used emerges from a science developed by men according to their own values and sense of reality. . . . When I write the word 'men' in this book, I am writing about some individuals, but also about the institution of masculinist politics, about men as a social category and dominant class" (pp. 3–4).—Editor.]

2. He does something further. He seeks principles of continuity, what O'Brien terms "some order of procession which transcends individual life spans in some self-regenerating way." Those principles have included hereditary monarchy; primogeniture; a political community that exists before we are born and remains after we die; and the notion of eternity (O'Brien, 1981).

3. The changeover from a matriarchal to a patriarchal family occurred over a period of 3,000 years and took place in different places at different times, as Barbara G. Walker, author of *The Woman's Encyclopedia of Myths and Secrets,* explained in an interview. In Egypt, both matriarchal and patriarchal families co-existed at the same time, she pointed out. Walker's guess is that the changeover occurred in the first millennium B.C. in most of the civilized world. The concept of adultery arrived with the patriarchal family.

4. We may not yet have the best handle on exactly what it is about woman's procreative power that men envy. Philosopher Mary Daly warns against womb envy theories, which "trick women into fixating upon womb, female genitalia, and breasts as our ultimately most valuable endowments." Fixating on women's procreative organs, either to disparage or glorify them, is an expression of fetishism, she adds. She argues that what men really envy is "female creative energy in *all* of its dimensions" (Daly, 1978, p. 60). Elizabeth Fisher also cautions that women are enslaved by being worshiped as mothers or breeders. "When woman is worshiped for her 'natural powers,' woe betide her humanity" (Fisher, 1979, p. 241, p. 252).

5. Corea, 1980. Because of the patriarchal view of a woman's body as a passive vessel, as matter upon which the male acts, many men have now, as they did centuries ago, a distorted view of the human reproductive process. They cannot imagine the female body *doing* anything. But it does. For example, the woman's cervical mucus plays an active role in fertilization.

The secretions in the female reproductive tract also capacitate sperm. That is, they initiate physiologic changes in the sperm so the sperm is capable of penetrating the egg. . . .

As the sperm is guided to the site of fertilization, the woman's reproductive tract appears to cull or select sperm. . . . Also, the fluid in the woman's oviduct may play an important role in the separation of fertilized eggs that are developing into embryos.

Because gynecologists see the woman's body as a passive vessel, when they want to find out when or if a woman ovulates, it does not occur to them to ask the woman. But many women know. They can feel it when the egg bursts from the follicle (mittleschmerz). For centuries women like those of the Cherokee nations detected ovulation by observing changes in their cervical mucus. Women can learn that now. . . .

When physicians in IVF programs want to pinpoint ovulation, they do not explore the possibility that the woman who is ovulating can give them any information. Instead, they measure hormones in her urine and scan her ovaries with ultrasound machines such as the Kretz Combison 100 sector scanner to make a "diagnosis" of ovulation.

References

Allen, Sally G. and Joanna Hubbs. 1980. "Outrunning Atalanta: Feminine Destiny in Alchemical Transmutation." *Signs*. 6(21): 210–229.

Bettleheim, Bruno. 1968. *Symbolic Wounds: Puberty Rites and the Envious Male*. Collier Books. New York.

Campbell, Joseph. 1964. *The Masks of God: Occidental Mythology*. The Viking Press. New York.

Corea, Gena. 1985. *The Hidden Malpractice*. Harper & Row. New York.

———. 1980, July. "The Cesarean Epidemic." *Mother Jones*.

Cummings, Richard. 1966. *The Alchemists: Fathers of Practical Chemistry*. David McKay Co., Inc. New York.

Daly, Mary. 1978. *Gyn/Ecology*. Beacon Press. Boston.

Ebon, Martin. 1978. *The Cloning of Man*. New American Library. New York.

Fischer, Elizabeth. 1979. *Women's Creation*. McGraw-Hill Book Company. New York.

Fletcher, Joseph. 1974. *The Ethics of Genetic Control: Ending Reproductive Roulette*. Anchor Press/Doubleday. Garden City, New York.

Francoeur, Robert T. 1970. *Utopian Motherhood*. Doubleday and Co., Inc. Garden City, New York.

Gillie, Oliver. 1983, May 29. "Could a Man Be a Mother?" *The Sunday Times* (London): 14.

Grossman, Edward. 1971. "The Obsolescent Mother." *The Atlantic Monthly* 227(5).

Guitton, Jean. 1967. *Feminine Fulfillment*. Paulist Press Deus Books. New York.

Hinkle, Warren. 1980, May 13. "Why Eldridge Cleaver Is a Wife-beater." *San Francisco Chronicle*.

Lederer, Wolfgang. 1968. *The Fear of Women*. Harcourt Brace Jovanovich, Inc. New York.

Lichtman, Wendy. 1982. *The Boy Who Wanted a Baby*. The Feminist Press. Old Westbury, New York.

O'Brien, Mary. 1981. *The Politics of Reproduction*. Routledge & Kegan Paul, Ltd. London and Boston.

O'Faolain, Julia and Laura Martines, eds. 1973. *Not in God's Image*. Harper & Row. New York.

Raymond, Janice. 1979. *The Transsexual Empire*. Beacon Press. Boston.

Roberts, Peter. 1981, July 31. "Some Men Keen to Volunteer as Mothers." *The Age*.

Rubin, Bernard. 1965, Aug. "Psychological Aspects of Human Artificial Insemination." *Archives of General Psychiatry*. 13.

Sherman, J. K. 1973. "Synopsis of the Use of Frozen Human Semen since 1964: State of the Art of Human Semen Banking." *Fertility & Sterility.* 24(5): 397–412.

Stannard, Una. 1977. *Mrs. Man.* Germainbooks. San Francisco.

Walker, Barbara G. 1983. *The Woman's Encyclopedia of Myths and Secrets.* Harper & Row. San Francisco.

The Ethics of Sex Preselection

Mary Anne Warren

In . . . "Sex Preselection: Eugenics for Everyone?"[1] Dr. Helen B. Holmes argues that it is morally wrong to preselect the sex of one's children, or even to wish to do so. (She does not, however, believe that it ought to be legally banned). In the first part of the article, Holmes provides a comprehensive overview of the current state of the art of sex preselection. She then summarizes the rather depressing facts about the prevalence of son-preference throughout the world: In almost every culture, the majority of prospective parents, women as well as men, would rather have a male firstborn child (or only child, if they plan to have just one) and/or more males than females. Finally, she presents a number of moral arguments against the development and use of either pre- or postconceptive methods of sex preselection. Since Holmes has done an excellent job of presenting the factual background, I will confine my comments to the moral arguments.

Holmes' view is that sex preselection is a sexist act, although it is sometimes inappropriate to blame individual parents for their desire to preselect their children's sex. Moreover, she argues that if the use of new medical technologies for preselecting sex were to become widespread, the consequences for women would probably be harmful. I will argue that, on the contrary, sex preselection is not necessarily a sexist act, though it may be so in many instances. Furthermore, I doubt that it is possible to know in advance what the long-term social consequences of sex preselection will be, or that these consequences will be, on balance, detrimental to women or society as a whole. That there is a risk of harmful consequences is enough to justify continued research and monitoring of the social and psychological effects of sex preselection; but it does not justify a wholesale condemnation of the practice.

Is Sex Preselection Sexist?

Sexism is usually defined as wrongful discrimination on the basis of sex. Discrimination based on sex may be wrong either because it is based on false

From James M. Humber and Robert F. Almeder, eds. *Biomedical Ethics Reviews-1985*. Clifton, N.J.: Humana Press, 1985, pp. 73–89. Reprinted by permission of the publisher.

and invidious beliefs about persons of one sex or the other or because it unjustly harms those discriminated against. For now, let us concentrate upon the claim that sex preselection is sexist because it is invariably motivated by sexist beliefs.

Tabitha Powledge presents the argument for this claim in its simplest form. In her view, sex preselection is "the original sexist sin," because it makes "the most basic judgment about the worth of a human being rest first and foremost on its sex."[2] In this form, her argument is unsound; it is false that all persons who would like to preselect the sex of their children believe that members of one sex are inherently more valuable. Some people, for instance, would like to have a son because they already have one or more daughters (or vice versa), and they would like to have at least one child of each sex. Others may believe that, because of their own personal background or circumstances, they would be better parents to a child of one sex than the other. On the surface, at least, such persons need not be motivated by any invidious sexist beliefs. They may well believe that women and men are equally intelligent, capable, and valuable; they may even be feminists, dedicated to the elimination of restrictive sex roles and sexist discrimination of all sorts.

It may, however, be argued that the desire to preselect sex is always based on covertly sexist beliefs. Michael Bayles notes that the desire for a child of a particular sex is often instrumental to the fulfillment of other desires, such as the desire that the family name be carried on. Such instrumental reasons for sex preference, he argues, are always ultimately based upon irrational and sexist beliefs. For instance, in many jurisdictions it is no longer true that only a man can pass his family name to his children; hence, he says, it would be irrational (in those jurisdictions) to prefer a son for this particular reason. Even the desire to have a child of each sex is, according to Bayles, irrational, because there are no valid reasons for supposing that this would be better than having several children of the same sex. He considers the case of a man who already has two daughters and would like to have a son as well, "so that he could have certain pleasures in childrearing—such as fishing and playing ball with him".[3] This man would be making a sexist assumption, since he could perfectly well enjoy such activities with his daughters.

John Fletcher also argues that the desire to preselect a child's sex (except for certain medical reasons) can only be based on irrational and sexist beliefs. Holmes apparently agrees with Fletcher's conclusion:

> *Prima facie* examination of any argument for sex selection cannot overcome the unfair and sexist bias of a choice to select the sex of a child. The desire to control the sex of a child is not rational, since any claim that is made for the parents' preference for one sex can be demonstrated to be provided also by the other sex.[4]

Fletcher is not opposed to sex preselection when it is done in order to avoid the birth of a child with a sex-linked disease, such as hemophilia. Women who are genetic carriers of a sex-linked disease often choose to abort male fetuses because males, unlike females, will have about a 50% chance of suffering from the disease. This is not a sexist reason for preselecting sex, although, as Holmes points out, even this use of sex preselection has some morally troubling aspects. (For one thing, it requires the abortion of some perfectly normal male fetuses; for another, it entails the birth of some female children who are themselves carriers of the genetic disease.) The question is whether there are any other nonsexist reasons for sex preselection.

Holmes speaks of the situation of women in the rural parts of northern India. The society is a harshly patriarchal one in which the birth of a male child is celebrated but the birth of a female is regarded as a severe misfortune. Son-preference is traditionally so strong that, up to about the end of the last century, the members of some tribes killed virtually all of their female infants.[5] Although infanticide is no longer openly practiced, female children still have a higher death rate than males, because they are more often neglected, underfed, or denied essential medical care.[6] Women in this society sometimes say that they are reluctant to bring a female child into a world in which she will be abused and devalued, as they themselves have been. Holmes notes that their preference for sons would seem to be morally correct on utilitarian grounds. I would add that their son-preference is not necessarily a sign of sexism on their part. To accuse such women of sexism because they act upon their understanding of the intense sexism of their society would be a case of blaming the victim. Their motivations are at least partly altruistic and do not appear to be in any way irrational. Thus, although the use by such women of selective abortion or other methods of sex selection to produce sons must be seen as a symptom of sexist institutions and ideology, there is not necessarily anything in its motivation that would justify calling it a sexist action—even one for which the women in question are personally blameless.

Another highly pragmatic reason for son-preference in northern India (and many other parts of the world) is that a son is an economic asset, whereas a daughter usually is not. Because of sexist discrimination in the job market, a daughter will almost certainly earn far less than a son. If the family is well-to-do, she is apt not to enter the job market at all. Thus, she will not be able to contribute as much to her family's economic support. Furthermore, the cost of providing her with a dowry is likely to be extremely high. Without a large dowry she will probably be unable to marry, and thus will be apt to remain dependent upon her family indefinitely. If she does marry without a dowry that is considered suitably large (or, indeed, even with such a dowry), she may be tormented or murdered by her husband or inlaws. Under these conditions, it would be difficult to show that the desire to have sons rather than daughters is irrational. It would surely be wrong to condemn the decision of a couple not to have children because they judge that they cannot afford to raise them. Why, then, should we condemn their decision not to have daughters for the same reason?

If son-preference is rational in rural Punjab, and not necessarily a sexist action, then it will be difficult to argue that this is not also true in much of the rest of the world. Wherever son-preference is especially pronounced, it is because, in large part, of powerful economic motivations. Even in societies that provide some social support for the aged, sons are often an important part of old-age security—more so than daughters, whose earning capacity is generally far less. For this reason, son-preference is often (though not always) stronger among the poorer classes. Giurovich, for instance, found that son-preference is stronger among lower-class Italian couples, primarily because sons are seen as more conducive to the family's upward economic mobility.[7] Even among (some groups of) Americans, son-preference has been found to correlate negatively with socioeconomic class, suggesting that here, too, economic factors may be among the motivations for it.[8]

It will not do to argue, as Fletcher does, that such economic motivations for son-preference are irrational because, "Few jobs exist that women cannot perform as well or better than men when performance is the criterion for evaluation (p. 343)."[9] Although this is certainly true, the fact remains that women's average earning capacity is far from commensurate with the true value of their work. As everyone knows, the average full-time employed women in America earns just 59% of what the average man earns, and the average women with a college degree still earns less that the average man with only a high school education. Poor women, especially if they have children, have few opportunities of escaping poverty. The morally appropriate social response to this situation would be to remove the economic incentives for son-preference through such measures as the elimination of unjust discrimination against women in education, hiring, and promotion, the provision of more adequate unemployment, old-age, and disability support for all persons, and the reduction of economic differentials through a more just distribution of wealth. But until such social changes occur, it is not necessarily irrational for poor people to seek to better their economic status through the preselection of sons.

Is it nevertheless immoral for them to do so? It might be argued that in opting for sons for economic reasons, parents are, in effect, seeking to exploit the sexism of their society for their own economic gain. Yet we cannot condemn their actions for this reason alone, unless we are also prepared to condemn the actions of women who earn a living through (for instance) modeling in bikinis for soft drink commercials. Such women may profit from sexist attitudes and institutions, but they are more often victims than victimizers; and they often have very few economically comparable options. If their actions, or those of parents who preselect sons for economic reasons, are immoral, it can only be because of their unintended social consequences.

Before turning to the consequentialist arguments against sex preselection, I would like to consider some other apparently nonsexist reasons for sex-preference. Even in the industrialized nations, prospective parents may have sound reasons to prefer that their children, for their own sake, be male. Women are still far from enjoying the full range of freedoms and opportunities available to men. On the average, they not only earn much less but also work longer hours, because regardless of whether they have jobs, they are still expected in most cases to shoulder heavier domestic responsibilities. Male violence and the threat of male violence still turn the lesser size and upper-body strength of females into a serious liability. The threat of rape still curtails women's freedom of movement. As long as these many forms of sexist oppression persist, I think that it is wrong to suggest that women are performing a sexist action if they seek to have male children in order that the latter may enjoy the freedoms that women are still denied.

I am not, of course, suggesting that most women reason in this way; still less that most women ought to. Many prospective mothers would be equally content with a child of either sex, and many others would prefer to have a daughter. Of these, some are planning to raise a child without a male partner and believe that under the present conditions they would have more in common with a child of their own sex, and thus (they hope) a better relationship with her. A son could share most of their particular interests or activities, but he could not share the basic experience of being female in a society that still values males more highly. However much he may sympathize with the plight of women, he will still be a member of the more privileged sex. Although such expectations may prove mistaken in particular cases, I see no grounds for condemning them as either sexist or irrational.

Other women may prefer to have daughters because they fear that, in Sally Gearhart's words,

> . . . if they have sons, no amount of love and care and nonsexist training will save those sons from a culture where male violence is institutionalized and revered. These women are saying, "No more sons. We will not spend twenty years of our lives raising a potential rapist, a potential batterer, a potential Big Man."[10]

Men, as a group, are far more apt to resort to serious violence against other persons (and, for that matter, against nonhuman animals) than are females. We need not speak of war, into which men are often conscripted against their will; it is enough to glance at the statistics on individual acts of violence. In the United States, for instance, males commit five times as many murders as females.[11] Rape and child molesting are primarily (though not exclusively) male crimes, and most battered spouses are female victims of male violence. The question is whether it is morally wrong to take account of such proven statistical differences between the sexes in deciding whether and how to make use of the new methods of sex preselection.

Most feminists would agree that it is usually unjust to discriminate against individuals of either sex on the basis of merely statistical differences between the sexes. Individuals have the right to be judged on their own merits, not condemned by association with some group to which they happen to belong. But choosing to have a daughter rather than a son, on the grounds that females tend to be less violent, is not a case of injustice against an individual person. The son one might have had instead might or might not have turned out to be violent, but since he does not exist, there is no way to evaluate him as an individual. Furthermore, since he does not exist, he cannot have been treated unjustly; he will not suffer from his nonexistence. This is most clearly true when preconceptive methods of sex selection are used. But even sex-selective abortion cannot be regarded as an injustice against an individual person, because, as I have argued elsewhere, fetuses are not yet persons and do not yet have a right to continued existence.[12]

Consequentialist Objections

Numerous speculations have been made about the long-term consequences should an effective means of sex preselection become widely available. Some writers have welcomed sex preselection as a voluntary means of reducing the birth rate and the number of unwanted children born in the attempt to get one of the "right" sex. Others, including Holmes and Fletcher, argue that the results are likely to be primarily detrimental. They fear that females may be psychologically harmed by the implementation of son-preference. Equally disturbing are the possible social consequences of sex ratio increases, i.e., increases in the relative number of males. An undersupply of women might result in their being increasingly confined to subordinate "female" roles and/ or subjected to increased male violence. Let us look first at these possible negative results of sex preselection.

Birth Order Effects

Throughout most of the world, a majority of prospective parents would prefer a male firstborn child. And firstborns, it has often been claimed, enjoy certain social and psychological advantages, perhaps because they have, for a time, a monopoly on their parents' attention. There have been hundreds of studies purporting to prove or disprove linkages between birth order and such personal traits as initiative, creativity, anxiety, affiliation, dependence, conservatism, rebelliousness, authoritarianism, mental illness, criminality, and alcoholism. The results are enormously complex and frequently contradictory. However, among the most consistent findings are that firstborns tend to achieve more in terms of formal education and career, and to be more dependent and affiliative.[13] Adler argued that each birth order position carries with it characteristic advantages and disadvantages. In his view, firstborns tend to be more responsible, conservative, and achievement-oriented, but may also suffer from anxiety and other mental problems because of the traumatic experience of "dethronement" by the birth of a younger sibling.[14] Robert Zajonc has argued that firstborn children tend to be more intelligent than laterborns because of the progressive degradation of the family's "intellectual environment" supposedly produced by the birth of each additional child.[15]

If either of these theories about the psychological effects of birth order were empirically well supported, there might be good reason to fear that increases in the relative number of male firstborns will have a detrimental effect upon women. However, the evidence for these theories is, at best, highly ambiguous. The isolation of birth order effects from the effects of socioeconomic status, ethnicity, religion, family size, urban versus rural back-

ground, and other social variables represents an extremely difficult method-
ological problem, and one that has not been resolved in most of the studies
that have been done. In many of the early studies that found firstborns to be
superior in intelligence, motivation, and achievement, there were no controls
for family size. Obviously, firstborns are more apt to come from small families
than laterborns. In most of the industrialized nations, parents of large families
tend to have less money and education and to score lower on standard tests of
intelligence than parents of smaller families. Thus, where family size is not
held constant, comparisons between first- and laterborn children are biased.
The latter have, on the average, less privileged socioeconomic backgrounds,
and any psychological differences found are as likely to be a result of this
factor as birth order itself. Where sample groups of first- and laterborns are
matched for family size and socioeconomic status, most (though not quite all)
of the apparent superiorities of the firstborn disappear.[16]

The birth order debate continues, with some psychologists presenting new
evidence of the influence of birth order upon personality and others debunk-
ing the idea. But at present, the weight of the evidence seems to support a
skeptical view. In 1983 two Swiss psychologists, Cecile Ernst and Jules Angst,
published an exhaustive review of the birth order research of the past four
decades. Their conclusion is that nearly all of the reports of significant birth
order effects are a result of errors in the design of studies and the statistical
analysis of the data.[17] They believe that there are some general differences in
the socialization process undergone by firstborns and laterborns, i.e., firstborns tend to be better cared for in infancy and to be more advanced in
linguistic development. But they conclude that these differences "do not seem
to leave indelible traces that can be predicted."[18] They do not deny that being
a first, middle, last, or only child may have great importance for the personal
development of some individuals, but only that it has any general and lasting
significance. Birth order theories, they argue, ignore the fact that each child
has a unique genetic constitution that influences his or her intelligence and
personality, and that consequently "each child in a sibship will interact in a
novel way with the environment, and, from the first day on, will mold it and
be molded by it in a highly individualistic way."[19]

Other Psychological Harms

What about the fact that many females will know that their parents chose to
have sons first? Roberta Steinbacher asks, "What are the implications of
being second born, and knowing at some early age that you were planned-to-
be-second?"[20] It might seem self-evident that girls will suffer a loss of self-
esteem from the knowledge that their parents chose to have a son first. And
Fletcher argues that even a firstborn girl is apt to be damaged if she learns
that, whereas she was not sex-selected, her younger brother was. Addressing
the parent who already has a daughter and is considering a sex-selected son,
Fletcher says,

. . . put yourself in your daughter's place. How will she respond to your reasons why you went to the fertility clinic to start a pregnancy with baby brother, when you did not do the same with the conception of her? What reasons will you give her? . . . You would not let her continue believing that only boys can be police, firefighters, or surgeons, would you? . . . You conclude that if you would not neglect her need to aspire equally to almost any job that a man might do, you will sabotage that parental duty by preselecting sex.[21]

This argument rests upon the assumption that there can be no nonsexist reasons for preselecting sex—or none that a female child can be expected to understand. But surely one need not believe that only boys can grow up to be police or firefighters to want a son as well as a daughter. One might, for instance, believe that children are apt to develop a better understanding of persons of the opposite sex if they have an opposite-sex sibling. Or one might believe that the best way to raise a nonsexist child is to raise her in the company of an opposite-sex sibling whom one does not treat any differently. Even if these beliefs are false, they are not obvious instances of sexism. Nor is it obvious that a girl would be apt to suffer psychological harm as a result of learning that her parents preselected a son because of such beliefs.

But what of the girl who learns that her brother was sex-selected for reasons that are sexist, e.g., because her father wants a male heir? No doubt she may be hurt by this knowledge. Yet, if her parents are sexist in their current behavior, if they treat her as worth less than her brother because of her sex, then the discovery that his sex was preselected can only come as one more confirmation of what she must already know. On the other hand, if her parents are not biased in their current treatment of her brother and her, then this particular discovery need not shake her conviction that she is equally valued—although, of course, it might. Every female must eventually come to terms with the sexist biases of her society. It would be difficult to prove that the implementation of son-preference through sex preselection will do much extra damage to female psyches.

Sex Ratios and the Status of Women

Very few studies have been made of the relationship between sex ratios and sex roles. The only well-developed theory in this area is that presented by Marcia Guttentag and Paul Secord.[22] Guttentag and Secord argue that women tend to be disadvantaged in both high and low sex ratio societies—although not necessarily any more so than in societies with a 50:50 sex ratio. On their theory, high sex ratio societies tend to impose rigid restrictions upon the sexual behavior of women and to confine them to the domestic role. Low sex ratios, on the other hand, tend to contribute to male misogyny and the devaluation of both women and marriage. This is because when there is an "oversupply" of women, men become reluctant to commit themselves to long-term relationships with a single woman. In such circumstances, women are apt to become dissatisfied with the terms of marriage and to seek other means of achieving economic security; hence, feminist movements may appear. According to Guttentag and Secord, whichever sex is in short supply is likely to gain an advantage in "dyadic power," i.e., power within two-person heterosexual relationships. Yet men are usually able to limit women's freedom even when sex ratios are low, because they have the advantage in "structural power," i.e., control of the economic, legal, and other key social institutions.

On this theory, high sex ratios may be either good or bad for women, depending upon the structural power that women already have. If women are economically dependent and lack basic legal rights and protections, they cannot make use of whatever dyadic power they might otherwise gain as a result of their scarcity value. But if they have a degree of economic independence and legal autonomy, then they may be able to take advantage of this dyadic power to drive a better bargain in relationships with men. This benefit applies primarily to heterosexual women. Guttentag and Secord say very little about nonheterosexual women, except that lesbianism is apt to be more severely discouraged in a high sex ratio society. Insofar as compulsory heterosexuality is a basic part of the oppression of women, this must be seen as an additional danger of sex ratio increases.

However, as Holmes points out, we cannot assume that the differences between typical high and low sex ratio societies are actually caused by sex ratios. It may be that the causal relationship tends to run in the opposite direction. Rather than high sex ratios causing women's confinement to the domestic role, societies that confine women to the domestic role may tend to have high sex ratios because many parents conclude that raising females is less worthwhile than raising males, and therefore practice sex selection through female infanticide or the neglect of female children. The high sex ratios may be relatively harmless in themselves. They might, conceivably, even be beneficial to women, in the context of a society that allows them very few opportunities to lead a decent life outside of the wife-and-mother role.

Even if it is true that in the past high and low sex ratios have tended to have the social consequences that Guttentag and Secord describe, it would be a mistake to assume that in the future the results will be the same. One may speculate that women in the more severely patriarchal societies will be apt to suffer a further loss of freedom should sex preselection lead to a significant increase in sex ratios; without substantial structural power, women cannot benefit from their own increased "value." Yet nothing in this scenario is inevitably predetermined. Improved education and movements toward socialism and democracy tend to facilitate the loosening of traditional constraints upon women, and might tip the balance in favor of sexual egalitarianism even in the face of declining sex ratios. The power of women's liberation movements throughout the world is another unpredictable factor. I suspect, however, that the growth of mass communication will make it increasingly difficult for women to be kept ignorant of their own oppression and the need to struggle against it.

Women in the more industrialized and/or less severely patriarchal nations probably have somewhat less need to fear increased oppression as a result of sex ratio increases. Not only is the relative increase in the number of males apt to be smaller, but because women often have greater (though still inadequate) opportunities for economic independence and political influence, they may be able to successfully defend those rights already won while continuing to improve their legal and economic status. This is not predetermined either; the forces of reaction are strong, and the gains that women have already made may be lost, with or without sex ratio increases. Nevertheless, sweeping predictions of a loss of freedom for women should sex ratios increase are unjustified.

Are We on a Slippery Slope?

Another consequentialist objection to sex preselection is that it may lead to the predesigning of children in other respects than sex. Holmes notes that some parents may be more concerned about a child's hair color or IQ than about its sex. She asks, "If we are going to custom design our children, for which traits is there moral justification?" Her reply is that "There are no such traits. Any specification means that we are not genuinely interested in adding a unique person to our home." There are two strands of argument here. One is a version of the slippery slope argument: We should reject sex preselection because it will lead to other forms of positive eugenics, which are objectionable. The other is that we should reject all forms of positive eugenics, because any attempt to predesign a child indicates a refusal to treat that child as a unique individual. Both arguments are questionable.

All slippery slope arguments presuppose that people cannot (learn to) make certain distinctions that the arguer considers vital; if the relevant distinctions can be made, then there is no reason to suppose that acceptance of the one form of behavior will lead to acceptance of the other. Such arguments fail if either (1) people can make such distinctions, or (2) these distinctions do not have the significance that the arguer takes them to have. In this case, both conditions apply. Many people who do not object to sex preselection would object to the preselection of hair color or IQ, because they perceive that these cases involve quite different considerations. Most of the arguments for and against sex preselection would not normally apply to the preselection of hair color, which usually has much less social significance than sex. Preselecting for intelligence would raise much more serious moral questions, because intellectual ability has a much more direct effect upon a person's life prospects than hair color normally does. These questions can and must be treated separately.

I am puzzled by the suggestion that all forms of positive eugenics are indicative of an unwillingness to perceive a child as a unique individual. Positive eugenics includes all attempts to select for certain traits that are positively desired, as opposed to selecting against certain undesirable traits, such as hemophilia or Down's syndrome. Positive eugenics tends to evoke the image of dictatorial governments predesigning people to serve their own nefarious ends, or of parents predesigning children to fit their own entirely selfish preferences. It is easy to forget that some forms of positive eugenics might serve children's own interests. Suppose, for instance, that there was a perfectly safe preconceptive or prenatal procedure that would endow a child with excellent vision or an increased life expectancy. I can see no a priori reason to deny that such a procedure might provide a real benefit to future persons. Why should we assume that parents who wish to provide their chilren with such benefits are uninterested in adding a unique individual to their home? As in the case of sex preselection, their reasons might be selfish or irrational, but they might also be altruistic and well reasoned.

Positive eugenics may be feared for a number of reasons: It might be abused for immoral purposes; it might prove to have unforeseen side effects; it might divert medical resources from more important purposes; and, above all, the advocacy of eugenics has been historically associated with vicious racist doctrines. These are sound reasons for proceeding cautiously, with full public disclosure and extensive public discussion of each new or proposed procedure—just as should be done in every other area of medical technology. They are not, however, reasons for a blanket rejection of all such procedures. Many possible eugenic procedures will prove too expensive or too dangerous to be worth pursuing. But each must be evaluated on its own merits. If we refuse to make the essential distinctions, insisting that all forms of positive eugenics must be accepted or rejected as part of a single package, then we may inadvertently contribute to the very sorts of abuses that we fear.

Will More Women Be Born Poor?

Some observers have predicted that if sex preselection becomes readily available, the poorer classes will become increasingly male, since son-preference is often strongest among the most economically deprived.[23] On the other hand, if the new methods of sex preselection continue to be expensive, or if governments, fearing their social consequences, seek to ban their use, sex preselection may become a prerogative of the relatively wealthy. In that case, it will probably be the upper classes that experience the greatest increase in sex ratios. As Steinbacher points out, this would mean "that increasing numbers of women in the future are locked into poverty while men continue to grow in numbers in positions of control and influence."[24]

This is perhaps the most damning of all the consequentialist objections to sex preselection. The detrimental effects of a further "masculinization of wealth" would be difficult to overestimate. Increased wealth and power in the hands of men could only result in the aggravation of the entire range of injustices against women. Yet we cannot move directly from this fact to the conclusion that the development and use of sex preselection is morally objectionable. What is morally objectionable is that it should be made available only to the wealthy. If we want to avoid some of the worst social consequences of sex selection, we must either suppress it completely (which is probably impossible), or seek to make it equally available to all social classes. It is much too early to predict that the latter goal will prove impossible.

The Possible Benefits

The possible benefits of sex preselection are just as difficult to predict as are the possible harms. I agree with Holmes that sex preselection should not be lauded as a means of reducing the birth rate. We cannot be sure that fewer children will be born if parents are able to preselect sex; some parents may have more children if they can be assured that they will be of the preferred sex. Nor do we know that decreases in the relative number of women will have the effect of reducing birth rates. In those cases in which pronatalism remains strong, high sex ratios may only result in each women being expected to have more children. If a shortage of women were to result in polyandrous marriages, women who received support from several men might find it possible—and perhaps necessary—to have more children than would be feasible in a monogamous marriage. Fertility drugs might even be used to increase the number of multiple births.

A more realistic possibility is that governments would take steps to prevent sex selection from resulting in a severe shortage of women. Whereas any absolute prohibition would probably be unpopular and ineffective, a variety of less severe measures might be employed. Couples might be forbidden to use sex preselection to produce sons until they have already produced at least one daughter; or tax penalties or other disincentives might be used to reduce the attractiveness of all-male families. Ways might even be found to reduce economic discrimination against women, thus reducing son-preference. Thus, the long-term effect of sex selection upon birth rates is quite unpredictable.

Moreover, as Holmes points out, there are better ways of promoting voluntary reductions in the birth rate than by encouraging the use of sex selection to produce sons. Free universal access to contraception and abortion is essential (and nonexistent in much of the world), but will be insufficient unless combined with more far-reaching social reforms. Improved economic security, education, and health care, and expanded opportunities for women outside of the maternal role have consistently proven effective in lowering birth rates. These measures are desirable on independent moral grounds and should be supported even by those who doubt that overpopulation is a real problem.

I also agree with Holmes that we cannot be certain that parents will be happier if they are able to choose the sex of their children. No doubt some will be happier and others will only be disappointed when their sex-selected children fail to live up to their expectations. Getting what one wants is never a guarantee of happiness—although it is usually more conducive to happiness than not getting what one wants.

There are, however, two predictable benefits of sex preselection that do much to counterbalance its possible ill effects. The most important is that fewer children will be doomed to abuse or neglect because they are of the "wrong" sex—in most cases, because they are female. It is true that even a wanted girl or boy may suffer from unrealistic parental expectations. But wanted children are less likely to be deliberately deprived of food, affection, and necessary medical care; and fewer wanted children die from such neglect. We will never know how many short and miserable lives will be avoided through sex preselection, but the data on different mortality rates for female children in northern India and many other parts of the world suggest that the number will be quite significant. In my mind, this potential benefit is at least as weighty as any of the potential harms that Holmes describes. I doubt that any of the possible benefits to be gained through discouraging the development and use of new methods of sex preselection is worth condemning even a few children to rejection and neglect.

Sex preselection will also provide at least some women with a new means of resistance to patriarchy. It is part of the oppression of women that they have generally had little choice but to bear and raise sons, thereby perpetuating the ruling sex/class. Women may soon have the option of refusing to do this, without avoiding motherhood altogether or abandoning their male children, as the legendary Amazons were said to do. Other women, less optimistic about the prospects for change, may resist patriarchy by refusing to add to the female underclass. The freedom to preselect the sex of one's children is far less vital to women's interests than the freedom to decide whether to bear a child or not; yet having the former option will still be important to some women. Granted, some women may be forced by their husbands or families to have sons when they would prefer daughters, just as some are forced to complete pregnancies they would prefer to abort, or to abort those they would prefer to complete. But the option of sex choice will still have value for those women with the desire and the opportunity to use it.

Conclusion

I have not argued that the net effects of sex preselection are bound to be beneficial. They may well prove to be detrimental, just as Holmes fears. My primary point is rather that we cannot possibly know in advance what the effects of sex preselection will be, and that we ought not to condemn it on the basis of what can be little more than speculation. Were it possible to prove that sex preselection is, in every instance, a sexist act, then it could be condemned without proof of a high probability of serious harm. But if, as I have argued, there are many nonsexist reasons for son-preference or daughter-preference, then sex preselection can be morally condemned only if the consequentialist arguments against it are very strong. Because these arguments are not particularly strong, because there are probable compensatory benefits as well as possibly ill effects, and because the possibility of net losses does not justify categorical condemnation, the presumption must be in favor of moral, as well as legal, toleration. Should the feared detrimental effect of preselection begin to materialize at some future time, then will be the time to reassess this moral stance.[25]

Notes

1. *Biomedical Ethics Reviews—1985,* James M. Humber and Robert F. Almeder, eds. (Humana Press: Clifton, NJ, 1985), pp. 38–71.

2. Tabitha Powledge, "Unnatural Selection: On Choosing Children's Sex," in *The Custom-Made Child? Women-Centered Perspectives,* Helen B. Holmes, Betty B. Hoskins, and Michael Gross, eds. (Humana Press: Clifton, N.J.: 1981), p. 197.

3. Michael B. Bayles, *Reproductive Ethics* (Prentice-Hall: Englewood Cliffs, N.J.: 1984), p. 35.

4. John C. Fletcher, "Is Sex Selection Ethical?" in *Research Ethics,* Kare Berg and Knut Erik Tranoy, eds. (Alan R. Liss: New York, 1983), p. 347.

5. Kanti B. Pakrasai, *Female Infanticide in India* (Editions India: Calcutta, 1981).

6. Barbara D. Miller, *The Endangered Sex: Neglect of Female Children in Rural North India* (Cornell University Press: Ithaca, N.Y., and London, 1981).

7. G. Giurovich, "Sul desiderio dei coniugi di avere figle e di avere figle di un data sesso" (On the wish of married couples to have children and to have children of a specified sex), *Atti Della 16 Riunoine Scientifica della Societa Italiana di Statistica* (Rome, 1956).

8. Lee Rainwater, *Family Design* (Aldine: Chicago, 1965), p. 131.

9. Fletcher, p. 343.

10. Sally Gearhart, "The Future—If There Is One—Is Female," in *Reweaving the Web of Life: Feminism and Nonviolence,* Pam McAlister, ed. (New Society: Philadelphia, 1982), p. 282.

11. National Commission on the Causes and Prevention of Violence, *Violent Crime* (George Braziller: New York, 1969).

12. Mary Anne Warren, "On the Moral and Legal Status of Abortion," *The Monist* 57 (1973), pp. 43–61, and "Do Potential People Have Moral Rights? *Can. J. Phil.* 7 (1977), pp. 275–289.

13. Bert N. Adams, "Birth Order: A Critical Review," *Sociometry* 35 (1972), pp. 411–439, at p. 411.

14. Alfred Adler, *Understanding Human Nature* (Greenberg: New York, 1927); "Characteristics of the First, Second, and Third Child," *Children* 3 (1928); and *What Life Should Mean to You* (Little, Brown: Boston, 1931).

15. Robert B. Zajonc, "Dumber by the Dozen," *Psychology Today* 8 (January, 1975), pp. 37–43, and Robert B. Zajonc, Hazel Markus, and Gregory B. Markus, "The Birth Order Puzzle," *J. Pers. Soc. Psychol.* 37 (1979), pp. 1325–1341.

16. Cecile Ernst and Jules Angst, *Birth Order: Its Influences on Personality* (Springer-Verlag: Berlin, Heidelberg, and New York, 1983), p. 45.

17. Ibid., p. 13.

18. Ibid., p. 187.

19. Ibid., p. 242.

29. Roberta Steinbacher, "Futuristic Implications of Sex Preselection," in *The Custom-Made Child? Women-Centered Perspectives,* Helen B. Holmes, Betty B. Hoskins, and Michael Gross, eds. (Humana Press: Clifton, N.J., 1981), p. 187.

21. Fletcher, p. 343.

22. Marcia Guttentag and Paul F. Secord, *Too Many Women? The Sex Ratio Question* (Sage: Beverly Hills, Calif., London and New Delhi, 1983).

23. Amitai Etzioni, "Sex Control, Science, and Society," *Science* 161 (1968), pp. 1107–1112, at p. 1109.

24. Steinbacher, p. 188.

25. The arguments in this article are further developed in the author's book, *Gendercide: The Implications of Sex Selection* (Rowman & Allanheld: Totowa N.J., 1985).

VI

CONSTITUTIONAL RIGHTS, LAW, AND PUBLIC POLICY

The articles in this part address questions of legal rights and legal regulation of reproductive technology. The first two articles debate whether the Constitution of the United States contains provisions that should be interpreted as recognizing a right (related to the right of privacy) to seek to have children through reproductive technology. If it should, then laws and governmental policies restricting reproductive technology would have to be narrowly defined and supported by compelling state interests. If not, then reproductive technology could be restricted for less weighty reasons.

In the first article, law professor John Robertson argues that existing Supreme Court decisions that extend constitutional protection to a wide range of procreative and family matters should be seen as implying protection for reproduction through reproductive technology as well. Countering this position, law professor George Smith and lawyer Roberto Iraola argue that these cases extend protection not to procreation itself, but only to more limited interests of remaining fertile, preventing conception, and terminating pregnancy. While these articles may debate seemingly technical points of constitutional interpretation, the implications of such arguments for practice are far-reaching, as is obvious to anyone who has followed the public controversy over abortion for the past several decades.

The remaining two articles in this part take up a particular legal issue: the proper legal status of parenting through contract. The options open to the law include not only (1) entirely banning the practice but also (2) criminalizing only some variants or elements of the practice (such as banning advertising or the payment of money to the mother in so-called commercial surrogacy), (3) allowing the practice but not enforcing contracts,[1] (4) allowing the practice and enforcing contracts, or (5) recognizing other sorts of regulatory schemes, such as assimilating parenting through contract to other practices, such as adoption.

Lawyer Noel Keane was the first, and has remained for over a decade the most prominent, public promoter of commercial parenting through contract. In the excerpt given below from an early law journal article, Keane argues that parenting through contract does not violate the law or public policy, and so its contracts should be recognized as valid and enforceable. He attempts to counter objections that commercial parenting through contract violates adoption laws and laws against baby-selling, that it is not in the child's best interests, and that it involves unacceptable commercialization of reproductive processes.

Even if the contract is enforceable, the question still arises as to what sort of remedy is appropriate for breach of the contract, such as the mother's refusal to surrender the child or the father's refusal to accept it.[2] Should a father be forced to accept a child born through contract? Would that be in the child's best interest? Should a mother be forced to surrender the child or should she only be required to pay damages? The latter is normally the case in personal service contracts. Should contracts for bearing and surrendering children be an exception? Keane addresses these and other complications that could arise in carrying out the arrangements.

In the final article in this part, philosopher Rosemarie Tong describes and evaluates various approaches that the law could take to parenting through contract and concludes that its commercial form should be banned, while its altruistic form, such as a woman's gestating a child for her sister without payment, should be legal and recognized as a form of adoption. Much of Tong's analysis is presented in terms of disputes among liberal, Marxist, and radical feminists, but the considerations she raises can be seen more generally to concern conflicts between values of free choice, avoidance of economic exploitation, and avoidance of other forms of exploitation. Tong identifies and weighs not only the effects of the four approaches on women, but also their significance for children and for our social consciousness in general.

Key to Tong's conceptual analysis is an argument that gestation, rather than a relationship of genes, is the most important consideration that should determine who has a right to parent a child. Thus, Tong's analysis and practical conclusions should be considered in connection with many of the articles that have preceded it in this anthology, especially the articles by Krimmel and Radin, all of Part III (on the meaning and significance of having children), and all of Part V (on the significance of reproductive technology for women). Parts of the article by Alpern comment directly, if briefly, on Tong's arguments concerning the primacy of pregnancy.

Notes

1. An unenforceable contract is one that a court of law will not recognize as binding in deciding the outcome of disputes. Generally, contracts for actions that are illegal or against public policy will not be enforced by the courts.

2. Actual instances of such refusals are presented below in the case studies "The Case of Baby M: Parenting through Contract When Everyone Wants the Child" (refusal to surrender) and "Parenting through Contract When No One Wants the Child" (refusal to accept).

Noncoital Reproduction and Procreative Liberty

John A. Robertson

Normative analysis of the legal structure of the new reproduction begins with a discussion of procreative liberty. IVF is now widely accepted, though a few years ago there were strong objections to it. Today, however, many people would support a ban on certain IVF activities, such as gamete and embryo donation and surrogacy. Since legal restrictions on use of noncoital reproductive techniques might preclude persons from the only reproduction possible for them, their procreative liberty would be limited significantly. Yet all liberty can be limited when its exercise substantially burdens others. Accordingly, we [offer] a discussion of the scope of procreative liberty and the extent of constitutional protection for noncoital conception and its collaborative variations.

The Nature and Scope of Procreative Liberty

"Procreative liberty" denotes freedom in activities and choices related to procreation, but the term does not tell us which activities fall within its scope. A crucial distinction is between actions designed to *avoid* procreation and those designed to *cause* procreation. In many societies cultural duties to procreate exist. In the United States, however, individuals and couples have no legal duty to procreate. The burdens of unwanted pregnancy and childbearing are deemed so substantial that any competent person—married, single, adult, minor—may choose to abort up to the fetus' viability and use contraceptives to avoid pregnancy.

The right to procreate—to do those things that will lead to biological descendents—is equally or even more significant to persons, yet has not received the explicit legal recognition that the avoidance of procreation has. The absence of explicit law is significant, for it shows how widespread and

From section II of "Embryos, Families, and Procreative Liberty: The Legal Structure of the New Reproduction." *Southern California Law Review* 59 (1986), pp. 939–1041. Reprinted with permission of the *Southern California Law Review*.

deep is the social understanding of the right to reproduce through sexual intercourse. While sterilization, fornication, and marriage laws have prevented some persons from reproducing, no law has prohibited or penalized married couples from having children as often as they like and can.

Extracorporeal conception and manipulation of the fertilized egg forces us to consider several new questions about the scope of the right to reproduce when that right, lodged as it is in the community's background assumptions, has itself received little critical scrutiny. Do persons with the right to reproduce coitally also have a right to do so noncoitally, if coital reproduction is not possible? May they enlist gamete donors and surrogate gestators to overcome their infertility? May they choose to limit their participation to discrete, unconnected reproductive roles, such as gamete or embryo donor or surrogate? Questions of posthumous procreation, embryo storage, and selection of offspring characteristics also arise.

Determining the scope of the right to procreate—and hence of reproductive liberty involving extracorporeal human embryos—depends on exploration of two issues that have never been isolated in this way. The first is the extent to which the basis for valuing reproduction applies when conception occurs noncoitally or collaboratively. The second concerns the meaning and scope of responsibility in reproduction, and thus the circumstances in which reproduction can justifiably be limited.

The first question requires us to examine the moral or value basis for according reproduction such high value. Reproduction is the creation of biological descendants through gametic fusion with a partner, gestation by the female, and usually rearing by one or both of the procreators. Creating and rearing biological descendants is immensely meaningful for individuals and for society. The case for according persons a large degree of liberty in creating and rearing biological descendants is plausible and appealing, and, at least within marriage, has been widely accepted.

It would seem, then, that freedom to procreate noncoitally should also be recognized, since it may be the only way for the person to reproduce. By the same token, the use of sperm, egg, embryo, or uterus donors may also be necessary for the person to have or rear biological descendants. While the possibility of harms unique to IVF procreation should be explored, a plausible argument to extend procreative liberty to transactions involving the extracorporeal embryo can be made.

This understanding of procreative liberty, however, can be distinguished from reproductive roles played by persons who are not themselves attempting to acquire offspring of their own. For the donor or surrogate, participation in partial reproductive roles, such as gamete or embryo donor, or gestator, may have less of the meaning that gives reproduction its significance, and therefore need not be as fully protected.[1] Similarly, the liberty to have one's heirs conceived or transferred to a uterus posthumously, which gamete and embryo storage makes possible, seems less compelling than the liberty to have heirs during one's life. Extension of the scope of procreative liberty thus raises questions about life, death, and one's continuity with the natural order. Analogies and similarities to current practices abound, but none is identical. Whether the dissimilarities are morally significant must await further experience and the evolution of shared understandings about the personal and social importance of the procreative interests at stake.

There is also normative uncertainty about the scope of reproductive responsibility—a second issue in need of clarification. May a person's freedom to acquire children for rearing or to engage in other activities with reproductive significance be limited to protect offspring and others? Reproductive decisions affect offspring and may lead directly to burdens for others. Yet there have been few efforts to assure reproductive responsibility, and the idea of reproductive responsibility is seldom addressed in countries without a population problem. In developed countries most people are free, if they have a partner, to reproduce when and as often as they like.

IVF will force elucidation of the concept of reproductive responsibility, for actions done to create or manipulate fertilized eggs may directly hurt offspring or others. In assessing reproductive responsibility in use of noncoital technologies, concerns about overpopulation, producing handicapped children, imposing rearing costs on others, maternal behavior during pregnancy, and the ability to parent competently must be distinguished. The limits of acceptable behavior will depend on the burdens and benefits of particular techniques and on the emerging meaning of reproduction as these techniques filter into common use.

Constitutional Recognition of a Right to Procreate

The legal structure of noncoital reproduction will reflect these questions concerning the meaning and scope of procreative liberty. The current legal situation is marked by an absence of direct regulation and uncertainty about the extent to which fetal research, adoption, and artificial insemination by donor (AID) laws apply to embryo manipulation and to donor and surrogate transactions. Further regulation limiting IVF and noncoital options is certainly a possibility. Discussion of the constitutional right to procreate will illuminate the underlying normative problems, indicate the scope of possible state intrusion, and thus define the freedom to make noncoital and collaborative reproductive decisions.[2]

The Right to Noncoital and Donor-Assisted Reproduction

The starting point of analysis is the recognition that married persons (and possibly unmarried persons as well) have a right to reproduce by sexual intercourse. Although laws regulating fornication, cohabitation, and adultery have limited the freedom of unmarried persons to reproduce, laws limiting coital reproduction by a married couple have been notably absent. As a result, there are no cases that directly involve a married couple's right to coital reproduction.

In dicta, however, the Supreme Court on numerous occasions has recognized a married couple's right to procreate in language broad enough to encompass coital, and most noncoital, forms of reproduction. In *Meyer v. Nebraska,* for example, the Court stated that constitutional liberty included the right of an individual "to marry, establish a home and bring up children."[3] In striking down a mandatory sterilization law for habitual criminals in *Skinner v. Oklahoma,* the Court noted that the law interfered with marriage and procreation, which were among "the basic civil rights of man."[4] In *Stanley v. Illinois* the Court observed that "[t]he rights to conceive and raise one's children have been deemed 'essential,' 'basic civil rights of man,' and '[r]ights far more precious . . . than property rights.' "[5] The Court has noted that "freedom of personal choice in matters of marriage and family life is one of the liberties protected by the Due Process Clause of the Fourteenth Amendment."[6] An especially explicit statement of the right to procreate appeared in Justice Brennan's opinion in *Eisenstadt v. Baird:* "If the right of privacy means anything, it is the right of the individual, married or single, to be free of unwarranted governmental intrusion into matters so fundamentally affecting a person as the decision whether to bear or beget a child."[7]

The Court's statements have not distinguished carefully between conceiving and rearing a child, analyzed the interests behind this protection, or taken account of new reproductive technologies. Moreover, these statements arise in a context where government control over entrance to, and exit from, marriage is not in question, and where public policy may mandate government interference with the reproduction of mentally incompetent persons.[8] Yet it seems indisputable that even a conservative Supreme Court would find that married couples have a fundamental constitutional right to reproduce by coitus.[9]

One need only imagine the result if a state passed a law that limited a married couple's freedom to reproduce by sexual intercourse. Involuntary sterilization, mandatory contraception and abortion laws, laws limiting the number of children, or other laws restricting coital reproduction doubtlessly would be subjected to the same strict scrutiny that laws restricting abortion and contraception now receive. Such laws would be struck down unless some compelling ground for such a drastic restriction of marital freedom could be shown.[10]

If the Supreme Court would recognize a married couple's right to coital reproduction, it should recognize a couple's right to reproduce noncoitally as well. The couple's interest in reproducing is the same, no matter how conception occurs, for the values and interests underlying coital reproduction are equally present. Both coital and noncoital conception enable the couple to unite egg and sperm and thus acquire a child of their genes and gestation for rearing. Aside from religious views that see coitus and reproduction as inextricably linked, the particular technique used to bring egg and sperm together is less important than the resulting offspring. The use of noncoital techniques such as IVF or artificial insemination to unite egg and husband's sperm, made necessary by the couple's infertility, should then also be protected.

The need for a third party donor or surrogate to provide the sperm, egg, or uterus necessary for the couple to beget, bear, or otherwise acquire a child should, under these principles of procreative liberty, also fall within the married couple's procreative rights. Although not as directly entailed as noncoital conception, the assistance of a third party collaborator should be treated similarly. The donor assists the couple in reproducing by contributing a factor of conception or gestation that the couple lacks. The donor is essential if the couple is to rear a child that has a gametic or gestational connection with the couple. Since they are otherwise qualified to be parents, and would be free, if fertile, to reproduce as often as they wished, they should be free to procreate with the help of gametic or womb donors.

Unpacking the meaning of procreation by sexual intercourse, as IVF and noncoital conception require us to do, we see that the reasons and values that support a right to reproduce coitally apply equally to noncoital activities involving external conception and collaborators. While the case is strongest for a couple's right to noncoital and external conception, a strong argument for their right to enlist the aid of gamete and womb donors can also be made. Both enable a couple to rear a child that is the biological descendant of, or has been gestated by, one of them.

If the couple's right to reproduce were fully recognized, married persons would have the right to engage in a wide range of noncoital activities involving embryos, donors, and surrogates in their attempt to reproduce. They would have the right to determine the use of their gametes and the disposition of embryos created with those gametes.[11] They would also have the right to contract with others for the provision of gametes or embryos, or gestation, with the contract settling the parties rearing rights and duties in resulting offspring. While the state could regulate the circumstances under which parties enter into reproductive contracts, it could not ban or refuse to enforce such transactions altogether without compelling reason.[12] In short, the interests and values supporting the right to reproduce by sexual intercourse extend to external conception and the need to contract with donors, surrogates, and physicians for the creation, gestation, and rearing of children. While the state is not obligated to facilitate or provide the means to reproduce, it would need a compelling justification to interfere with noncoital reproductive choices made by freely consenting persons in the private sector.

Unmarried Persons

Although no law prohibits reproduction by unmarried persons, fornication, cohabitation, and paternity laws that penalize nonmarital coitus still exist in many states. Of more immediate concern is the reluctance of physicians and hospitals to make donor insemination and other reproductive options available to single persons. Access for unmarried persons takes on greater significance as single women and same sex couples seek to beget and rear children.

The argument for the right to reproduce coitally is clearest in the case of married persons but can also be made for unmarried persons. If their right to reproduce by sexual intercourse were recognized, then they too would have a right to noncoital and donor-assisted reproduction.

A strong argument that unmarried persons should have a right to reproduce coitally can be made.[13] Unmarried persons also have needs or desires to have and rear biological descendants, and may be as competent parents as married couples. They may not be able or willing to marry to satisfy this desire. Given the personal significance of reproduction, it would seem to deserve protection for unmarried as well as married persons.[14] Indeed, banning coital or noncoital conception by single persons seems absurd when unmarried sexual relations are common and when single women cannot be forced to use contraception or to abort after pregnancy has occurred.[15] Surely capable rearers should not be denied the opportunity just because they are unmarried.

While the argument for the right of single persons to reproduce coitally persuades many persons, it is not clear that it would be accepted by the Supreme Court. The single person's right to use contraception and to continue a pregnancy once begun does not necessarily entail a right to conceive in the first place. Preventing conception and pregnancy by requiring contraception and abortion interferes with bodily integrity in a way that preventing conception in the first place—by preventing access to the needed means—does not.[16] Like the distinction between reading pornography in the home and purchasing it to bring home, these distinctions might be appealing to a Supreme Court not disposed to extend the list of fundamental rights. While traditions of family and of reproduction within marriage make it difficult for the Court to deny the procreative liberty of married persons, it may be less willing to recognize the right of single persons to reproduce. For example, the Supreme Court has not yet held that fornication and marriage laws violate an unmarried person's right of privacy. In any event, if the right of single persons to reproduce coitally is recognized, then they too should have the right to reproduce through IVF and other forms of noncoital reproduction.

Limits on the Right to Noncoital Reproduction

If the foregoing analysis seems startling, it may be because we are unpacking the implications of a right that never, because of technology, had to be unpacked. If procreative liberty protects a wider swath of reproductive activities than one might have thought, limits on reproductive choice may nevertheless exist, either because the values behind reproduction are not significantly implicated or because valid state interests justify limiting the right.

Recognition of a right to reproduce noncoitally and to contract with donors and surrogates to that end leaves unanswered many questions raised by noncoital conception. Even if there is a right to use IVF to have and rear biological descendants, it may be that IVF activities not aimed at acquiring a child for rearing are not protected. For example, a married or single person's desire to play a partial reproductive role, such as providing gametes or gestation *tout court,* may not involve the underlying values that support a right to reproduce to such an extent as to deserve protection in its own right.[17] Similarly, the values underlying a right to reproduce may be too attenuated to deserve protection when posthumous disposition of stored gametes or embryos is at issue.[18] Nor may reproductive values be strongly implicated in a person's wish to manipulate the genes of extracorporeal embryos in order to select or control offspring characteristics. Whether such reproductive choices deserve constitutional protection will depend upon the evolving social and individual meanings attached to reproduction and its disaggregated components.

A second important limit on IVF and noncoital activities would be prevention of harm to other persons or to important state interests. The main concerns with IVF have centered around harm to extracorporeal embryos, offspring, family, and the human dignity of reproduction. While some of the debate concerns the meaning of harm in a reproductive context, this article concludes that most noncoital maneuvers pose a low risk of the kinds of harm that might justify prohibition of their use.[19] Thus, regulation to assure free, informed entry into donor and surrogate transactions might be justified to protect the autonomy of the parties, but a complete ban on collaborative arrangements would ordinarily not be justified.

Noncoital reproduction, however, does raise the possibility of symbolic harm. Its main impact may be on moral or religious notions about sexuality, reproduction, family, female roles, and similar value-laden concerns. Such concerns are of immense importance to individuals and society. In choosing values, persons and societies understand themselves as beings and groups with particular ethical or moral beliefs. Because these choices are so fundamental, individuals may vary widely in their choice of and commitment to such values. It is no surprise that activities that carry such symbolic weight are controversial and lead to efforts to enlist legal institutions to enforce one's views of the matter.

Constitutional protection for noncoital reproduction thus has enormous importance, for symbolic concerns without direct, tangible harm to others are usually insufficient to justify infringing the fundamental rights of persons with different views.[20] Views of the rightness or wrongness of particular means of conception might properly animate individual choices to avoid, seek, or provide such services. They also permit the state to refrain from funding or subsidizing the activity.[21] But they generally do not justify public action that interferes with the exercise of the right.

In short, IVF and noncoital reproduction illustrate the recurring dilemma of rights in a society of limited governmental powers. Recognition of fundamental rights is essential in the constitutional scheme, yet it permits activities that may run counter to the values that a majority holds and may even lead to changes in those values. Yet the community through law may not stop the exercise of those rights, even though an impact on its value structure may occur. Noncoital reproduction is thus left to the moral discretion of patients, physicians, and other actors in the private sector.

Notes

1. The recipient of the donation, however, may have the full procreative interest, even if the donor does not. Thus, persons desiring to reproduce may have a right to receive gametes and gestation from others, even if the others have no independent right to provide those services. *See* infra text accompanying notes 11–13.

2. Whatever the constitutional posture of procreative liberty, persons in the private sector will remain free to make decisions concerning IVF and their participation in it. *See* infra text accompanying note 21.

3. 262 U.S. 390, 399 (1923).

4. 316 U.S. 535, 541 (1942). San Antonio Indep. School Dist. v. Rodriquez states that "[i]mplicit in the Court's opinion is the recognition that the right of procreation is among the rights of personal privacy protected under the Constitution." 411 U.S. 1, 34 n. 76 (1973).

5. 405 U.S. 645, 651 (1972) (citations omitted) (brackets in original).

6. Cleveland Bd. of Educ. v. LaFleur, 414 U.S. 632, 639–40 (1973) (citations omitted).

7. 405 U.S. 438, 453 (1972) (emphasis omitted). Only four members of the Court concurred in Justice Brennan's opinion. See also Bowers v. Hardwick, 106 S. Ct. 2841, 2851 (1986) (Blackmun, J., dissenting) ("We protect the decision whether to have a child because parenthood alters so dramatically an individual's self-definition, not because of demographic considerations or the Bible's command to be fruitful and multiply.")

8. See Buck v. Bell, 274 U.S. 200, 207 (1927); see also *In re* Grady, 85 N.J. 235, 251–52, 426 A.2d 467, 475 (1981) (courts can order sterilization under parens patriae jurisdiction). Recognition of the state's right to sterilize mentally incompetent persons implicitly supports the notion of the married couple's right to reproduce. These cases assume that persons have a procreative right not to be sterilized, and they examine whether mental retardation allows the right to be overridden. Although the grounds or source of the person's right is never examined, it could be justified as necessary to protect against unwanted physical intrusion and to protect the ability to reproduce if one later marries.

9. The claim of a married couple's right to reproduce coitally is a claim of substantive due process—a claim that unwritten rights exist and are appropriately identified by the Supreme Court within the confines of the fourteenth amendment.

10. The point is that state restriction of coital reproduction would be tested by a standard more rigorous than a rational basis test. Extraordinary situations like the need to reduce population because of severe over-population or food shortages might meet such a standard, . . . but a moral dislike of the way people are choosing to reproduce would not. Another conceivable ground for limitation might be when a person knowingly and avoidably conceives and brings to term a severely handicapped child and passes the costs and burdens of rearing that child to others.

11. Thus, existing fetal research, adoption, and AID laws that limit noncoital reproductive options are of doubtful constitutionality, and may be struck down if challenged. Similarly, legal presumptions about who is the rearing father and mother in situations involving donor gametes and surrogates may also fall, once the full implications of procreative liberty are recognized. . . .

12. Refusal to enforce reproductive contracts and prohibitions on money payments would amount to an interference with procreative liberty, since it would prevent

couples from obtaining the donor assistance that they need to acquire a child genetically or gestationally related to them. . . .

The right to contract for reproductive assistance asserted here may be compared
with the right of persons contemplating marriage to regulate by contract the relation
between them and a future divorce settlement. Both reproductive and prenuptial
contracts illustrate the social movement from status to contract in family and reproductive relations. . . . Recognition of such a contract right also raises the question of why
contracts to adopt children made before or after conception but before birth would not
be valid, or why parties should not be free after birth to make private contracts for
adoption directly with women who want to relinquish their children. The logic of my
argument is that persons, at least if married, have a right to acquire a child for rearing
purposes, and may resort to the medical or social means necessary to do so. Although
IVF and its variations preserve a genetic or gestational link with one of the rearing
parents, the right at issue may not be so easily confined. It may be that the law of
adoption needs to be rethought in light of the right to contract for noncoital reproductive assistance.

13. The argument for a single person's right to procreate sexually must be distinguished from the argument for the right of a single person to have sex with consenting
others and the right to avoid reproduction. Recognition of the unmarried person's
right to avoid procreation through access to birth control and abortion does not necessarily imply either a right to procreate or a right to have sex with consenting others.
Sexual liberty would not necessarily entail reproduction (merely sex with contraception), and a right to reproduce would not necessarily entail sexual freedom beyond the
sexual or other acts required for reproduction.

14. While poor, young, single mothers who are unemployed or lack skills arguably
may not be well situated to raise families, unmarried persons with means clearly could
be. Indeed, many poor, single women are capable mothers, and more single parents
than ever now raise children. Since unmarried status or single parenthood is not in
itself grounds for termination of parental rights, unmarried status is, arguably, a poor
reason to prevent conception or the means to achieve it.

15. A single person may have a right to go to term once she has conceived, i.e., a
woman cannot be forced to have an abortion even if she is single. But this right may be
based on a right of bodily integrity, rather than on a right to reproduce. Similarly, a
single woman who has given birth cannot be forced to relinquish a child just because
she is single. But in this case it would be a heavy intrusion to separate mother and child
on the basis of unmarried status when her parenting capacity is clear. Also, a single
person is constitutionally guaranteed the right to access to contraceptives in order to
avoid the burdens of reproduction. But these cases do not demonstrate that a single
person cannot be penalized for fornication. If so, the state could deny IVF and other
noncoital reproductive services to single persons.

16. The distinction is admittedly strained. In the one case, the state is forcing one
type of burden on the woman, and in the second, another type of burden altogether.
But difference in type of burden seems less important than the significance or magnitude of the burden. On this score there appears to be no morally cognizable difference
between the two.

17. This example focuses attention on the interests that make reproduction so
highly valued and on whether they are present when gestation and rearing without a
gene link occur. Indeed, it is not clear that we would say that such persons have
reproduced. In the reverse case, a gene link without gestation and rearing, we might

accurately say that reproduction has occurred. For example, an anonymous sperm donor has reproduced himself when a child is born from his donation even if there is never any contact between them. It would not follow, however, that the choice to give or withhold the sperm is part of protected liberty, for some additional interest could be required before a reproductive incident is constitutionally protected. The case of rearing or gestating without the hereditary link may have those other incidents and thus merit constitutional protection even though the avoidance or creation of an hereditary link alone does not. . . .

18. This issue involves an assessment of the importance to people of the knowledge that a biological descendant will come into being and live after one has died. . . . The right to transmit property to embryos and children born posthumously of stored gametes is a separate matter.

19. However, prohibition in particular instances might be justified. For example, the offspring's interest in knowing her genetic roots may justify a ban on collaborative reproduction that does not maintain records concerning the gamete source.

20. There is no way to understand cases such as Roe v. Wade, . . . Eisenstadt v. Baird, . . . Griswold v. Connecticut, . . . and a host of others other than as standing for the proposition that symbolic or moral evaluation of protected conduct without more does not justify state interference with the conduct. The community's power to enforce or impose morality stops at the threshold of another person's fundamental rights.

21. Since procreative liberty is (like most constitutional rights) a negative—not a positive—right, it obligates the state to refrain from interference with reproductive arrangements among consenting adults and physicians. It does not obligate the state to fund these activities or allow the activities in state institutions, any more than the state is obligated to fund abortions or contraception. . . . Nor is the private sector obligated to offer IVF services. Hospitals may refuse to allow IVF or may restrict the reproductive transactions that it allows. Doctors and institutions conducting IVF may set their own limits on what they will permit. The power of the private sector suggests that patient-physician relations may be as important as constitutional limitations in determining the development and impact of the new reproduction. . . .

Equal Protection for Whom?

George P. Smith III and Roberto Iraola

Traditional Equal Protection Analysis

. . . When a statute creates a classification resulting in disparate treatment of similarly situated people, the equal protection clause[1] compels courts to examine the justification for the classification. The level of scrutiny to be employed, however, will depend on the interest at stake. Traditionally, the legislative classification will be upheld if it is "reasonable, not arbitrary," and if it rests "upon some ground of difference having a fair and substantial relation to the object of the legislation. . . ." However, if a fundamental right is involved, a more critical examination of the classification is required. A higher level of scrutiny then demands that "the statutory classification . . . be not merely *rationally related* to a valid public purpose but *necessary* to the achievement of a *compelling* state interest."

The AID [artificial insemination with donor sperm] statutes make an express classification between married and unmarried women. Accordingly, the next step in the analysis is determining whether the right affected by the classification is fundamental. If the right is "explicitly or implicitly guaranteed by the Constitution," it will be deemed fundamental, and the strict scrutiny standard will apply. Or the strict scrutiny standard will apply if the classification involves a suspect class.

But equal protection arguments are an inappropriate basis for those seeking to protect informal, illicit relationships.[2] Legal distinctions between married and unmarried persons are justified when the state seeks to protect and regulate marriage as a social institution, as well as to maintain and validate legitimate individual interests, such as property, taxation, contracts, and torts, which are inherent in every marital relationship.

Recently, a number of commentators have suggested that an unmarried woman's right to AID may derive from a liberal reading of Supreme Court decisions establishing fundamental rights to procreation and privacy.[3] The following discussion summarizes the points of view presented in those cases.

As society evolves and changes, so do many of its values. Autonomy, self-

From sections III & IV of "Sexuality, Privacy and the New Biology," *Marquette Law Review* 67 (1984), pp. 263–291. Reprinted with permission of the Marquette Law Review.

representation, personhood, identity, intimacy, and dignity are all essential to privacy. The extent to which these essentials play a role in shaping sexual, procreational autonomy must surely remain flexible; attempting to define them with precision would challenge and erode any efficacy they might enjoy. The right of the state to control and to shape the behavior of both individuals and groups regarding the birth of children is always an area of high emotion and concern.

The majority view on privacy holds that private conduct between consenting adults or, for that matter, personal conduct of any nature, should be regulated only to the extent necessary to prevent harm to others.[4] Thus conformity is not a priority and is certainly not a value worth pursuing. The opposing view argues that the business of the law is to suppress vice and immorality.[5] Advocates of this view reason that if violations of society's moral structure are indulged and promoted, the whole basis of society would be undermined.

Arguably, under the majority view, the state would be justified in acting to control personal decision making in the areas of artificial insemination and surrogation for unmarried women. The requirement of harm to others is met because society could suffer economic harm by incurring expenses associated with the maintenance and education of a fatherless child born of artificial insemination. Similarly, the prevention of harm theory could be invoked in surrogation where the state, by attempting to prevent such acts, seeks to maintain the dignity and continuity of the traditional family.

A Basic Right to Procreate?

Buck v. Bell[6] was the first case to address what has now come to be regarded as a fundamental right to procreate. In *Bell* the Supreme Court upheld a Virginia statute that permitted the sterilization of state institution inmates who suffered from hereditary forms of insanity or imbecility. The opinion, authored by Justice Holmes, was written before the fundamental right-compelling state interest standard was developed. Thus, it must be determined whether the Court's opinion implicitly recognized the existence of a compelling state interest, or whether the Court refused to classify procreation as a fundamental right. The latter appears to be the case; it has been suggested that the Court's emphasis on the state's right to promote the general good or welfare approximates a rational basis standard of judicial review.[7]

In *Skinner v. Oklahoma*[8] the Supreme Court again considered the validity of compulsory sterilization laws. Unlike the *Bell* Court, which did not find an equal protection violation, the *Skinner* Court struck down an Oklahoma sterilization statute on equal protection grounds. The statute provided for the sterilization of habitual criminals, that is, persons convicted of three or more felonies. However, the statute did not consider felonies which arose from the violation of prohibitory laws, revenue acts, embezzlement, or political offenses. In its opinion, the Court first recognized that marriage and procreation are fundamental to both the existence and survival of mankind. It then observed, however, that for purposes of criminal sterilization, a classification distinguishing larcenists from embezzlers represented a form of invidious discrimination. Consequently, the Court subjected the classification to strict scrutiny and found it violative of the equal protection clause.

Although a number of subsequent Supreme Court decisions have cited the *Skinner* case as validating, if not in fact creating, a constitutional right to procreate,[9] it is important to recognize the precise contours of that right. In both *Bell* and *Skinner,* the Court confronted sterilization statutes. Sterilization, unlike other methods of control over human reproduction, is irreversible. Thus, in discussing the procreative "right" affected by Oklahoma's Habitual Criminal Sterilization Act, the *Skinner* Court aptly observed that this "right [is] basic to the perpetuation of a race. . . ."[10] Given this background, it is apparent that the procreative right recognized in *Skinner* was simply a right to remain fertile, and not an uninhibited right to engage in potentially procreative conduct.

Searching for a Fundamental Right to Sexual Privacy

Neither the rationale of *Buck v. Bell* nor *Skinner v. Oklahoma* applies to the insemination issue, creating a new right in the area. Nowhere does the Constitution mention a right to privacy. Nor is any right of sexual freedom to be found within the ambit of procreative rights recognized by the Supreme Court. Nor, for that matter, has the Court fashioned a general right of personal privacy which is sufficiently broad to permit sex outside marriage.[11] However, in *Griswold v. Connecticut*[12] the Supreme Court recognized a constitutionally protected zone of privacy and invalidated part of a Connecticut statute forbidding the use of contraceptives by married persons.[13] The protection of this aspect of procreative autonomy "was largely subsumed within a broad right of marital privacy"[14] which "stressed the unity and independence of the married couple and forbade undue inquiry into conjugal acts."[15] But it cannot be argued from this that there must exist a corresponding fundamental right to reproduce or to use artificial reproductive technology.[16] As Justice Goldberg made emphatically clear in his concurring opinion, *Griswold* "in no way interferes with a State's proper regulation of sexual promiscuity or misconduct."[17] Thus, the constitutionality of Connecticut's statutes prohibiting adultery and fornication remained beyond dispute.

In *Eisenstadt v. Baird*[18] the Court was confronted with a Massachusetts statute which prohibited the distribution of contraceptives to unmarried persons. In holding that the statute violated the equal protection clause of the fourteenth amendment, the Court observed that, "[if] the right of privacy means anything, it is the right of the *individual,* married or single, to be free from unwarranted governmental intrusion into matters so fundamentally affecting a person as the decision whether to bear or beget a child." Accordingly, the *Eisenstadt* Court fleshed out the procreative skeleton of *Griswold* at a time when *Griswold* appeared confined to the so-called "sacred" precincts of the matrimonial bedroom chambers. However, this decision did no more than refine a qualified right to procreative autonomy blurred by the *Griswold* Court's emphasis on the marital relation.[19]

In *Roe v. Wade*[20] the Court squarely addressed an integral part of the individual's right to procreative autonomy. In *Roe* an unmarried woman challenged the constitutionality of the Texas criminal abortion laws. The Court articulated a new source of privacy derived from the fourteenth amendment's standard of personal liberty and inherent restrictions upon state action. It held that this right was sufficiently broad to embrace a decision made by a woman to terminate her pregnancy.[21] The Court went on to state, however, that it was not recognizing "an unlimited right to do with one's body as one pleases. . . ."

The final case of interest is *Carey v. Population Services International.*[21] In *Carey,* the Court invalidated a New York statute regulating the sale and distribution of contraceptives to minors and stated that "at the very heart of [the] cluster of constitutionally protected choices" recognized in the previous privacy cases[23] is "the decision whether or not to beget or bear a child. . . ." As the following discussion illustrates, this decision is particularly instructive on the question of the unmarried woman's right to artificial insemination because it examines the previous privacy cases and delineates the extent of the individual's right to procreative autonomy.

Although it has been suggested by some commentators that since a woman has a right to terminate her pregnancy and to use contraceptives, a fortiori, the conduct required to bring about those procreative choices must also be protected,[24] the Court's opinion in *Carey* indicated that this is simply not the case. First, with regard to contraception and abortion, the Court made it clear that it is the "individual's right to decide to *prevent conception* or *terminate pregnancy*" that is protected. Such unequivocal language lends little or no support to the argument that a concomitant right to conceive is also protected. Second, the Court emphasized that its decision did not encompass any constitutional questions raised by state statutes regulating either sexual freedom or adult sexual relations. This reading of *Carey* is supported by a later decision of the Court in which it stated that if the "right to procreate means anything at all, it must imply some right to enter the only relationship in which the state . . . allows sexual relations legally to take place."[25] The lesson from the Court's decisions in *Skinner, Griswold, Eisenstadt, Roe,* and *Carey* is plain: "procreative autonomy includes both the right to remain fertile and the right to avoid conception,"[26] but nothing more.

The Level of Scrutiny and the State's Justification for Action

Since the unmarried woman's decision to be artificially inseminated does not fall within the ambit of any recognized fundamental right, state statutes limiting this procreative technology to married women may "be sustained under the less demanding test of rationality. . . ."[27] Under this test, the distinction drawn must merely be "rationally related" to a "constitutionally permissible" objective.[28] In employing this rather relaxed standard, courts must be sensitive to the fact "that the drawing of lines that create distinctions is peculiarly a legislative task and an unavoidable one."[29]

Absent a suspect classification or the infringement of a fundamental right, the Supreme Court has recognized that legislation "protecting legitimate family relationships," as well as both the regulation and protection of the family unit, are "venerable" concerns of the state.[30] Statutes limiting the availability of artificial insemination to married women fall squarely within this classification.

As early as 1888, the Court recognized marriage as "the foundation of the family and society, without which there would be neither civilization nor progress."[31] Recently, the Court observed that "a decision to marry and raise the child in a traditional family setting must receive . . . protection."[32] Thus, although certain aspects of an individual's right to procreative autonomy have been lawfully separated from the familial and marital relationship, the Court has also implicitly recognized that, whenever possible, childrearing should take place within the traditional family unit.[33] An unmarried woman's decision to seek artificial insemination goes against the tide of these pronouncements.

Adoption laws offer an instructive analogy. Like statutes regulating artificial insemination, adoption statutes are rooted in state law. Although all states currently allow adoption by unmarried adults, it occurs only in rare cases. In *Adoption of H.*,[34] both an unmarried middle-aged woman and a young couple sought to adopt a thirteen-month-old child. In rejecting the unmarried woman's application, the court observed:

> Adoption by a single person has generally and in this Court's experience been sought and approved only in exceptional circumstances, and in particular for the hard-to-place child for whom no desirable parental couple is available. In the universal view of both experts and laymen, while one parent may be better than none for the hard-to-place child, joint responsibility by a father and a mother contributes to the child's physical, financial, and psychic security as well as his emotional growth. This view is more than a matter of present convention, anthropologists pointing out that the institution of marriage, which is a method of signifying commitment to such joint responsibility, evolved in response to the need for two-parent care of children.

This observation applies with equal force to the artificial insemination of unmarried women.[35] Indeed, if a state may reasonably regulate unmarried adults in their quest to adopt children, it may be contradictory to suggest that the state could not regulate an unmarried individual's use of a procreative technology designed to bring children into the world.

More importantly, however, the unmarried woman's access to artificial insemination and, thus, surrogation, directly undermines "[t]he basic foundation of the family in our society, the marriage relationship. . . ."[36] The desirability of having a child reared within a traditional family unit has been repeatedly recognized by the courts.[37] Moreover, it is clear that "[w]ithin the traditional model, marriage serves as the genesis of the family. . . ."[38] Accordingly, both the inherent procreative potential of this union and the stability to the social fabric it provides would be dealt a fatal blow by either permitting unmarried women to be artificially inseminated or permitting them to act as surrogate mothers.[39] Equally unpersuasive is an argument that a state is painting with too broad a brush when it limits AI [artificial insemination] to married couples. Although the Supreme Court has failed to formulate a concrete definition of the family, *Moore v. City of East Cleveland*[40] "represents the only clear extension of protection [routinely afforded the nuclear family] to a quasi-familial group."[41] In *Moore* a zoning ordinance which limited an area to single family dwellings was challenged by a woman who shared her home with her two grandsons. The Court recognized that the extended family occupies a place in American tradition similar to that of the nuclear family and, thus, is to be guaranteed protection by the Constitution. As the procreation and privacy cases illustrate by analogy, although a mother and her offspring may find protection within the nuclear family structure, this does not imply a right to freely bring about that condition, nor does it demonstrate that the limitations placed on AI with respect to unmarried women are in any way irrational. Thus, an expanded definition of family is required in order to contend that statutes limiting AI to married women are not rationally related to a constitutionally permissible objective. The line of demarcation may be drawn imprecisely, but the Constitution is not offended "simply because the classification 'is not made with mathematical nicety or because in practice it results in some inequality.' "[42]

Conclusion

The legal system, by protecting relationships such as kinship and formal marriage, promotes not only the interests of the parties involved, but the interests of society in social and political structures which ensure a long-term individual view of liberty. As one legal commentator remarked:

> [T]he structure of marriage and kinship responds to that social interest by maximizing the interest of children and society in a stable family environment; by ensuring a socialization process and an attitude toward personal obligation that maximizes democracy's interest in the voluntary "public virtue" of its citizens; by maintaining marriage and kinship as legally recognizable structures that mediate between the individual and the State, thereby limiting governmental power; and by maintaining sources of objective jurisprudence that will ensure stable personal expectations and encourage generality of laws, thereby minimizing the arbitrary power of the state. In these ways, the structure of formal family life emphasizes that sense of

"ordered liberty" necessary to achieve individual liberty as a long range objective.[43]

In judicial decisions affording familial and marriage relationships a higher degree of constitutional protection, tradition has played a pivotal role. In the procreative field, the Supreme Court has carved out a limited degree of autonomy for the individual. As this article has demonstrated, a woman's fundamental right to privacy or procreation does not encompass a right to AI or to surrogation. Accordingly, statutes limiting the use of this reproductive technology need only be rationally related to a constitutionally permissible state interest. The state's desire to raise children in the *traditional* family setting and, at the same time, promote the institution of marriage and the family is an unquestionably permissible, if not laudable, objective. Thirty years ago, Justice Frankfurter cautioned: "Children have a very special place in life which law should reflect. Legal theories and their phrasing in other cases readily lead to fallacious reasoning if uncritically transferred. . . ."[44] State legislatures, in limiting the practice of artificial insemination to married women, have taken this advice to heart. The extended use and application of this procedure through surrogation must be strictly controlled by legislative design. Surrogation should be limited to married women who have gained their husband's consent, and then, only under proper medically supervised conditions. As a medical aid to infertility, surrogation should be allowed only as an adjunct to medical treatment of the impediment and not as a popular or novel experiment.

A legislative program designed to validate, and thereby license, the procedure of surrogation for married women, as well as the married surrogates participating therein, should seek to not only protect the health and well-being of the issue born, but also to assure the safety of the surrogate. Ideally, such a legislative program should include provisions shaping the rights and determining the extent of the contracting parents' liabilities in the surrogate contract vis-a-vis the infant. Due consideration should be given to shaping the sphere of responsibility for various types of error which intermediaries, such as doctors and lawyers, might commit in facilitating the process. In addition, the specific policy matters coincident with the administration of a structured surrogation program should be implemented by an administrative body or licensing board. The Surrogate Parenting Associates, Inc., of Kentucky could serve as a model for legislative reform in other states. Their policies and standards for evaluating and processing requests for surrogate mothering are both comprehensive and equitable in their design and utilization.

The new reproductive biological techniques are of enormous significance for humanity and demand a comprehensive inquiry into the parameters of future development. The legislative branch of government is far better equipped to deal with this inquiry than the executive or judicial branches. Thoughtful study and cautious planning are needed now before the growing complexities overwhelm, confuse, and confound the role of the rule of law in meeting the challenges of the brave new world of tomorrow.

Notes

1. [The equal protection clause of the Fourteenth Amendment to the Constitution stipulates that no state shall "deny to any person within its jurisdiction the equal protection of the laws."]

2. Hafen, *The Constitutional Status of Marriage, Kinship, and Sexual Privacy— Balancing the Individual and Social Interest,* 81 Mich. L. Rev. 463, 541 (1983).

3. *See generally* Annas, *Fathers Anonymous: Beyond the Best Interest of the Sperm Donor,* 14 Fam. L.Q. 1 (1980); Kritchevsky, *The Unmarried Woman's Right to Artificial Insemination: A Call for an Expanded Definition of Family,* 4 Harv. Women's L.J. 1, 26–39 (1981); Shaman, *Legal Aspects of Artificial Insemination,* 18 J. Fam. L. 331, 344–46 (1979); Comment, *Artificial Insemination and Surrogate Motherhood—A Nursery Full of Unresolved Questions,* 17 Willamette: L.J. 913, 935 (1981). *See also* Robertson, *Procreative Liberty and the Control of Conception, Pregnancy and Childbirth,* 69 Va. L. Rev. 405, 405–36 (1983).

4. H.L.A. Hart, Law, Liberty and Morality 57 (1963).

5. P. Devlin, The Enforcement of Morals 7 (1965).

6. 274 U.S. 200 (1927).

7. Note, *Legislative Naivete in Involuntary Sterilization Laws,* 12 Wake Forest L. Rev. 1064, 1071 (1976). Writing for the *Bell* Court, Justice Holmes observed: "We have seen more than once that the public welfare may call upon the best citizens for their lives. It would be strange if it could not call upon those who already sap the strength of the state for these lesser sacrifices, often not felt to be such by those concerned, in order to prevent our being swamped with incompetence. It is better for all the world, if instead of waiting to execute degenerate offspring for crime, or to let them starve for their imbecility, society can prevent those who are manifestly unfit from continuing their kind." 274 U.S. at 207.

8. 316 U.S. 535 (1942).

9. Comment, *Artificial Human Reproduction: Legal Problems Presented by the Test Tube Baby,* 28 Emory L.J. 1045, 1056 (1979). Indeed, this commentator suggested that *Skinner* has been incorrectly interpreted since "the *Skinner* Court neither denied the state's right to sterilize nor established a constitutional right to procreate. Rather, the Court expressly declared that the scope of the state's policy power was unaffected by its holding." . . .

10. *Skinner,* at 536. Writing for the Court, Justice Douglas stated: "The power to sterilize, if exercised, may have subtle, far-reaching and devastating effects. In evil or reckless hands it can cause races or types which are inimical to the dominant group to wither and disappear. There is no redemption for the individual whom the law touches" (541).

11. Hafen, supra note 2, at 538.

12. 381 U.S. 479 (1965).

13. Id. at 485. The Court observed that "specific guarantees in the Bill of Rights have penumbras, formed by emanations from those guarantees that help give them life and substance." *Id.* at 484 (citation omitted). Thus, it is those "[v]arious guarantees [which] create [the] zones of privacy." Id.

14. Note, *Eugenic Artificial Insemination: A Cure for Mediocrity?,* 94 Harv. L. Rev. 1850,1867 (1981).

15. *Developments in the Law—The Constitution and the Family,* 93 Harv. L. Rev. 1156, 1183 (1980).

16. Comment, supra note 9, at 1058.

17. *Griswold,* 381 U.S. at 498–99 (Goldberg, J., concurring). But Professor Tribe states that since *Griswold* recognized as valid individual decisions not to bear a child, read as such and considered with *Skinner,* it forces the conclusion that whether or not one's body is to be the source of new life, "must be left to that person and that person alone to decide." L. Tribe, American Constitutional Law 923 (1978).

18. 405 U.S. 438 (1972).

19. "It has been suggested that the Court's opinion was lacking in candor, for it stated in broad dictum a major extension of the 'privacy' right which could have justified its decision, while purporting to rest on a strained conclusion that the statute involved failed even the minimal rationality test." *Developments in the Law,* supra note 114, at 1184 (footnotes omitted).

Under an expansive liberal interpretation, *Eisenstadt* has been seen as extending the right of privacy to all sexual activities of whatever nature. See Wilkinson & White, note 12, at 589. . . .

A more conservative and narrow construction views *Eisenstadt* as merely recognizing a freedom to decide issues related to the birth of a child. See, e.g., Neville v. State, 290 Md. 364, 374, 403 A.2d 570, 575 (1981); People v. Onofre, 51 N.Y.2d 476, 498, N.E.2d 936, 946, 434 N.Y.S.2d 947, 957 (1980) (Gabrielli, J., dissenting); State v. Santos, 413 A.2d 58, 68 (R.I. 1980).

20. 410 U.S. 113 (1973).

21. Id. at 153. This right, however, is not absolute and the degree of involvement allowed is contingent upon the length of the pregnancy. . . .

22. 431 U.S. 678 (1977) (plurality opinion).

23. In addition to the privacy cases already discussed in this article, the Court cited Cleveland Bd. of Educ. v. La Fleur, 414 U.S. 632 (1974); Loving v. Virginia, 388 U.S. 1 (1967); Prince v. Massachusetts, 321 U.S. 158 (1944); Pierce v. Society of Sisters, 268 U.S. 510 (1925).

24. Kritchevsky, supra note 3, at 27–28.

25. Zablocki v. Redhail, 434 U.S. 374, 386 (1978).

26. *Developments in the Law,* supra note 15, at 1185.

27. Maher v. Roe, 432 U.S. 464, 478 (1977).

28. Lindsey v. Normet, 405 U.S. 56, 74 (1972).

29. Massachusetts Bd. of Retirement v. Murgia, 427 U.S. 307, 314 (1976).

30. Weber v. Aetna Casualty & Sur. Co., 406 U.S. 164, 173 (1972) (citation omitted).

31. Maynard v. Hill, 125 U.S. 190, 211 (1888).

32. Zablocki v. Redhail, 434 U.S. 374, 386 (1978).

33. See generally Parham v. J.R., 442 U.S. 584 (1979); Wisconsin v. Yoder, 406 U.S. 205 (1972); Pierce v. Soc'y of Sisters, 268 U.S. 510 (1925); Meyer v. Nebraska, 262 U.S. 390 (1923).

34. 69 Misc. 2d 304, 330 N.Y.S.2d 235 (1972).

35. One commentator has argued that the AI [artificial insemination] process in fact makes "it less likely that the parent will be indigent or emotionally unfit to care for the child. . . . First, because the procedure of AI itself is expensive, its use would tend to be limited to the nonindigent. Second, prospective AI mothers . . . receive screening and counseling to ensure that they are fit to become parents. . . . Third . . . use of AI guarantees that the child be born into a home that sincerely wants it, and there is no reason to believe that this is less true in the single parent than the dual parent

home. . . . [F]inally, since a woman refused AI remains free to choose to conceive through sexual intercourse, any state rationale arguing that eliminating AI will protect it financially or will protect children is irrational." Kritchevsky, supra note 3 at 29.

36. Smith v. Organization of Foster Families for Equality & Reform, 431 U.S. 816, 843 (1977).

37. *See* supra note 33.

38. *Developments in the Law,* supra note 114, at 1270.

39. One commentator recently suggested that a clearer understanding of the family-marriage-procreation cases can be attained by focusing on the right to freedom of intimate association underlying those decisions. Karst, *The Freedom of Intimate Association,* 89 Yale L.J. 624 (1980) at 625. According to Professor Karst, procreation is considered fundamental because it "strongly implicates the values of intimate association, particularly the values of caring and commitment, intimacy, and self-identification." Id. See also Note, supra note 14 at 1869. None of these values is present in the unmarried woman's desire to AI, thus lending further support to a state's legitimate interest in limiting AI to married women.

40. 431 U.S. 494 (1977).

41. *Developments in the Law,* supra note 15, at 1272.

42. Dandridge v. Williams, 397 U.S. 471, 485 (1970) (quoting Lindsley v. Natural Carbonic Gas Co., 220 U.S. 61, 78 (1911).

43. Hafen, supra note 2 at 559.

44. May v. Anderson, 345 U.S. 528, 536 (1953) (Frankfurter, J., concurring).

Legal Problems of Surrogate Motherhood

Noel P. Keane

The development of new reproductive technologies, such as artificial insemination, poses a variety of legal questions which often cannot be readily resolved in terms of traditional legal doctrines and categories. Those who employ technically feasible but legally unrecognized solutions to marital or reproductive difficulties often must act without being certain of the legal consequences. Such a state of affairs cannot be reconciled with the recent recognition of a constitutional right of privacy which protects decisions with respect to marriage and reproduction.

This article concerns the legal issues raised by the practice of surrogate motherhood by means of artificial insemination. This refers to an arrangement between a married couple who is unable to have a child because of the wife's infertility and a fertile woman who agrees to conceive the husband's child through artificial insemination, carry it to term, then surrender all parental rights in the child. Often, the surrogate mother receives compensation for her services. The final step in the process is typically the father's acknowledgment of paternity and adoption, with his wife, of the child. Through surrogate motherhood, a couple desiring a child need not wait an indefinite number of years for an adoptable baby, as generally happens at the present time. The married couple obtains a child who is the husband's biological offspring—a child for whose existence both husband and wife can feel responsible.

Despite the arrangement's simplicity and advantages for all concerned, surrogate motherhood is fraught with legal difficulties. In most, perhaps all states, a contract providing for surrogate motherhood is probably void. In some states, payment for parental consent to the adoption of a child is a crime. Moreover, the child itself may be considered illegitimate, and some courts have even taken the view that artificial insemination, except between husband and wife, is adultery. The applicable law, whether statutory or decisional, was not fashioned with surrogate motherhood in mind.

If the surrogate mother is married, additional difficulties arise at the adoption stage. In some states, adoption by the donor and his wife may be blocked by an irrebuttable presumption that a child born to a married couple is the

From *Southern Illinois University Law Journal* 1980 no. 2, pp. 147–169. Abridged. © 1980 by the Board of Trustees of Southern Illinois University. Reprinted with permission.

legitimate offspring of that couple. The donor-husband and his wife would be unable to adopt the child in such a state, unless direct private adoption is available. Other states regard this presumption as rebuttable, thereby offering a friendlier forum for the adoption proceedings. . . . Overall, however, the law is at best awkwardly adapted, and at worst, hostile to the surrogate motherhood arrangement. . . .

Statutory and Public Policy Impediments to Compensating the Surrogate Mother

Among the most serious impediments to surrogate motherhood arrangements are statutes in effect in some states which make it a crime to make payments to a (biological) parent in connection with the adoption of his child. Although the evident purpose of these statutes is to prevent the "sale" of infants as if they were property, their language is sufficiently broad—or overbroad—to forbid compensation for a surrogate mother. Thus a California statute makes it a misdemeanor to pay or offer to pay a parent in return for the placement of his child for adoption, or his consent to, or cooperation with the child's adoption. A Michigan statute forbids payment of any money or other consideration in connection with placing a child for adoption or the release of parental rights, except as approved by a court. Parties are required to file an accounting of all fees and expenses which are subject to court approval.

A respected Michigan judge with considerable experience in the domestic relations area has expressed his informal opinion that only the direct medical expenses of the surrogate mother—not the value of her services in carrying the child or even her foregone income—could be approved by the court.[1]

Although such statutes are rarely enforced, their very existence deters surrogate motherhood arrangements. Apart from the possibility of criminal prosecution, such statutes render surrogate motherhood contracts void and unenforceable under the doctrine that contracts requiring an illegal act are unenforceable by any party.

A contract is deemed unenforceable if it contravenes the law or a known public policy. Even without a statute, a court may hold, as did the Georgia Supreme Court, that a contract calling for payment to a mother in return for placing her child for adoption is unenforceable on public policy grounds.[2] If a surrogate motherhood contract is unenforceable, the married couple would be without recourse if the surrogate mother aborted the husband/father's child or decided to keep it, and the surrogate mother would likewise be unable to enforce payment if the married couple failed to pay her.

Unless surrogate mothers can be offered meaningful compensation for their services, very few children will be brought legally into the world in this manner. Pregnancy and childbirth are hazardous, time-consuming, painful conditions which few women can be expected to experience for the sake of someone else unless they receive meaningful compensation. The irony is that the masculine counterpart to surrogate motherhood—the "surrogate fatherhood" of a sperm donor in the AID situation—is apparently lawful in all jurisdictions, enjoying explicit legislative recognition in some, despite the fact that the semen is usually paid for and the sperm donor assumes none of the risk and burdens that an "ovum donor" does.

Public Policy—The Child's Best Interest

Statutes like those in Michigan and California serve a legitimate purpose insofar as they forbid the sale of infants as if they were chattels. Children are not the property of their parents[3] and cannot be made the subject of barter.[4] Due to the scarcity of adoptable babies—a scarcity aggravated by the increased availability of abortion and contraceptives as well as other circumstances—the baby black market is flourishing. Prohibitory legislation may well be justified, although it is often difficult to enforce. Surrogate motherhood, though, is radically different from baby-buying and presents a situation which was never envisaged by the legislatures that enacted the penal statutes now in force. As applied in such situations, their impact is harmful and, as discussed below,[5] their constitutionality is questionable.

Policy reasons underlying the antipathy to payment for adoption are largely inapplicable to the surrogate situation. The principal reason for this policy is undoubtedly a desire to protect and promote the family, which the courts have often identified as the foundation of society. An Illinois decision, *Willey v. Lawton,*[6] held that an agreement between the natural parent and the adopting parents, whereby the latter agreed to pay the natural parent for adoption of the child, was unenforceable as contrary to public policy. The court reasoned that the bartering away of children for a property return "tends to the destruction of one of the finest relations of human life," the parent/child relation. There is merit in the court's decision considering the particular facts of the case. The former husband of a woman who had remarried was in arrears in paying child support, and the couple contracted with the delinquent husband to forego the arrearages and pay $5,000 in return for his consent to their adoption of the child born to the divorced parties during their marriage. Thus an established parent/child relationship between the biological and custodial father and his legitimate child would have been disrupted, and the father's motive in consenting to adoption could only have been economic duress overbearing his desire to keep the child.

In the typical baby-buying situation, an involuntarily pregnant unwed mother gives birth to an illegitimate child whose biological father usually takes no interest in it. Even if the mother desires to keep the child, she is often financially unable to do so. An intermediary whose motives are strictly mercenary brings "buyer" and "seller" together on the basis of the buyer's urgent desire for a child and the seller's financial exigency. Both "adoptive" parents are biologically unrelated to the child, which is removed from the single mother who, despite her perhaps difficult circumstances, may well represent a rudimentary but real "family" for the child. The "adoptive" parents' fitness is not ascertained by anyone, and the biological mother may well experience guilt and pain over relinquishing her child, especially in these circumstances. At least in some cases, a potential parent/child relationship is precluded for reasons unrelated to the child's well-being or the true desires of its biological mother.

Surrogate motherhood is different. A married couple desiring a child which the wife is incapable of bearing herself enters into the arrangement, not to "buy" a biologically unrelated baby, but to bring a child into existence by conscious prearrangement which is, as far as biologically possible, their "own." Without entering into an adulterous sexual relationship which might impair the marriage, the husband arranges to become the child's biological father. The surrogate mother, on her part, consciously chooses to bear a child for another couple with the understanding that she will consent to their adoption of it. The decision to give up the child for adoption is not the product of the adverse circumstances of an unplanned pregnancy. When the child is born, there is already a home prepared for it with its biological father and his wife. The potential for feelings of guilt or loss on the biological mother's part is minimized, though not eliminated.

Realistically, the only true "family" whose future is at stake is the one the child is predestined to enter—that of the childless married couple—not the nominal, intentionally temporary "family" represented by the surrogate mother. Clearly, surrogate motherhood, like AID, *strengthens* the family insofar as it offers a solution for couples whose marriage may well be endangered by a desire for children which is frustrated by one spouse's reproductive incapacity. Whatever implications surrogate motherhood has for the family in the abstract, it means joy and fulfillment for certain real, flesh-and-blood families approaching despair over their inability to realize their parental aspirations.

Commercializing Aspect and Black Market Statutes

Ringing denunciations of baby-buying and declarations that children are not property may make stirring reading, but it is difficult to specify precisely why the "commercialization" of a surrogate motherhood arrangement is inconsistent with public policy. In a commercial society, "commercialization" is the usual way in which many individual needs are satisfied. There is no doubt that the financial return may motivate the surrogate mother to make her reproductive capacity available to others. Any broker or intermediary who brings the interested parties together could also act from motives of pecuniary gain, although he may also be acting incidental to a role such as attorney or physician, serving his client's best interests as he sees them.[7] What is important, however, is that the adoptive parents are no more acting upon economic considerations than are married couples who elect to have children.[8] The involvement of third parties whose actions are influenced by the profit motive may well justify regulation of surrogate motherhood agreements,[9] but not their prohibition.

The application of the anti–black market statutes to surrogate motherhood contracts poses a number of problems on the issue of what, if anything, may be paid to the surrogate mother without contravening the statutes. Under the Michigan statute, medical and other "expenses" may apparently be paid, but nothing beyond that. One authority is of the opinion that the surrogate's foregone wages cannot be paid,[10] but this is not clear from the statutory language. If the object of the statute is to prevent anyone from "profiting" from an adoption, it should not be necessary to proscribe payments which merely compensate the surrogate mother's income loss. In a Nevada decision, the issue arose as to whether a newspaper had libelled an attorney by referring to his arrangement of an adoption in which the biological mother was paid for foregone wages as a "black-market" sale of the child.[11] The court stated: "Under any reasonable construction of the term, 'black market sale' contemplates a sale contrary to regulations with a profit calculated either to compensate for the risk of apprehension or to match the buyer demand which has created the market." The court held that a jury could properly decide, as it did, that compensation for lost wages did not turn the transaction into a sale, stating:

> Appellants contend that the compensation paid for loss of wages amounted to a profit and constituted the transaction a sale. In absence of statute the determination of whether such compensation was proper rested in the first instance with the jury. We shall not disturb their determination, implicit in their verdict, that such compensation did not constitute the transaction a sale. There is nothing to indicate that the payment permitted the mother to profit from childbirth. To the contrary, it would seem to have been intended simply to prevent her confinement from resulting in pecuniary loss.

One difficulty in applying these statutes to surrogate motherhood contracts is that they relate only to the final phase—the adoption—of a contract which has other important provisions. The surrogate mother is not paid primarily for consenting to the adoption of the child. The services performed which justify substantial compensation consist rather of pregnancy and parturition, together with the risks and limitations which these experiences entail. These statutes do not purport to make it a crime to pay someone for becoming pregnant or having a baby. This omission, of course, confirms that surrogate motherhood was never the intended target of the anti–black market statutes. What the surrogate mother has to offer is what the sterile wife of the biological father unfortunately lacks: the biological capacity to reproduce. The essence of the surrogate motherhood contract is to redress the injustice of nature in conferring this capacity on certain individuals who are able but unwilling to assume parental responsibilities while denying it to others who are willing but unable to do so. Thanks to artificial insemination, the solution of the biological problem is technically simple. What complicates the situation is the legal significance that the state has placed on the fact of biological parenthood. Because the custody of and parental responsibility for the child of an unmarried mother is automatically assigned to her upon the child's birth, it is necessary to terminate her parental rights and bestow them on the biological father and his wife through adoption of the child by the latter. Yet this final stage of the surrogate arrangement is apparently interdicted by the anti–black market statutes.

Because "the statutes prohibiting black-market transactions are normally couched in terms of a prohibition against receiving compensation for child placement,"[12] surrogate motherhood contracts appear to be proscribed by the statutory language if it is read literally. But it is certain that surrogate motherhood was not within the contemplation of the legislators who enacted these statutes, and surrogate motherhood contracts present few of the evils of baby-buying. Where statutory language is of doubtful meaning, a reasonable construction must be given to effect the purpose of the statute; the spirit of the statute should prevail over the strict letter to avoid unjust applications and absurd consequences. Additionally, as these statutes carry criminal sanctions, they should be narrowly interpreted. Ambiguities with respect to the ambit of criminal statutes should be resolved in favor of lenity. Finally, even if such statutes render surrogate motherhood contracts technically illegal, it may not follow that they are invariably unenforceable. The rule that contracts requiring an illegal act are unenforceable is not inflexible, and courts must look to the legislative intent before invalidating such agreements. No specific legislative intent to invalidate surrogate motherhood contracts can be shown, since such arrangements have only recently come to the attention of the public, and courts should await explicit legislative direction before invalidating these voluntary agreements among adults.

Enforcing the Surrogate Motherhood Contract

Even if surrogate motheroood contracts were lawful and enforceable, the unique features of the arrangement would still present difficulties in the event of a breach. If the biological father and his wife breached the contract, as by refusing to pay the agreed-upon compensation or adopt the child, the surrogate mother could simply give the child up for adoption and sue the married couple for the compensation due. Such a turn of events should be rare, since couples entering into such arrangements are likely to be motivated by a strong desire for a child, especially if it is the offspring of the husband. In any event, their breach presents no novel legal problems.

Breach by the surrogate mother, in contrast, poses a difficult problem in finding an appropriate remedy.[13] If she breaches by refusing to submit to artificial insemination, the married couple could probably sue for recovery of any compensation already advanced to her, but beyond that their remedies are uncertain. Money damages (apart from restitution of money advanced) would almost certainly be inadequate: the couple's out-of-pocket pecuniary losses should be recoverable but are likely to be small. The real loss suffered is the distress and disappointment of the frustration of their parental aspirations, but damages for emotional distress are usually not recoverable in contract actions. An alternative possibility is an action in tort for intentional or negligent infliction of mental or emotional distress. However, even if such a suit is successfully brought, it may well be that the defendant cannot satisfy a substantial money judgment: rich women are unlikely to contract to become surrogate mothers.

The alternative remedy, available where money damages are not an adequate remedy, is specific performance, i.e., an order that the breaching party perform as she has promised. As regards a pre-birth breach, however, it is very unlikely that [a] court would order a woman to submit or resubmit to artificial insemination, to become pregnant and to give birth to a child. The general rule is that courts will not order specific performance of contracts for personal services because of the impracticality of assuring satisfactory performance. In this situation, enforcement problems would be monumental. The reluctant surrogate might surreptitiously practice contraception, or engage in activities detrimental to the health of the fetus, or even arrange to be impregnated by someone other than the husband of the sterile wife. Clearly the contract could not be enforced short of taking the surrogate into custody. In case of pre-birth breach by the surrogate mother there is, unfortunately, little that can be done.

The situation is not necessarily the same where the surrogate mother, having given birth, decides to keep the child and refuses or retracts her consent to its adoption. Such cases have already occurred.[14] In these circumstances, specific performance should be feasible, since all that is needed is to order the surrogate to consent to the adoption and deliver the child into the custody of its other biological parent. If the controversy arises without regard to a contract, it reduces to a dispute between the two biological parents of an illegitimate child. Currently most courts look with disfavor upon prenatal releases of parental rights or consent to adoption by the expectant mother, one area where reform is imperative to accommodate the special circumstances of surrogate motherhood. Such a release and consent, given in the context of a deliberate pre-pregnancy decision to bear a child for another, should be not only lawful but irrevocable. Present law regarding revocation of consent varies widely from state to state, but the tendency in most jurisdictions "is to hold that the natural parent may not withdraw his consent to the adoption without careful scrutiny by the courts."[15] Because of the infant's tendency to form psychological ties with the parent who has custody, prompt resolution of the custody dispute is a matter of urgency. It would be desirable if, upon a prima facie showing of a surrogate motherhood contract containing consent to adoption, custody of the child were transferred to the biological father pending a final custody decision made on an expedited basis. . . .

Conclusion

Surrogate motherhood is growing in popularity because it meets the urgently felt needs of those who resort to it better than any of the alternatives as they see them. As a consensual arrangement it is as worthy of legal protection as many others which, formerly suspect, are now taken for granted. Subject to reasonable regulation, it deserves to take a place among the growing array of methods available to individuals for the ordering of their own marital and reproductive lives. Doctrines fitted to other circumstances should not be allowed to bar the legality or enforcement of surrogate motherhood agreements.

Notes

The author wishes to acknowledge and express appreciation to Robert C. Black for his efforts and assistance toward completion of this paper.

1. Letter to Margaret Pfeiffer from Executive Judge James H. Lincoln, Wayne County Juvenile Court, March 2, 1977.

2. Downs v. Wortman, 228 Ga. 315, 315, 185 S.E.2d 387, 388 (1971).

3. Hooks v. Bridgewater, 111 Tex. 122, 131, 229 S.W. 1114, 1118 (1921).

4. Parks v. Parks, 209 Ky. 127, 132, 272 S.W. 419, 422 (1928).

5. [Keane's discussion of the constitutionality of parenting contracts is not included here. For a debate on constitutional issues, see in this anthology Robertson, "Noncoital Reproduction and Procreative Liberty," and Smith and Iraola, "Equal Protection for Whom?"—Editor.]

6. 8 Ill. App. 2d 344, 132 N.E.2d 34 (1956).

7. For a discussion raising possible problems of professional ethics where attorneys act as adoption brokers, see Podolski, "Abolishing Baby Buying: Limiting Independent Adoption Placement," 9 *Fam. L.Q.* 547, 552–53 (1975).

8. "Economic" reasons for having children include the use of children as a source of consumable entertainment, as vehicles of conspicuous consumption and vicarious achievement; and as a means of preserving property, even after death, through inheritance. See R. Cooperstein, *Some Notes on the Reproduction of Human Capital* (1974). Psychoanalytically oriented authorities contend that parental self-love flowing from self-validation through reproduction is the original source of the parents' love for their child. See J. Goldstein, A. Freud & A. Solnit, *Beyond the Best Interest of the Child*, 16–17 (1973). It may be a good thing that parental motivation is ordinarily not subject to official scrutiny.

9. For some proposals for regulation, see Comment, "Contracts to Bear a Child," 66 *Cal. L. Rev.* 611, 621–22 (1978).

10. See note 1 and accompanying text, supra.

11. Las Vegas Sun, Inc. v. Franklin, 74 Nev. 282, 329 P.2d 867, (1958).

12. "Black-Market Adoptions," 22 *Catholic Law*, 48, 50 n. 12 (1976).

13. For an excellent overview of contract remedies law, see Farnsworth, "Legal Remedies for Breach of Contract," 70 *Colum. L. Rev.* 1145 (1970).

14. See "Agreement by Couple to Pay Girl for Having Baby," *The Times* (London), June 21, 1980, at 1, 2. The article noted that the British courts would consider the arrangement "pernicious and void." [See also in this anthology the case studies "The Case of Baby M: Parenting through Contract When Everyone Wants the Child" and "Parenting through Contract When No One Wants the Child."—Editor.]

15. H. Clark, *The Law of Domestic Relations in the United States*, 627 (1968).

The Overdue Death of a Feminist Chameleon: Taking a Stand on Surrogacy Arrangements

Rosemarie Tong

Ever since the Baby M case, I have been troubled about surrogacy arrangements. These arrangements concern me whether the contracted mother (oftentimes inappropriately referred to as "surrogate" mother) is or is not genetically related to her child; and whether her decision to serve as a contracted mother is commercially motivated or not.[1] Is a surrogacy arrangement simply another reproductive option for infertile couples—a felicitous, technological mode of collaborative reproduction? Or is it a tragic manifestation of some of our worst cultural trends, the tendency to believe that all relationships—including the most intimate ones—can be (1) initiated and terminated at will and (2) bought and sold for the right price? Does a surrogacy arrangement further liberate or further oppress women? Does it serve or disserve the best interests of children?

I have changed my position on surrogacy arrangements so often that I recently felt kindred to a chameleon that was crawling on one of the plants in my New Orleans hotel room. Perhaps it was this surreal experience that convinced me not only to deliver my old greenish-brown suit to the Salvation Army but also to take a definite stand on what legal policies ought to regulate surrogacy arrangements. What I propose to do in the following article is (1) to outline the arguments on behalf of the four major legal remedies that have been proposed for surrogacy arrangements and (2) to comment on each of these remedies, identifying those that are most likely to best serve women's interests. Specifically, I will argue that since the woman who gestates a child *is* the mother of that child, (1) commercial surrogacy should be recognized for what it is—the selling of a relationship—and dealt with accordingly; and (2) non-commercial, or altruistic surrogacy should be recognized for what it is—a form of adoption—and dealt with accordingly.

From *Journal of Social Philosophy,* 21 (1990), 40–56. Reprinted by permission from the *Journal of Social Philosophy* (Fall/Winter 1990).

Part One: Proposed Legal Remedies for Contracted Motherhood

I. Non-Enforcement of Surrogacy Arrangements

In the original Baby M case, District Judge Harvey R. Sorkow had ruled that it was in Baby M's best interest to enforce the terms of the contract William and Elizabeth Stern had made with Mary Beth Whitehead. In overturning Judge Sorkow's ruling, the New Jersey Supreme Court proclaimed that contracts for mothers cannot be enforced because they are against public policy for at least two reasons.[2] First, they may lead to the exploitation of financially needy women; and second, they are a disguised form of baby-selling.[3]

To proclaim that a contract for a mother is unenforceable is to say that if the contract is breached by either the contracted mother or the contracting couple, the State will leave the parties as it finds them. So, for example, if the contracting couple fail to pay the contracted mother her fee, the State will not help her collect it. Or if the contracting couple refuse to take the child from the contracted mother, the State will not force them to do so. Instead, the State will require the contracted mother either to maintain her parental relationship with the child or to put the child up for adoption. In the former case, she may be entitled to child support from the genetic father; and in the latter case, she may be entitled to his financial assistance. Alternatively, if the contracted mother refuses to give the child to the contracting couple, the genetic father will not be able to secure custody based on the *contract* he and his wife made with her. Neither will he and his wife be able to legally force the contracted mother to waive her abortion right or to maintain a program of proper diet and exercise during pregnancy.[4] Because there is a great deal of concern for contracted infants, however, the State will not leave them as it finds them. Rather the State will use the "best interests of the child" standard—the custody test that is employed in divorce cases—to determine who contracted children's social parents should be.[5]

II. Enforcement of Surrogacy Arrangements through Contract Law

Unconvinced that contracts for mothers are against public policy, some commentators have urged that these contracts be recognized as collaborative-reproduction agreements. All disputes between contracted mothers and contracting couples should be regarded as breaches of contract to be remedied either by a specific performance or damages approach.[6]

1. Specific Performance:
Beause specific performance forces the parties to a contract to fulfill its terms, it eliminates the kind of uncertainty that characterizes less formal human arrangements. Uncertainty is always difficult for human beings to handle, particularly when their most precious dreams are at stake. For a contracting couple to wait nine months for a child, not knowing whether the

contracted mother will finally relinquish him or her to them, is agonizing. So too it is agonizing for a contracted mother to gestate a child for nine months, not knowing whether the contracting couple will accept him or her upon "delivery."

Significantly, specific performance is not the preferred way to enforce personal service contracts. For example, if Johnny Carson refuses to come on stage and perform, no court is going to force him to do his monologue. Under such circumstances, Johnny is not apt to be very funny. Analogously, a contracted mother will achieve less than optimal results if she forces a contracting couple to take the child she has borne for them but whom they no longer want. Similarly, a contracting couple will achieve less than optimal results if they force a contracted mother to follow reasonable medical instructions during her pregnancy; to carry the fetus to term unless doing so endangers her life; and/or to surrender the child to them no matter how much she loves him or her. But because a contracted child is separable from his or her contracted mother in a way that Johnny's wit is not separable from him, supporters of the contract approach observe that the State may nevertheless force the contracted mother to relinquish the child to the genetic father. Since she has contributed at most the same amount of genetic material as the father has,[7] and since genetic fathers, "unwillingly deprived of access to their children suffer from 'feelings of regret and self-betrayal' akin to those that contracted mothers feel when similarly deprived,"[8] the promises the contracted mother knowingly and willingly made to the contracting couple arguably work to their advantage.

2. Damages Approach:

Unconvinced that specific performance is the appropriate remedy for breach of a personal service contract, some legal commentators have stressed the advantages of a damages approach. Imagine, for example, a contracted mother who "gets religion." As a result, this "born-again" woman reneges on her contract, viewing it as the foreign act of a former, false self—an unborn Christian who led her true self astray. Since specific performance of her promise to serve as a contracted mother would force her to confront her old unredeemed self repeatedly, the State should, on this view, permit her another way to make good on her contract—namely the paying of damages.[9] What the supporters of the damages approach offer the parties to a contract for motherhood, then, is a choice. They may honor the contract, but do violence to their sense of self on the one hand; or breach the contract, pay damages, but emerge with their sense of self intact on the other hand.

Whatever the theoretical merits of the damages approach, however, it lacks several practical advantages. Since contracted mothers are generally less wealthy than contracting couples, they will have difficulty paying the damages assessed against them; and, even if they are able to pay the assessed damages, the money will not adequately compensate the childless contracting couple. Likewise, money will not adequately compensate a contracted mother who is left with a child that she never intended to parent.

III. Criminalization of (Commercial) Surrogacy Arrangements

Some legal theorists have argued that the best remedy for commercial surrogacy is simply to ban it. In 1985 the United Kingdom passed the Surrogacy Arrangements Act. Reasoning that it is not in the best interests of a child to be born of parents "subject to the taint of criminality," the House of Lords decided not to enforce criminal sanctions against contracting couples and contracted mothers.[10] Rather, they decided to penalize the people who serve as the "middlemen" in commercial surrogacy negotiations. Lawyers, physicians, and social workers are subject to fines and/or imprisonment if they

(a) initiate or take part in any negotiations with a view to the making of a surrogacy arrangement,

(b) offer or agree to negotiate the making of a surrogacy arrangement, or

(c) compile any information with a view to its ease in making, or negotiating the making of, surrogacy arrangements.[11]

In addition, publishers, directors, and managers of newspapers, periodicals, and telecommunications systems are subject to fines and/or imprisonment if they accept ads such as "womb for hire" or "couple willing to pay royally for host womb."[12]

The authors of the Surrogacy Arrangements Act apparently relied on the principle of legal moralism according to which a person's liberty may be restricted to prevent immoral conduct on his or her part. They argued not that surrogacy arrangements are necessarily harmful but that they are necessarily immoral:

> . . . [e]ven in compelling medical circumstances the danger of exploitation of one human being by another appears to the majority of us far to outweigh the potential benefits, in almost every case. That people would treat others as a means to their own ends, however desirable the consequences, must always be liable to moral objection.[13]

Several United States jurisdictions have expressed a readiness to follow the United Kingdom's lead.[14] In fact, Michigan has already passed a law making it a felony to serve as a "surrogate broker," the penalty being a maximum $50,000 fine and five years in prison.[15]

IV. The Assimilation of (Non-Commercial) Surrogacy Arrangements into Adoption Law

Since a ban on commercial surrogacy is not a ban on non-commercial surrogacy, and since there is little difference between making arrangements to adopt a mother's baby as soon as she knows she is pregnant and making arrangements to adopt a *contracted* mother's baby even before it has been conceived, some legal theorists argue that the same rules that govern adoption should govern surrogacy arrangements.[16] Adoption rules permit payment but only for the pregnant woman's reasonable medical expenses. They also provide for a "change of heart" period. The adopting couple may pull out of the negotiations at any time before or, lately, even after the adoption papers are signed;[17] and the biological mother has several days, weeks, or even months to decide whether she really wants to relinquish her child.[18]

The adoption approach harmonizes with the long-standing legal view that the woman who gives birth to a child is that child's mother. Thus, lawyer George Annas argues that whether or not the contracted mother is genetically related to her child, the State should recognize her as the child's legal mother because of her gestational contribution to him/her, and because "she will definitely be present at the birth, easily and certainly identifiable, and available" to care for the child.[19] Unless it can be proven that a contracted mother is truly unfit, she should be awarded sole custody of the child if she decides not to relinquish him/her for adoption.

To the objection that to give custodial advantage to the contracted mother is unfair to the contracting couple, supporters of the adoption approach reply that it is no more unfair to the contracting couple than the kind of disappointment would-be adoptive parents sometimes sustain. From the very beginning of the adoption negotiations, would-be adoptive parents know that if the gestational mother ultimately decides not to give up her child for adoption, they will go home to an empty nursery. Thus, provided that a contracting couple know from the outset that the contracted mother may void the contract at any time, no injustice is done them in the event that she decides to keep her child.

To the further objection, that the adoption and contracted motherhood cases are disanalogous because in the case of contracted motherhood the man who wishes to adopt the child is also the genetic father of the child, supporters of the adoption approach argue that genetic linkage is not the determining criterion for parenthood. What genetic linkage to a child gives a man or a woman is a limited right to *establish* a relationship with a child, where "relationship" means any mode of nurturance from the most physical to the most psychological. Thus, the fact that a man's sperm constitute 50 percent of the genetic material necessary for conception does not make him 50 percent owner of any resultant child. Likewise, the fact that a woman's egg constitutes 50 percent of the genetic material necessary for conception does not make her 50 percent owner of any resultant child. Children are not possessions; rather they are the kind of beings with whom relationships can be forged, and at birth the only direct relationship a child has is with the woman who has gestated him/her. Although this gestational relationship is not an interpersonal one, it is one that shows that the contracted mother was committed enough to the fetus to bring it to term.[20]

Part Two: Feminist Assessments of the Proposed Legal Remedies for Surrogacy Arrangements

I. Assessing the Non-Enforcement of Surrogacy Arrangements

The first remedy for surrogacy arrangements—a "hands-off" policy—is simply an affirmation of a status quo that few, if any, feminists wish to affirm. Realizing that the State will "let the chips lie where they fall," some people will not risk surrogacy arrangements. Others, however, will on the assumption that nothing is likely to go wrong. But optimism notwithstanding, "things" frequently do go wrong when there are *profits* to be made. First, the temptation to employ slipshod or bogus medical evaluations and psychiatric counseling is large. That no one at the profit making Infertility Center of New York bothered to question Mary Beth Whitehead about her ability to relinquish a baby suggests that the Center may have been overly eager to supply the well-to-do Sterns with a "compatible surrogate" (the physical resemblance between Elizabeth Stern and Mary Beth Whitehead has not gone unnoticed).[21] Second, the temptation to minimize the risks and to exaggerate the benefits for the contracted mother is also large. In *The Sacred Bond: The Legacy of Baby M,* author Phyllis Chesler reports that contracted mothers are not usually well prepared for the possibly traumatic experience of relinquishing a baby. Indeed, they are frequently put in "support groups," the overall purpose of which is to enable them to repress their feelings.[22] Finally, the temptation to charge contracting couples as much as possible and to pay contracted mothers as little as possible is also large. Although some surrogacy agencies refuse to enroll indigent women into their programs,[23] other agencies prefer such women. Indeed, John Stehura, president of the Bionetics Foundation, Inc., believes that a contracted mother can never be poor enough. Since the going rate for contracted mothers is high even by middle-class American standards, he has urged surrogacy agencies to move either to poverty-stricken areas of the United States where a mother can be contracted for one-half the standard fee of $10,000 or, better, to the Third World where a mother can be contracted for one-tenth the standard fee.[24]

Clearly, there is reason to think that women's (and children's) best interests are not ultimately served by the State's refusal to regulate at least *commercial* surrogacy. Not only do surrogacy agencies routinely violate the spirit, if not the letter, of informed consent requirements, courts frequently award custody to the contracting couple for the wrong reasons. Just because one parent is more wealthy than another parent does not mean that s/he qualifies as the better parent. Nevertheless, courts often give custody to the parent who can provide his/her child with a higher material standard of living. Thus, the fact that a contracted mother is typically poorer than the contracting couple is a fact that will work to her disadvantage in a custody hearing.[25] So too is the fact that she signed the contract in the first place. Indeed, in the Whitehead/Stern dispute over Baby M, Judge Sorkow observed that the day she signed on the dotted line, Mary Beth Whitehead proved her "unfitness" as a mother.[26] In any event, custody disputes, especially if they terminate in an unwieldly set of visitation rights, are not likely to be in the child's best interest if her/his parents are unwilling to collaborate peacefully and joyfully as s/he grows towards adulthood.

II. Assessing the Enforcement of Surrogacy Arrangements through Contract Law

To claim that not enforcing surrogacy arrangements disserves contracted children and contracted mothers in particular is not necessarily to claim that enforcing such contracts serves them. Rather, it is to observe that a firm stand has to be taken on surrogacy arrangements. They must either be banned or be regulated; and if they are to be regulated, they must be regulated in ways that serve women's and children's interests.

Interestingly, liberal feminists believe that the best way to regulate surrogacy arrangements is through contract law. Although they concede that society is not required to enforce any and all contracts—say, a contract to kill someone, or a contract to sell one's self into slavery, or a contract to sell one's soul to the devil—liberal feminists insist that, given widely-accepted interpretations of Constitutional law, two or more consenting adults have a right to contract with each other to procreate a child collaboratively. However, only some of these collaborators—namely, the sperm and egg contributors—will have what amounts to property rights over their co-produced child. What is clear on this line of reasoning is that William Stern, for example, had as much claim to Baby M as Mary Beth Whitehead initially had. He contributed the sperm; she contributed the egg. Similarly, the "father" who sued for joint custody of his and his ex-wife's frozen embryos had as much right to destroy them as she had to preserve them.[27] Finally, the contracted mother who sued for joint custody of the child she had gestated had no cause to sue since she was genetically unrelated to the child.[28] What is also clear on this line of reasoning is that surrogacy arrangements do not constitute "baby-selling." When a contracted mother relinquishes her genetic child to a contracting couple for a fee, she is no more "selling" that child than they are "buying" that child. Rather, she is simply waiving and transferring her property rights to that child, while the genetic father is reaffirming his.

But even though liberal feminists do not think that surrogacy arrangements are wrong in general, they concede that they can be wrong in particular. To the degree that a surrogacy arrangement violates women's Constitutional rights, says feminist lawyer Lori B. Andrews, it is wrong. According to Andrews, any contract to which a contracted mother is a party must be worded so that she is free during her pregnancy (1) to engage in self-chosen activities; (2) to refuse or accept proposed medical treatments; and (3) to abort or not abort the contracted child. Under no circumstances, says Andrews, should the contracted mother be liable for damages or subject to a court suit in the event that the fetus spontaneously aborts, is delivered stillborn, or is born with defects.[29]

Andrews also believes that no matter how correctly worded a contract is, a contracted mother need not heed it unless she has given her informed consent to it. Physicians and psychologists must clearly outline to would-be contracted mothers all of the physical and psychological risks that attend surrogacy arrangements. But, cautions Andrews, too much information of the wrong kind, as well as too little information of the right kind, can undermine a woman's reproductive freedom. Andrews notes, for example, that several years ago the city of Akron, Ohio passed an ordinance that required physicians to inform women seeking abortions that the fetus is sentient (able to feel pain) and that the abortion procedure is often dangerous.[30] "Speculative," often times misleading, information caused numerous women to change their abortion decision from "yes" to "no." What concerns Andrews is that, fearing liability suits or worse, some physicians and psychologists will exaggerate the risks that attend surrogacy arrangements. As a result, the medical establishment will deprive fertile women of a new way to profit from their reproductive abilities and infertile women of a new way to secure a deeply-desired child.

Unconvinced by liberal feminist arguments (including those of Lori Andrews), Marxist feminists argue that when a woman consents to sell her reproductive services to an infertile couple, her consent is about as real as the "consent" a woman gives when she sells her sexual services to a client. Unable to get a decent job, a woman will sometimes sell the only thing she has which does seem to have any value: her body. To say that a woman "chooses" to do this, says the Marxist feminist, is simply to say that when a woman is forced to choose between poverty and exploitation, she sometimes chooses exploitation as the lesser of two evils. Thus, Marxist feminists oppose commercial surrogacy and recommend a ban on it.

Not surprisingly some liberal feminists have questioned the logic behind a ban that has as its apparent object only *commercial* surrogacy. Why, asks Andrew, is it exploitation to serve as a contracted mother if a woman is paid but *not* if she is not paid? Andrews reasons that if contracted motherhood is not inherently exploitative but becomes so only when women are economically coerced into it, then "our focus should not be on banning payment, but on making sure the surrogates get paid more."[31] Although we can *imagine* situations in which a woman would become a contracted mother in order to avoid destitution or worse, says Andrews, in point of fact most women who become contracted mothers do so not because they have been "tricked into it" or because they need food, clothing, or shelter, but because they want "luxuries" such as children's education, a redecorated house, or a second car.[32]

In response to Andrews' objections, Marxist feminists note that her view of economic exploitation is simplistic. Andrews argues that if commercial surrogacy is exploitative, it is exploitative only because contracted mothers are paid too little. For example, for her $10,000 fee Mary Beth Whitehead was required to "assume all risks, including the risk of death, which are incidential to conception, pregnancy, childbirth, including but not limited to postpartum complications," with no compensation whatsoever in the event of a first-trimester miscarriage, and a mere $1000 if she aborted on Mr. Stern's demand.[33] But Marxist feminists believe that had Whitehead been offered $1,000,000 and $100,000 respectively rather than $10,000 and $1,000 respectively, her decision to be a contracted mother would have been no less coerced. Indeed, as Mary Gibson has observed, it would probably have been more coerced, for the better the terms of a surrogacy arrangement, the more difficult it is for a poor woman to say "no" to its "undue inducements."[34]

Agreeing with Marxist feminists that commercial surrogacy ought to be banned, radical feminists broaden the Marxist feminist analysis of exploitation to include cases of non-economic exploitation. Relying on an analogy between prostitution and contracted motherhood, radical feminists note, for example, that when a well-to-do college graduate decides to work as a high-priced call girl, her choice is not necessarily free. Women, says the radical feminist, are socialized to meet male sexual wants and needs as a matter of duty and pride. Just as prostitutes are not born but made by a society that teaches girls that, if all else fails, they can always gain attention or money by offering their bodies to men, contracted mothers are not born but made by a society that teaches girls that they are *better* than boys because they are so generous, so willing to share all that they have including their bodies. Although many radical feminists believe that biological motherhood is a highly valuable activity, some radical feminists caution that appeals for contracted mothers often constitute a "Compassion Trap" for women. Appeals are made to generous, loving, altruistic women to give "the gift of life" to sorrowing, lonely, childless couples; and the fact that approximately one-third of all women who answer this appeal have either had an abortion or given up a child for adoption strengthens radical feminists' suspicion that deep and dark forces are driving women to "choose" contracted motherhood even when it may not be in their best interests to do so.[35]

Whatever power this much of the radical feminist case has against contracted motherhood, liberal feminists observe that *if* it is true that women are "brainwashed" into becoming *contracted mothers,* then they are also "brainwashed" into becoming *regular mothers.* Therefore, radical feminists "should not forbid women to be mothers through alternative reproduction without forbidding them to be mothers through normal reproduction as well."[36] But even if no one is "brainwashing" women to be mothers—contracted or regular—liberal feminists may lack a convincing response to another objection some radical feminists have raised against surrogacy arrangements: namely, that in the name of gender equality, such arrangements privilege a possible relationship over an actual one, an abstract intention over a concrete experience. What liberal feminists should see when they look at contracted motherhood, asserts Phyllis Chesler, is not gender equality but another victory for man, the mind, culture, and reason *over* woman, the body, nature, and emotion, the primitive, chaos and anarchy. Chesler observes that in surrogacy arrangements "the *idea* of fatherhood" triumphs over "the *fact* of motherhood."[37] William Stern conceives of Baby M in his thoughts and implants that idea in Mary Beth Whitehead's womb where it is supposed to grow apart from her—as if she were indeed only an "incubator." Whereas gestational motherhood is supposedly only a "natural" event, contracted motherhood is supposedly a "civilized" event. Ideas, intentions, and words are incanted over Mary Beth Whitehead's blood, sweat, and tears until, as Chesler puts it, Elizabeth Stern emerges as Baby M's father and William Stern as her true mother.[38]

III. Assessing the Criminalization of (Commercial) Surrogacy Arrangements

The Marxist and radical feminist cases against commercial surrogacy (and perhaps also against non-commercial surrogacy, a point to which I shall return) strike me as stronger than the liberal feminist case for commercial surrogacy. It is difficult to view commercial surrogacy as anything other than baby-selling. Supporters of commercial surrogacy frequently argue that contracted mothers are not selling their children but simply renting out their wombs.[39] But this is a distinction that does not make a difference. No matter what society terms commercial surrogacy, the contracted mother relinquishes her child, the contracting couple take him/her home, and money passes hands. One distinction that may make a difference, however, is that often at least one member of the contracting couple is genetically related to the child (usually the man). On the ownership model of parenthood, this man cannot buy what he already owns. But in point of fact, when he pays the contracted mother to waive and transfer her parental rights to her child, he is buying something that he did not previously own; namely, her *relationship* to her child.

Now it may be the case that even if there is something immoral about buying and selling babies, or *relationships* to babies, there is nothing particularly harmful about doing so. Since I am steeped enough in liberal tradition to believe that unless an individual is harming someone in the secular sense of the term "harm," the State should leave him/her alone, this is an objection that I cannot ignore. Critics of the Warnock Committee, the United Kingdom Committee that criminalized commercial surrogacy, claim that it undermined the work of the Wolfenden Committee, the United Kingdom Committee that de-criminalized homosexuality and prostitution some thirty years ago on the grounds that:

> [The law's] function . . . is to preserve order and decency, to protect the citizen from what is offensive or injurious, and to provide sufficient safeguards against exploitation and corruption of others. . . . It is not . . . the function of the law to intervene in the private lives of citizens, or to seek to enforce any particular pattern of behavior. . . . There must remain a realm of private morality and immorality which is, in brief and crude terms, not the law's business.[40]

In banning commercial surrogacy, say the critics, the Warnock Committee has once again invaded the realm of private morality, seeking to enforce *one* particular kind of family structure "in which the nurturing obligation of the birth mother is primary (if not virtually exclusive) and inviolable."[41]

Although I am certainly not interested in mandating one particular family structure, I am interested in preventing harm to women and children. Since there is evidence that surrogacy arrangements, at least in their commerical form, harm contracted mothers and contracted children, I think that a ban on commerical surrogacy needs to rely only on the harm principle. The principle of legal moralism is otiose.

The harms that contracted mothers typically suffer are the ones discussed above. For what amounts to very little money for a nine-month, twenty-four-hour-a-day "job," the contracted mother risks and usually experiences a variety of physical but especially psychological harms. The harms to contracted children are the ones alluded to but not discussed above. Without any possibility of saying "yes" or "no" to their parents' surrogacy arrangements, contracted children are often subject to more physical and psychological harms than "regular" children are. Since contracted mothers supposedly have no interests in their fetuses other than financial ones, they may engage in more fetus-threatening behavior (drinking, smoking, "shooting" drugs) than "regular" mothers do. But even if a contracted child is born healthy, s/he may experience some stresses and strains that "regular" children do not. For example, s/he may experience the kind of harm an adopted child sometimes experiences—not understanding why his/her biological parent(s) would not or could not keep him/her. And if the contracted child is not born healthy, s/he may experience what is the greatest harm any child can experience: rejection. In the notorious Malahoff/Stiver case, for example, Judy Stiver agreed to be artificially inseminated by Alexander Malahoff and to gestate the subsequent embryo for $10,000. The child was born microcephalic and mentally retarded. The Malahoff couple not only refused to take the baby, they claimed that Malahoff was not the father, insisting that a blood test would prove their claim. As a carnival touch, the results of the blood test were announced on the Phil Donahue talk show. They showed that Malahoff was indeed not the genetic father. Judy Stiver then admitted that she had had sexual intercourse with her own husband at about the same time as she was artificially inseminated with Malahoff's sperm. As the upshot of the sad affair, the Stivers reluctantly took custody of their child.[42] To be a child that no one wants is a tragic burden, and one that no child should be deliberately called into existence to shoulder.

In addition to harming particular contracted mothers and contracted children, surrogacy arrangements (especially the commercial ones) harm women and children in general. Destructive divisions are set up among women. Economically-privileged women are pitted against economically-disadvantaged women. Relatively-rich women hire relatively-poor women to meet their reproductive needs, adding childbearing services to the child-rearing services which economically-disadvantaged women have traditionally provided to economically-privileged women. Another destructive division is one which radical feminist Gena Corea envisions—namely, between childbegetters, childbearers, and childrearers. According to Corea, society is specializing and segmenting reproduction as if it were simply a form of production. In the future, no one woman will beget, bear, and rear a child. Rather, genetically-superior women will beget embryos *in vitro;* strong-bodied women will carry these "test-tube babies" to term; and sweet-tempered women will rear these newborns from infancy to adulthood.[43]

Although it is not easy to articulate the harm that surrogacy arrangements do to children in general, a number of traditional and feminist philosophers have managed to do so. Several years ago, economists Elisabeth Landes and Richard Posner proposed a free market in babies. As they saw it, if infertile people want babies and if fertile people are willing to help them get what they want, then the State should permit the former people to pay the latter people for their help. There is, they insisted, no true analogy between a baby market and a slave market. When a contracting couple "buys" a baby from a con-tracted mother, that baby can look forward to the life not of an abused slave but of a privileged child. Thus, Landes and Posner challenged their critics to specify the purported immorality and/or harm of commercial surrogacy.[44]

Traditional philosopher J.R.S. Pritchard met Landes and Posner's chal-lenge head on. To permit a market in babies is to "commodify something—life—which should not be treated as a commodity."[45] Over the years, babies would come to be viewed as no more special a purchase than an equally costly purchase—say, a new car. Parents' love for their children would no longer be unconditional; rather, it would depend on whether or not their children were "good" products.[46] In a worst-case scenario, parents might trade-in their defec-tive "models" for the latest "models" science and technology have to offer.

Another traditional thinker, Herbert Krimmel, raises similar points against commercial surrogacy. He believes that it is wrong, and I will add harmful, for a contracted mother to procreate a child *with the intention* to abdicate personal responsibility for him or her upon birth because:

> The procreator should desire the child for its own sake, and not as a means to attaining some other end. Even though one of the ends may be stated altruistically as an attempt to bring happiness to an infertile couple, the child is still being used by the surrogate. She creates it not because she desires it, but because she desires some-thing from it.[47]

The fact that the contracting couple desire the child for its own sake, insists Krimmel, does not negate the fact that the contracted mother desires it for her own, arguably ulterior motives (money). For anyone to procreate a child with no desire for a personal relationship with him/her is to procreate in a morally irresponsible manner. Why have a child if not to know and love him/her? To serve simply as the means to one's own ends: security in old age, help around the house, a Ken or Barbie doll?

Interestingly, on Krimmel's line of reasoning it is the contracted mother and not the contracting couple who merits moral censure. After all, they do desire to know and love the baby. But this good end does not, suggests essayist Roger Rosenblatt, cancel out the bad means they have used to secure a baby. When William and Elizabeth Stern paid Mary Beth Whitehead to gestate Baby M, says Rosenblatt, they were not simply paying her for gestational services, "services" that seem morally neutral when described abstractly. Rather the Sterns were paying Whitehead "to experience maternal love, the forced separation of that love, and a whole range of feelings in the process that are not ordinarily put up for sale." The Sterns were wrong to want to buy—and Whitehead was wrong to agree to sell—an emotional as well as physical relationship to Baby M, and the "transaction fell through because neither buyer nor seller had a grasp of the commodity in the first place."[48]

To be sure, as some feminist philosophers have observed, the problem with Krimmel's and, to a lesser extent, Rosenblatt's arguments is that they tend to blame one or more of the "victims." Rather than asking who the evil person is (most often a woman), Rosenblatt and Krimmel should instead be asking what forces motivate an infertile couple to do almost anything to procreate a child genetically related to them, and what motivates a fertile woman to gestate a child for someone else. Still, Krimmel's and Rosenblatt's main point is unaffected. Because children are not parties to the contracts that have brought them into existence, special care must be taken not to treat them as commodities that people may or may not relate to at will.

Significantly, points similar to those of Krimmel and Rosenblatt have been made by philosophers Hilde and James Nelson. They argue that when parents bring a child into existence, they "create a vulnerability."[49] Having created a person with a set of basic needs, one parent, for example, may not let another parent, however willing, assume full child-rearing responsibilities because both parents owe a "debt" "*to the child.*"[50] It may be okay with mom if dad doesn't spend any time with junior, but it may not be okay with junior if dad absents himself from his life. Similarly, even if the contracting couple is only too happy to rear by themselves the child they contracted for, it is still the contracted mother's job to help rear her child unless she is unable to do so.[51] It makes no difference that the contracted mother believes that the contracting couple will meet her child's needs and well, for as Nelson and Nelson see it, the contracted mother "herself is the only person she can bring to *perform* the required services."[52] Parents, no less than children, are not interchangeable. One is not necessarily as good as, and certainly not the same as another. Comment Nelson and Nelson:

> . . . To engineer a situation in which the biological father can discharge his responsibility daily, but the mother cannot, is to put her under an obligation to the child that she does not intend to meet. Apart from making deceitful promises to Nazis, there would seem to be few cases where we can legitimately act in such bad faith.[53]

What the above arguments demonstrate, I think, is that the general and specific harms caused by commercial surrogacy are not *private* but *public* harms, and ones that may be serious enough to warrant limits on individuals' liberty. People do have a right to privacy, including a right to procreate using "artificial" means if necessary. However, as lawyers Alexander Capron and

Margaret Radin note, the right to privacy is a negative not a positive liberty.[54] In recognizing a freedom *from* State interference in making procreative choices, the Supreme Court did not also recognize a corresponding right *to* State assistance in implementing those procreative choices.[55] Just because an infertile couple has a right to contract a mother does not mean that the State has a duty either to permit that couple to pay her or, in the event that they cannot afford her "services," to pay her itself. To the objection that since few women are willing to gestate other people's children for free, the right to use a contracted mother without the right to pay her for her "services" is useless, the Michigan Appellate Court has already replied that:

> [T]he Constitution does not guarantee that all infertile couples desiring surrogate motherhood will find willing surrogates any more than it guarantees that all infertile couples desiring adoption will find available children to adopt. The wife's infertility, not the state's prohibition against payment to the surrogate, prevents the couple's exercise of their right to bear and beget children.[56]

Whatever the merits of this line of reasoning, I think that there is no right to pay for a *relationship* to a child. Unless we are ready to resolve standard custody cases by awarding the child to the parent who is willing to pay the most money for a relationship with him/her, I submit that we should ban commercial surrogacy as a harmful practice.

IV. Assessing the Adoption Approach for (Non-Commercial) Surrogacy Arrangements

Given the fact that non-commercial surrogacy may, as Nelson and Nelson suggested above, be as harmful to the child as commercial surrogacy is, it may seem inconsistent not to ban it together with commercial surrogacy. My reasons for not urging a ban on non-commercial surrogacy, however, are similar to the reasons why I think a ban on selling organs but not on donating organs is correct. Even in a disutopian society, some contracted mothers are already utopian—that is, not only generous enough to help an infertile couple gestate a child but also imaginative enough to fulfill their parental duties to that child. Likewise, some contracted couples are generous enough to extend their families to include the contracted mother as well as the contracted child (sociologist Barbara Rothman has urged contracting couples to treat their child's contracted mother as if she were his or her *aunt*).[57] Moreover, some contracted couples are honest enough to realize that at the moment of birth the contracted mother is more their child's parent than they are. Initially, what makes a parent a parent is not the mere *intention* to be a parent, nor even the fact that without one's *genetic material* no child would have been conceived, but the fact that without one's *lived commitment* to that child no child would have been *born*.

  The general advantage of an adoption approach to non-commercial surrogacy, then, is that is permits well-motivated people to move a few steps toward truly collaborative reproduction. Moreover, the *feminist* advantage of an adoption approach to non-commercial surrogacy is that it acknowledges a relationship whose moral significance traditional philosophy has ignored— namely, the gestational relationship. In constructing a case for the priority of gestational connection over genetic contribution, feminist philosopher Sara Ann Ketchum has made five points. First, as soon as scientists and technologists develop gene-splicing and chromosome-splicing techniques, it will be possible to procreate children with enormously complex genetic backgrounds. Who, then, say Ketchum, will count as the genetic parents of these children? Will only the donors who contributed the *most* genes or chromosomes to the child count as his/her parents? Or will the donors who contributed only one less gene or chromosome than the highest donors also count as his/her parents? Or will all the donors count as the child's parents, no matter how many or how few genes or chromosomes they contributed to him/her. After all, had even one gene or chromosome been different, the child of whom we speak would not have been the same child. Second, insists Ketchum, our intuitions suggest that at least in the case of rape, it is implausible to regard genetic connection as conferring parental rights. Third, as some radical feminists (for example, Mary O'Brien) see it, men valorize *genetic* fatherhood because there is no such experience as gestational fatherhood. O'Brien points out that men's experience of reproduction is indirect for at least three reasons:

(a) because the physical and temporal continuity between the sperm and the resulting child takes place outside the man's body, the seed is "alienated,"
(b) since the basic labor of reproduction—pregnancy and birth—is necessarily performed by a woman, when a man appropriates a child (even his genetic child), he is appropriating the product of someone else's labor;
(c) whereas a woman's connection to a particular child is proven in the act of birth, a man's connection to a particular child is always arguable since the child he wishes to call "his" may be the product of a liaison between another man and his wife/girlfriend.[58]

Fourth, says Ketchum, to identify genetic connection as the essential criterion for parenthood is to suggest that this abstract relationship with a child is more important than such concrete relationships as gestation and child care. Fifth, and finally, observes Ketchum, to stress genetic connection as the essential criterion for parenthood is to imply that adoptive parents are not *real* parents.[59]

But even if the negative case against the genetic criterion for parenthood is fairly strong, some positive argument needs to be made on behalf of the gestational criterion for parenthood. Lawyer George Annas argues that there are at least two moral reasons why a gestational mother should be legally presumed to have the parental right and responsibility to rear the child. First, because the gestational mother has made such a large "biological and psychological" investment in the child, she deserves to maintain her relationship with the child unless, I suppose, she abuses him or her.[60] Second, because the gestational mother "will of necessity be present at birth and immediately thereafter to care for the child," designating her the legal or "natural mother" of the child is more likely to protect his or her interests than any alternative arrangement.[61] What makes a person a parent, therefore, is the degree to which s/he has shown that her/his commitment to a child is more than a matter of mere intention.

Although the arguments against "nature" and for "nurture" as the determining criterion of parenthood are strong, a variety of critics are reluctant to downplay the genetic criterion. Among these critics are those who refuse to look at gestation and/or child-birth as lived relationships, as *active* encounters between a woman and a child. As these critics see it, pregnancy and childbirth are events that simply happen to a woman. She has little control over her body as it grows full with child, and even less control over it during the process of birth. But surely this view of pregnancy is rather "male." Although male gynecologists and obstetricians did not conspire to take charge of the birthing process, they did take over the work of female midwives, replacing their hands of flesh (female hands sensitive to female anatomy) with hands of iron (for example, obstetrical forceps). In addition, these male gynecologists and obstetricians wrote the official rules not only for giving birth but also for being pregnant: when to eat, sleep, exercise, have sex, and feel pain. Arguing against these rules, feminist poet Adrienne Rich writes that when they clash with a woman's lived experience—and they do so frequently—a woman does not know whether to trust the rules of the doctors or the sensations of her own body. Such self-doubting experiences can transform a pregnancy into a profoundly alienating experience. Indeed, Rich writes that this is precisely what happened in her own case:

> When I try to return to the body of the young woman of twenty-six, pregnant for the first time, who fled from the physical knowledge of her pregnancy and at the same time from her intellect and vocation, I realize that I was effectively alienated from my real body and my real spirit by the institution—not the fact—of motherhood. This institution—the foundation of human society as we know it— allowed me only certain views, certain expectations, whether embodied in the booklet in my obstetrician's waiting room, the novels I had read, my mother-in-law's approval, my memories of my own mother, the Sistine Madonna or she of the Michelangelo *Pieta,* the floating notion that a woman pregnant is a woman calm in her fulfillment or, simply a woman waiting.[62]

Were women in charge of pregnancy and childbirth, suggests Rich, these experiences would have *active* rather than *passive* meanings for them. Women would no longer sit passively, waiting for the birth event to seize hold of them. Rather, they would actively direct the birthing of their children, regaining control of the pleasures as well as the pains of the experience.

But even if Rich's view of pregnancy and childbirth is convincing, there may still be feminist reasons not to stress "nurture" over "nature" as the determining criterion of parenthood, and not to stress the "fact" of having had a child over the "decision" to have a child as that which makes a parent a parent.[63] First, I am not certain that the line between deciding to have a child and having had a child can only be crossed at the moment of birth. As they ready the nursery, for example, the contracting couple show that their decision to have a child is not a *mere* intention. Second, although it is wrong to trivialize the gestational connection as California Judge Parslow did when he equated gestating an embryo with providing day-care or "nanny" services for it,[64] it is also wrong to dismiss as entirely irrelevant genetic and/or intentional connections to a child. However primary the gestational relationship is, it is a relationship that is readily supplemented and gradually replaced by other caring acts of parental commitment—the kind of acts that a genetic father, for example, can do: feeding, rocking, diapering, and washing the baby. Moreover, one of the primary motivations for having a child is to see one's self live on in him or her. Although this motivation may be criticized as "narcissistic," Mother Nature may have been wise when she found a way for humans to concretely link the past with the future. Children, no less than adults, often derive comfort from the fact that they have mom's eyes or dad's smile. Third, emphasizing the gestational relationship may as easily harm women as benefit women. Lately, national attention has focused on a wide range of issues arising from actions taken by women during pregnancy that may have harmful consequences for their children. Among these issues are: (1) medical interventions (such as refusal of a recommended cesarean section or insulin treatment for gestational diabetes); (2) innovative therapies (such as fetal surgery); (3) prenatal diagnosis; and (4) lifestyle issues (such as alcohol or cocaine use during pregnancy). Given a worrisome social tendency to control women's pregnancies—even to punish women for things that go wrong during pregnancy—it may be politically inadvisable for women to emphasize the specialness of the gestational relationship.[65]

V. Conclusion

Although I have taken a stand on surrogacy arrangements, I am not altogether happy with it. I do not ordinarily favor bans, and I rather doubt that non-commercial surrogacy will produce many "auntlike" relationships. Moreover, I agree with Phyllis Chesler that there is something morally disquieting about viewing a non-commercial surrogacy transaction as just another form of adoption. As Chesler sees it, adoption should be regarded as a child-centered practice whereby adults, willing to give children the kind of love they need to thrive, take into their homes and hearts *already* conceived and/or existing children. Adoption, insists Chesler, should not be regarded as an adult-centered practice whereby children are *deliberately* conceived and brought into existence so that adults can have someone to love.[66] But be all of this as it may, I favor the commodification of children, custody fights that give priority to money, and contracts that give priority to genes even less. No wonder that some commentators have proposed "ectogenesis" as the ideal solution for surrogacy arrangements. Wouldn't it be wonderful, say the fans of ectogenesis, if we could substitute artificial wombs for natural wombs? Were a fetus gestated in an artificial placenta, s/he would be in relationship to *no* one at birth. An infertile couple could take her/him home without jeopardizing any one else's relationship to her or him.

My objection to this "technological fix" is not the traditional one—that there is something "unnatural" about ex utero gestation. Rather, it is a feminist objection. We make a mistake when we choose the easy "fix" of no relationship over the difficult task of sorting through a complex network of relationships—a network that includes in surrogacy arrangements not only the relationships between the contracted mother, the contracting couple, and the contracted child, but also the relationships between fertile and infertile people. The best solution to harmful surrogacy arrangements is not ectogenesis but a serious effort to address the large social problems that make them attractive: infertility, limited employment options for working class women (the class of women from which most contracted mothers come), and labyrinthine adoption laws.[67] Only when these social problems are solved will we be in a position to work towards truly collaborative reproduction: a state of affairs in which more than two people, able to fully share all parental blessings and burdens, together procreate a child whose best interests are paramount. For now, however, we need to be aware that collaborative reproduction is not just around the corner. We also need to be aware that although harmful surrogacy arrangements are a social problem, they are less of a social problem than is parenthood in general. Feminist philosophers are asking the questions that traditional philosophy has tended to neglect: (1) *Why* do adults want children? and (2) What must an adult *do* as well as *intend* to merit the title "parent?" I only hope that would-be parents (and already-been parents for that matter) have some good answers for these very hard questions.

Notes

1. Roger D. Kempers, MD, ed., "Surrogate Mothers." In *Fertility & Sterility,* Sept. 1986, p. 62S. To say that a woman who gestates a child is that child's *surrogate* mother is not true. She *is* that child's mother. She is not a "fill in" for the child's "real" mother.

2. "Excerpts from Decision by New Jersey Supreme Court in the Baby M Case," *The New York Times* (February 4, 1988), p. B6.

3. Ibid.

4. Lori B. Andrews, "The Aftermath of Baby M: Proposed State Laws on Surrogate Motherhood." In Richard T. Hull, ed. *Ethical Issues in the New Reproductive Technologies* (Belmont, CA: Wadsowrth, 1990).

5. Lori B. Andrews, "Alternative Modes of Reproduction." In Sherrill Cohen and Nadine Taub, eds., *Reproductive Laws for the 1990s* (Clifton, NJ: Humana Press, 1988), p. 384.

6. Andrews, "The Aftermath of Baby M: Proposed State Laws on Surrogate Motherhood," pp. 33–39.

7. There are two types of contracted mothers: those who gestate an embryo genetically related to them (so-called partial surrogacy) and those who gestate an embryo genetically unrelated to them (so-called full surrogacy). At present most cases of contracted motherhood are cases of partial surrogacy. A woman contracts to be artificially inseminated with the sperm of a man who is not her husband; to carry the subsequent pregnancy to term; and to turn the resulting child over to the man and his wife to rear. Because the child is genetically related to the contracted mother, at the time of transference she must relinquish her parental rights to the child; and because the child is not genetically related to the woman who wishes to rear the child, at the time of transference or some time later she must legally adopt him or her. In the future, an increasing number of cases of contracted motherhood may be cases not of partial but of full surrogacy. Full surrogacy involves an embryo transfer after in vivo or in vitro fertilization. A woman may be able to produce eggs but unable to carry a pregnancy to term. If she and her husband are able to conceive a genetic child in vivo, physicians can flush the resulting embryo out of her womb into the womb of the woman who has agreed to gestate it. However, if she and her husband are not able to conceive a genetic child in vivo, physicians will first remove one or more eggs from the woman's womb, fertilize them outside her womb with her husband's sperm in vitro, and then introduce the resulting embryo into the womb of the woman who has agreed to gestate it. Clearly, full surrogacy is technologically more complex than partial surrogacy, a factor that accounts for its current limited use.

8. Note, "Rumpelstiltskin Revisited: The Unalienable Rights of Surrogate Mothers," 99 *Harvard Law Review* (1986), pp. 1953–1954.

9. Anthony Kronman develops a similar case in "Paternalism and the Law of Contracts," 92 *Yale Law Journal,* pp. 780–784.

10. Department of Health and Social Security, United Kingdom, *Report of the Committee of Inquiry into Human Fertilisation and Embryology,* London, HMSO, July 1984, p. 47.

11. Surrogacy Arrangements Act 1985, United Kingdom, Chapter 49, 2. (1) (a) (b) (c).

12. Ibid., 3. (1)–(5).

13. Ibid., p. 46.

14. Andrews, "The Aftermath of Baby M: Proposed State Laws on Surrogate Motherhood," pp. 191–92.

15. Phyllis Chesler, *The Sacred Bond: The Legacy of Baby M* (New York: Times Books, 1988), pp. 197–203.

16. Andrews, "Alternative Modes of Reproduction," pp. 365–366.

17. Andrea Sachs, "When the Lullaby Ends," *Time* (June 4, 1990), p. 82.

18. Mary Beth Whitehead, "A Surrogate Mother Describes Her Change of Heart—and Her Fight to Keep the Baby Two Families Love," 26 *People Weekly* (October 26, 1986), p. 47.

19. George J. Annas, "Regulating the New Reproductive Technologies." In Cohen and Taub, eds., *Reproductive Laws for the 1990s,* p. 414.

20. For more reflections on this subject, see Sara Ann Ketchum, "Is There a Right to Procreate?" Presented at the Pacific Division Meetings of the American Philosophical Association, 1987 (unpublished).

21. Chesler, *The Sacred Bond: The Legacy of Baby M,* p. 21.

22. Ibid., p. 60.

23. Gena Corea, *The Mother Machine* (New York: Harper & Row, Publishers, 1985), p. 279.

24. Ibid., p. 214.

25. Kelly Oliver, "Marxism and Surrogacy," 4, no. 3 *Hypatia* (Fall, 1989), p. 103.

26. Chesler, *The Sacred Bond: The Legacy of Baby M,* p. 38.

27. Significantly, the courts thought otherwise in this case. Ultimately, the "mother" was awarded custody of the embryos. [See the case study below of *Davis v. Davis* in "Property or Persons?—The Status of Embryos in In Vitro Fertilization."]

28. Ellen Goodman, "Whose Child?" *Charlotte Observer* (Sunday, October 28, 1990), p. 3c.

29. Andrews, "Alternative Modes of Reproduction," p. 365.

30. Ibid., 369.

31. Ibid., p. 371.

32. Ibid.

33. "Surrogate Motherhood," 9, no. 1 *Philosophy and Public Policy,* pp. 3–4.

34. Mary Gibson, "The Moral and Legal Status of 'Surrogate' Motherhood," presented at the Eastern Division Meeting of the American Philosophical Association, 1988 (unpublished).

35. Patricia A. Avery, " 'Surrogate Mothers:' Center of a New Storm," *U.S. News and World Report* (June 6, 1983), p. 76.

36. Andrews, "Alternative Modes of Reproduction," p. 369.

37. Chesler, *The Sacred Bond: The Legacy of Baby M,* p. 31.

38. Ibid., p. 24.

39. For a full discussion of arguable distinctions between baby-selling and surrogate-parenting contracts, see "Note: Developing a Concept of the Modern Family: A Proposed Uniform Surrogate Parenthood Act," 73 *Georgetown Law Journal,* Part 2 (1985), pp. 1289–1295.

40. Report of the Committee on Homosexual Offenses and Prostitution, 1963, pp. 23–24.

41. Peggy C. Davis "Alternative Modes of Reproduction: Determinants of Choice," in Cohen and Taub, eds., *Reproductive Laws for the 1990s,* p. 428.

42. Peter Singer and Deane Wells, *Making Babies: The New Science and Ethics of Conception* (New York: Charles Scribner's Sons, 1984), pp. 103–104. [See the case study below, "Parenting through Contract When No One Wants the Child."]

43. Corea, *The Mother Machine,* p. 276.

44. Elizabeth Landes and Richard Posner, "The Economics of the Baby Shortage," 7 *Journal of Legal Studies* (1978), pp. 323–345.

45. J.R.S. Pritchard, "A Market for Babies?" 34 *University of Toronto Law journal* (1981), p. 352.

46. Nancy Davis, "Reproductive Technologies and Our Attitudes Toward Children," 7, no. 1 *From the Center* (Summer 1988), pp. 1–4.

47. Herbert T. Krimmel, "The Case Against Surrogate Parenting," 13, no. 5 *The Hastings Center Report* (October, 1983), p. 36.

48. Ibid.

49. Hilda Lindemann Nelson and James Lindemann Nelson "Cutting Motherhood in Two: Some Suspicions Concerning Surrogacy," 4, no. 3 *Hypatia* (Fall 1989), p. 91.

50. Ibid., p. 93.

51. Ibid.

52. Ibid.

53. Ibid.

54. Alexander Capron and M. J. Radin, "Choosing Family Law Over Contract Law as a Paradigm for Surrogate Motherhood," 16, no. 2 *Law, Medicine, and Health Care* (Spring, 1988), p. 3a.

55. *Maher* v. *Roe* 432, U.S. 464, 474 (1977).

56. *Doe* v. *Kelley,* 106 Mich. App. 169, 307 N.W. 2d 438 (1981) *app. denied* 459 U.S. 1183 (1983).

57. Barbara Katz Rothman, *Recreating Motherhood: Ideology and Technology in a Patriarchal Society* (New York: Norton, 1989), p. 255.

58. Mary O'Brien, *The Politics of Reproduction* (Boston: Routledge & Kegan Paul, 1918).

59. Sara Ann Ketchum, "New Reproductive Technologies and the Definition of Parenthood: A Feminist Perspective," presented at Feminism and Legal Theory: Women and Intimacy (a conference sponsored by the Institute for Legal Studies at the University of Wisconsin-Madison, 1987).

60. Sherman Elias and George J. Annas, "Noncoital Reproduction," 225 *JAMA* (January 3, 1986), p. 67.

61. George T. Annas, "Death Without Dignity for Commercial Surrogacy: The Case of Baby M," 18, no. 2 *Hastings Center Report* (1988), pp. 23–24.

62. Adrienne Rich, *Of Woman Born* (New York: Norton, 1979), pp. 38–39.

63. Nelson and Nelson, "Cutting Motherhood in Two: Some Suspicions Concerning Surrogacy," p. 87.

64. Goodman, "Whose Child?" p. 3c.

65. Lawrence J. Nelson and Nancy Milliken, "Compelled Medical Treatment of Pregnant Women: Life, Liberty, and Law in Conflict." In Hull, ed., *Ethical Issues in the New Reproductive Technologies,* pp. 224–240.

66. Chesler, *The Sacred Bond: The Legacy of Baby M,* pp. 109–146.

67. "Surrogate Motherhood," *Philosophy and Public Affairs,* p. 4.

VII

PROFESSIONAL RESPONSIBILITIES

Professionals who aid in the use of reproductive technology stand in potentially conflicting positions. Physicians, nurses, technicians, attorneys, psychological counselors, and others have professional responsibilities both to serve their clients and to protect certain values of society (the latter in virtue of society's recognition of the profession and the grant of self-regulation to it). Professionals also have their own moral and other personal convictions. Furthermore, professionals often practice in institutions, such as hospitals, to which they have further obligations. All these responsibilities, convictions, and obligations do not always concide. How are practicing professionals to understand and resolve the conflicts they encounter? The readings in this part address a number of specific issues in this complex area of problems.[1]

Professional organizations often formulate codes of ethics and other policies to guide their members in ethical practice and to inform and reassure the public that the profession is meeting its obligations to society. The first article below is from the American Fertility Society's guidelines, "Ethical Considerations of the New Reproductive Technologies," presented in 1986. The short excerpt given here, concerning certain elements of the practice of IVF, is a representative sample of the sort of analysis and guidance commonly offered in such documents.[2] In considering these documents, one must ask whether they are adequate to the many demands made of them. What is their authority, both in the sense of getting the answers right and in the sense of being binding on practitioners? Are the brief analyses they offer adequate, even if more thorough analysis is supposed to support them? Without more thorough analysis, how can one tell whether the committee's conclusions have been predetermined by the selection of its members?[3] On the other hand, how much philosophical inquiry should be demanded of professionals who are not trained as philosophers and who are fully engaged in their own area of expertise?

The other two articles in this part concern an apparent conflict between professional responsibility and the moral convictions of professional practitioners. The specific issue is whether a Catholic hospital, founded on values of the family and its union of marriage, love, sexuality, and procreative capacity, should provide maternity services to women who are giving birth in arrangements to parent through contract. For though the maternity services the hospital is being asked to provide are perfectly acceptable to it, parenting through contract, in which it will be playing a role, is not. On this issue, Leonard Weber argues that hospitals have a social responsibility to provide needed medical services, limited only by the morality of the medical services themselves, which in this case are morally unexceptionable.[4] Weber is particularly worried that hospitals not create the perception that they will provide medical services only to persons who are moral in their judgment. Ann Neale's response can be interpreted as largely agreeing with Weber's views on eligibility for medical services. But, Neale points out, hospitals cannot serve all medical needs, and the decision of policy as to the best use of limited resources should be based on moral as well as on economic, legal, and social considerations. Thus, a hospital can legitimately refuse to provide a medical service that, though in itself perfectly moral, is part of a larger activity that the hospital morally condemns.[5] Though these two readings concern conflict between an *institution's* moral commitment and its social responsibilities, similar arguments can be applied to the corresponding tensions between the social responsibilities and personal convictions of individual practitioners.

Notes

1. For further discussion of the many conflicting obligations of health care professionals, see Tom L. Beauchamp and Laurence McCullough, eds., *Medical Ethics: The Moral Responsibilities of Physicians* (Englewood Cliffs, NJ: Prentice-Hall, 1984).

2. In addition to the full American Fertility Society document, see also, for example, the series of statements on the ethics of reproductive technology by the American College of Obstetricians and Gynecologists, Washington, DC.

3. A list of members of the committee that drafted the AFS report is given in the List of Contributors.

4. This case thus contrasts with the case of abortion, which the Catholic church regards as in itself morally wrong.

5. In the actual case at issue in the debate between Weber and Neale, the hospital decided that its policy would be to not provide the services in question, but that physicians would not be required to determine or report whether a woman was serving in an arrangement to parent through contract.

Ethical Considerations of in Vitro Fertilization

Ethics Committee of the American Fertility Society

In Vitro Fertilization

Reservations

Several objections have been raised against the procedure. The first is that it separates procreation from sexual union, life-giving from lovemaking. The assumption of the objection is that, for the good of the child and the couple, the child should be conceived in an act of sexual love-making.

A second objection is speculative in character. It argues that the standard procedure involves the possibility that it might produce some deformed or retarded children and is therefore an immoral means, for it involves exposing others to potential risk without their consent. It is a procedure to benefit the parents, with the risks borne by the unconsenting child.

A third objection underlines the problem of containment; if the standard procedure is approved, we will be on a "slippery slope" and will inevitably proceed to the variants and accompaniments of IVF, some or all of which would be rejected by large numbers of people.

Fourth, it has been objected that infertility is not a life-threatening disorder. Use of IVF as a therapeutic modality for a condition that is not medically harmful tends to medicalize other basic human problems. Furthermore, if IVF is not a corrective procedure and if it basically bypasses the disorder that cannot be corrected by therapeutic modalities, then there are likely to be reservations from those concerned about health care costs.

The fifth concern is that IVF involves the use of expertise and resources to produce more offspring in an already overpopulated world.

Rationale

The overall basic rationale for the IVF procedure is that the benefits provided outweigh the risks both to the couple and to the offspring produced. From the facts currently available, the procedure produces normal, healthy offspring with a success rate that approaches the natural one. There is no known in-

From Chapters 13 & 18, *Fertility & Sterility*, Supplement 1, 46(3) (September, 1986). Abridged. Reproduced with permission of the publisher, The American Fertility Society.

creased risk to the parents or to the offspring. Therefore, IVF has become an accepted therapy for intractable infertility.

Deliberations

The Committee could find no persuasive evidence that the child and/or married couple suffer harm (the personal criterion) when IVF is used as a last resort. The analysis insisting on the inseparability of the life-giving and love-making dimensions is built on an excessively biologic notion of what is morally right and wrong. Furthermore, numerous commentators see IVF not as a substitute for sexual intimacy, but as an extension of it, and therefore as not involving the radical separation of procreation and sexual intimacy. (For an extended discussion of these reservations and objections, please see McCormick, 1984.[1])

As for risks, similar risks are run by couples in their ordinary sexual lives. Therefore, if the risks in IVF are not notably greater than those involved in sexual intercourse, the argument loses force. Factually, on the basis of experience so far, IVF involves no greater risk to the child.

The extension of reproductive technology into suspect areas is a legitimate concern. Yet, the response to such a concern is that possible abuse does not invalidate appropriate use. Furthermore, there is likely to be sharp pluralism about what constitutes abuse.

Finally, the Committee argued that the infertile couple should not be held responsible for the population problems of the world. Realistically, IVF would not affect such problems one way or another.

Recommendations

The Committee unanimously finds that basic IVF is ethically acceptable.

Preembryos from In Vitro Fertilization for Donation

Background

A preembryo from in vitro fertilization (IVF) for donation by definition has no lineal genetic relation to either party of the recipient couple. There are no data on this use of donor preembryos in human beings. However, the demand to adopt children suggests that there may be a use for this service; but, in contrast to basic IVF, it would seem that the demand for this service would be relatively less.

Medical Indications

The primary indications for the giving and receiving of a preembryo are rare. It would apply to a couple, the female partner of whom had one of the medical indications for a donor egg and the male partner of whom had one of the indications for the use of donor sperm.[2]

If no donor egg were available and if a donor preembryo became available, an indication of an alternative nature might arise for a patient who required a donor egg.

Donor preembryos might become available from several sources. The most likely is from preembryos in excess of those thought desirable for transfer to the donor for treatment of her own infertility. This situation might arise if nontransferred preembryos were cryopreserved for future use by the donor and subsequent events made such use undesirable or impossible; fresh preembryos might unexpectedly become available if after insemination some serious illness, accident, or even death prevented their intended transfer. In very rare circumstances, fresh preembryos might unexpectedly become available because of an unexpected result after insemination. For example, if previous experience with a patient with oligospermia or other abnormality predicted that only about a 25% fertilization rate could be expected, and on subsequent trials a large number of eggs, e.g., 12, happened to be available for insemination, all 12 might be inseminated with the hope of having the optimum three or four fertilized eggs for transfer. If the unexpected happened and all 12 eggs did, in fact, fertilize—a highly unlikely event—several preembryos would become available.

At the current level of operations, both of the just-mentioned circumstances would require prompt action for the viability of the preembryos to be preserved if facilities for cryopreservation were not immediately available.

Reservations About the Procedure

There are concerns about the possibility of genetic defects in the preembryo similar to those with donor sperm or a donor egg. Furthermore, the possibility of immunologic incompatibility must be considered, as with a donor egg.

There are ethical concerns pertaining to the use of third-party gametes for a couple, neither one of whom would have a lineal genetic relation to the offspring. This relationship is analogous to that of adoption, although that relationship is generally considered to refer to children already born. The ethical concerns include the potential effect on the families of the donor and the recipient and the possible effect on the child. The legal status of a donor preembryo is in a state of evolution, with a growing tendency to protect the conceptus under civil and criminal law.

Rationale for the Procedure

There are no risks to the donor other than those risks already accepted in the treatment of her own infertility and no risks to the recipient except the risk associated with transfer in the normal in vitro process. Thus, there are no substantial incremental risks to either the donor or the recipient in a donor preembryo program. Concerns about the genetic defects of the preembryo can be diminished with the use of a genetic screen of the sperm and egg donor. . . . However, this may not always be feasible, because the availability of a preembryo may be unanticipated. Concern about immunologic incompatibility is essentially the same as with the use of donor eggs in that with both donor eggs and donor preembryos, no transmission of genetic material occurs between the potential mother and the preembryo. However, based on animal experience and the limited experience in human beings, there would be apparently no immunologic consequences.

No data exist on the consequences of the use of donor preembryos to the individual or to society. It has been suggested that the use of donor preembryos is similar in concept to adoption and that the only difference is the time the adoption occurred. However, it needs to be noted that the situations are by no means parallel. In the case of traditional adoption, the adoption is accepted as a solution to an established unfortunate situation, i.e., an extant child without rearing parents. In the case of the donation of a preembryo, the donation is deliberate to allow the couple to bear a potential child and, particularly, to accommodate the desire of the potential mother for carrying a child to viability within her own uterus. It may be argued with some merit that from the point of view of the recipient couple, this experience more closely approximates the normal situation with human reproduction by allowing the couple to experience the pregnancy than does traditional adoption.

The question of the paternity of the donated preembryo has not yet been determined, but . . . courts have generally held that the gestational mother is the legal mother of the child.

Considerations and Recommendations of the Committee

Because of the general concern over the use of third-party gametes, the use of existing preembryos for donation remains controversial. There may be potential recipients or groups in the position to offer this service who find that the reservations to the procedure outweigh the benefits to the couple, i.e., that the procedure is not in the best interests of the persons integrally and adequately considered. In that circumstance, the recipient or group would not wish to participate in a donor egg program.

The Committee finds the use of preembryos from IVF for donation ethically acceptable. The Committee further agrees that several guidelines should apply. As with the use of donor eggs and sperm, there should be no compensation to the donors of the preembryo. This does not exclude the reimbursement of expenses and inconvenience in connection with the donation. Anonymity, as has been traditionally practiced with adoption, may be a desirable goal, but there seem to be no compelling data to exclude transfer of a donor preembryo among parties known to each other. To minimize the transfer of genetic defects, a donor preembryo should be derived from an egg and sperm from young donors. Furthermore, except for unexpected situations, both the sperm and egg donor should have gone through a genetic screen. . . .

Notes

1. McCormick, R. A. "Notes on Moral Theology," *Theological Studies* 45 (1984).

2. [These indications, mentioned earlier in the AFS's guidelines, include, for the female, absent or dysfunctional ovaries, lack of technical ability to retrieve eggs, and genetic defects, and for the male, impaired sperm production, complete gonadal failure, genetic defects, or other sorts of subfertility or infertility—Editor.]

Social Responsibility Demands Treating All Patients in Need

Leonard J. Weber

In deciding whether surrogate mothers should be permitted to deliver their babies in hospitals that are committed to the highest ethical standards, two different approaches can be identified. One focuses on the practice of surrogate motherhood itself (with all its questionable dimensions). The other approach examines the hospital's obligations to provide health care services to those in need. This article argues that the second approach is more appropriate and that, in this light, the denial of services to a woman because of her involvement in a surrogate motherhood arrangement is difficult to justify.

The question is not whether, or when, surrogate motherhood is ethically defensible. The appropriateness of delivering the child would not be an issue if serious ethical reservations about surrogate motherhood did not exist. (Some of the most important of these are identified by Ann Neale. See below, "Responsible Stewardship Requires Not Cooperating with Surrogacy.") The argument that a hospital should admit the surrogate mother is not a defense of surrogacy; it is not a neutral stand on the practice; and it is not a claim that surrogate motherhood involves issues of minor moral significance. It is, rather, an argument in defense of a particular understanding of the ethics of health care delivery.

Meeting Society's Needs

Clear identification of the most important ethical questions being addressed is important: What is the hospital's responsibility when someone in need of health services is engaged in behavior that is contrary to what the hospital represents? To what extent are hospitals justified in evaluating the behavior of those who are seeking health care? What is the individual hospital's role in contributing to a more just health care delivery system?

The concept of social responsibility is widely used in discussing business

From *Health Progress* 68, (March, 1987), pp. 38, 40–42. © 1987 *Health Progress*. Reprinted with permission.

ethics and can be used to clarify the role of health care organizations. It allows us to focus on the organization's purpose and to recognize that none of us lives or works in a vacuum; we are part of a society that has particular needs and problems, and we meet our obligations, or do not meet them, in the midst of that world. What we do rarely affects only individuals; it has social impact as well.

A socially responsible organization meets the needs of those it is designed to serve and promotes justice. A socially responsible hospital provides high-quality health care, respects individual dignity, and promotes justice in society. A hospital's responsibility goes beyond (although it includes) the obligation to serve those who come to it for care. This social responsibility includes evaluating its practices' impact on society (primarily in terms of health care) and promoting the common good.

Protection of Human Dignity

As the National Conference of Catholic Bishops has argued in its recent pastoral letter, *Economic Justice for All: Catholic Social Teaching and the U.S. Economy* (Washington, DC, 1986), the common good demands the protection of everyone's human rights. And the full range of human rights includes not only civil and poltical rights to freedom of speech, worship, and assembly, but also social and economic rights to food, clothing, shelter, education, and health care. If human dignity is to be protected, individuals and organizations must promote the kind of society in which these rights are all acknowledged and respected.

Social responsibility, defined as respect for all human rights, requires that society's resources be distributed according to need. Justice requires that everyone's basic needs be met. People do not "merit" or "earn" their right to the essentials of life; the fact that human dignity depends on these essentials justifies the claim to them.

The conviction that everyone has a basic human right to necessary health care and that health care resources should be distributed according to need suggests a particular attitude toward health care for surrogate mothers. Despite a hospital's effort to make a policy decision rather than a judgment of the individual woman, refusal to admit a surrogate mother clearly means that factors other than need are considered relevant in deciding whom to treat. Delivery services are a real need (regardless of how the woman became pregnant) and are not unethical per se. If a hospital refuses the woman admission, it is taking the stand that the surrogate arrangement is unethical and is not to be supported in any way.

But what is a hospital saying when it refuses to admit patients for necessary and ethically acceptable procedures because it believes their behavior— or the enterprise they are part of—to be unethical? Obviously, the hospital has strong objections to surrogacy, but it also is stating that the hospital may decide who is worthy of being treated. Hospital administrators, sponsors, or trustees may not intend to say that health services should be provided according to merit; in their own minds, they may have a different rationale. But such a decision will be heard and seen as a moral evaluation of the patient's life or behavior; the woman is being refused precisely because of her involvement in a practice judged unethical.

People are becoming more aware of the extent to which behavior choices affect health and health care needs. The use of tobacco, the abuse of alcohol and other drugs, certain eating patterns, lack of exercise, and particular types of sexual activity are all behaviors that are likely to affect health. And some of these behavior choices would be considered morally unacceptable by others.

Nevertheless, someone who is guilty of immoral behavior still has a basic right to health care, and a health care facility that attempts to evaluate someone's worthiness for care on the basis of an assessment of his or her behavior would systematically violate human dignity and the basic human right to health care.

Thus refusing admission to a surrogate mother might well contribute to a less just health care system. People have long acknowledged that everyone should be treated, including notorious criminals injured in their assaults on others, and wounded enemy soldiers.

Granted, the purpose of policies to refuse admittance to surrogate mothers is not to say that they should not be treated anywhere, and presumably, in an emergency, every facility would admit such patients. Nevertheless, a judgment is being made here that someone should not be admitted, and this judgment is based on an evaluation of a behavior or practice.

Our society, however, currently focuses on a person's responsibility for his or her condition. We hear references to "the deserving poor" (with the implication that many of the poor are undeserving); where people used to discuss the "overmedication" of the elderly, now they talk about "drug abuse" among the elderly; almost everyone has seen evidence of anger directed at those who have AIDS. This tendency to place responsibility on the one in need is a part of the present social context in which institutional decisions are made.

People commonly refer to the traditional concept of "cooperation" in an effort to sort out the responsibilities of someone associated with the morally unacceptable practices of others. That effort often can help clarify responsibilities. The concept needs to be used carefully, however, or we might focus so much on the evils of others, and on our need to separate ourselves from those evils, that we fail to recognize the evil that could result from this separation. The failure to provide for basic human needs without judging the worthiness of the one in need should not be excused or minimized by an appeal to the "cooperation" doctrine.

One of the most important reasons for hospitals to seriously consider whether to admit surrogate mothers is that this consideration provides the opportunity to clarify their approach to a variety of ethical issues. Often, ethical deliberation concentrates on a few clearly discernible ethical issues, such as those related to death and dying and reproduction. These issues are important, but the basic framework for addressing most issues of *institutional* responsibility should be social ethics—the principles of economic justice and human rights that the U.S. Catholic bishops, among others, have articulated so clearly. Health care organizations are an essential part of the U.S. economic system, and their primary social responsibilities are to be identified in terms of economic and social ethics. The concern for "cooperation with evil" should be voiced in the context of social ethics, not as a way of bypassing the hard questions of social responsibility.

Hospital Policy

Social responsibility requires hospitals to assess the impact on the common good if they *do* admit and care for the surrogate mother at the time of childbirth. Some might see this as an endorsement of the practice of surrogacy. Because of the deeply held belief that the right to health care should be separated from consideration of moral worthiness, however, the danger of the message of endorsing surrogacy is less than that of morally judging patients.

How, then, can hospital administrators, sponsors, and trustees prepare to react appropriately to the possibility of a surrogate mother being admitted? The above arguments suggest these summary points:

- Surrogate mothers should not be refused just because they are surrogate mothers.
- If a surrogate mother (or the attorney) makes the fact of surrogacy known, the hospital should inform her that she is welcome but that it will not change its normal practices to conform to the surrogate contract (e.g., that it will discharge the baby to the genetic mother, if that is the standard practice, and not to the contracting couple). Persons will be cared for without judging their behavior, but that does not mean that the hospital will conform to their desires.
- Hospitals should be prepared to explain, in the event of external publicity or internal questions, that childbirth services for surrogate mothers do not constitute an endorsement of the practice any more than the care of other persons constitutes an endorsement of their behavior.

The question that has occasioned this debate has provided an important opportunity to sort out various issues and responsibilities. Among these responsibilities, the obligation to develop a system that meets the health care needs of all without judgment should rank high.

Responsible Stewardship Requires Not Cooperating with Surrogacy

Ann Neale

Recently a committee of the American Fertility Society (AFS) released a report on ethical issues involved in a variety of new reproductive technologies. The committee expressed dismay at the lack of empirical evidence on how the surrogacy process works and how it affects the surrogate mothers, the couples, the families of both the surrogates and the couples, the resulting children, and society. They concurred with the prevalent assessment of surrogate motherhood that it is fraught with moral, legal, and social problems. The AFS recommended the procedure be limited to women for whom it is a medical necessity and then only in the context of a clinical experiment, with prior approval by a local institutional review board (IRB) or ethics committee and periodic review of the protocol by the IRB.[1]

Unsatisfactory Alternative

Three years ago the American Medical Association (AMA) house of delegates stipulated that surrogate motherhood "does not represent a satisfactory reproductive alternative for people who wish to become parents" and suggested that physicians not become involved in the financial or legal aspects of a surrogate motherhood arrangement.[2] The director of practice activities for the American College of Obstetricians and Gynecologists, while holding out the possibility that surrogacy in some situations could be acceptable, generally agreed with the AMA position that these arrangements do not appear to serve societal interests.[3]

The discussion on the ethics of surrogacy is enlightening and perhaps helpful to clinicians, potential surrogate mothers, and couples considering participation in such arrangements. Nevertheless, further discussion is necessary to guide the moral discernment of clinicians and organizations that are asked to provide services to those who have already undertaken a surrogate

From *Health Progress* 68, (March, 1987), pp. 39, 42–43. © 1987 *Health Progress*. Reprinted with permission.

arrangement. For example, hospitals at which obstetricians (whether they were involved in the surrogate arrangements or only in the surrogate mother's prenatal care) wish to deliver these women's babies have to decide whether to cooperate in the surrogate arrangement by delivering the babies.

The primary ethical objection to surrogacy involves the essence of the arrangement, which is the surrogate mother's abdication of responsibility for her child and the transfer of that responsibility to others. The surrogate mother is intentionally conceiving her child as an object for the benefit and use of others rather than as a gift of God to be wanted and loved for the baby's own sake.

This arrangement, which precedes conception, fundamentally challenges the meaning and purpose of parenting. Parenting has always entailed the notion of loving and caring for one's offspring. Surrogacy, and, by extension, cooperation in the delivery of a surrogate mother's child, mistakenly implies that children may be created to be given up.

Furthermore, surrogacy has potential negative social consequences. An obvious drawback is the commercialization of human reproduction, bordering on baby selling. Many commentators assert—and some evidence supports their claim—that surrogate mothers agree to these arrangements primarily for monetary reasons. One attorney who handles surrogate contracts in Southern California believes women motivated primarily by money are more likely to honor their surrogate contract, and therefore he accepts only such women into his program.[4]

The power exerted by the affluent "adoptive" couple over a less affluent woman to conceive and give up to them a child in exchange for money could lead to the exploitation of a needy woman. Surrogate mothers, who may begin to bond with the fetus during pregnancy and wish to change their minds, are under considerable financial and psychological pressure not to break their contract. The baby is also particularly vulnerable, potentially wanted by all or none of the parties, subject to their changing their mind or the baby's not being "perfect."

A moral judgment that, on balance, surrogate arrangements are not justified does not necessarily mean that hospitals should refuse to provide care for surrogates. The moral issues of whether to participate in formulating a surrogate arrangement and whether to cooperate after the fact by delivering the baby, although closely related, can be approached separately.

Nevertheless, in contrast to Leonard J. Weber's understanding of a hospital's social responsibility (see above, "Social Responsibility Demands Treating All Patients in Need"), I believe that the delivery of surrogate mothers' babies is ill advised. The serious, unresolved reservations the AFS and others express about surrogacy warrant hospitals' refusal to cooperate.

A responsible ethics of health care delivery requires a comprehensive assessment of the services rendered. On the basis of such assessments, hospitals often make considered judgments concerning which among an array of possible health services they will provide. Those considerations involve weighing the moral, legal, economic, and social implications of the technology or service in question. From this perspective a policy not to admit a surrogate mother for delivery can be compared with a university medical center's decision not to provide organ transplantation services. Such policies are the result of judgments about the acceptability or feasibility of providing the technology or service. The hospital's policy not to provide the service need not be construed as a negative moral judgment on the persons needing or wanting it.

The ethical, legal, and social questions raised by surrogate arrangements create a dilemma for hospitals concerning the admission of surrogate mothers. A hospital may be reluctant to cooperate in a practice about which most commentators have grave moral reservations; which could undermine the traditional notion of parenting and our professed unconditional valuing of children; which puts needy women and helpless infants in morally and legally vulnerable positions; and whose societal consequences are so uncertain. On the other hand, hospitals have a mission to deliver competent, compassionate care, not to evaluate the moral character of those they serve. Unwed mothers, the indigent, schoolteachers, and AIDS patients should receive expert and nonjudgmental care from all hospitals.

Responsible Stewardship

My argument rests primarily on the negative aspects of surrogacy as a practice, rather than on a judgment on the moral rectitude of persons involved in surrogate arrangements. From this perspective, a policy not to admit surrogate mothers can be seen as an expression of responsible stewardship in pursuit of what best serves the hospital's mission and the common good, rather than as a dangerous precedent likely to lead to unjustified discrimination against others in need of health services.

In working out a policy on surrogate motherhood, a hospital might discuss with its employees, medical staff, and patient population, not just the values at stake, but also technology assessment, resource allocation, and equity and access issues. Such a discussion should demonstrate that, on balance, the reasons for not admitting surrogate mothers (except those who arrive in labor or require services which only that hospital can provide) outweigh the reasons for admitting them.

One way to think about the problem is to ask on what basis, if any, a hospital could decide not to provide certain health care services. One clear basis is a moral repugnance for the service requested. Providers are not morally obliged to carry out procedures that violate their conscience or are not in society's best interest. For some health care providers, abortion is a case in point.[5] In the future, delivering babies who are a result of the technology of cloning could be another example.

Another basis for a policy decision not to provide a service is that the service is beyond the hospital's competence or ability to provide. For instance, many community hospitals do not provide sophisticated, resource-intensive technological care such as transplant surgery. Furthermore, even when a service is not beyond a hospital's technological competence, some choose not to provide certain services for reasons of community needs and resource allocation.

A provider also may refuse to provide certain services when no medical indication exists or when, indeed, the requested service is medically contraindicated. Professional integrity, patient well-being, and resource allocation are involved here.

Morally Defensible Policy

Any one or a combination of reasons spanning moral reservations about the procedure itself, patient and societal well-being, medical necessity, and resource allocation, then, in some instances could justify not providing a service. I suggest the following bases for a morally defensible hospital policy not to admit a surrogate mother for delivery, except in emergencies:

- The hospital's administrators, sponsors, and trustees believe all health care technologies and services should be thoroughly assessed, and hospital policy regarding the availability of those technologies and related services should reflect that assessment.
- The hospital's leaders believe surrogacy to be a seriously flawed practice that diminishes the meaning and purpose of parenting and the intrinsic value of children.
- The leaders have grave reservations about the impact of a surrogate arrangement on all parties, especially society.
- The leaders believe sufficient community discussion and attempts to formulate sound public policy on surrogacy have not taken place.
- The leaders concur with the AFS committee's recommendation that surrogacy not be widespread, but rather that it be carefully controlled and studied.

Such a policy could be based on the reasonable assumption that the parties involved in the surrogate arrangement should work out all details in advance, including the delivering obstetrician and hospital.[6] The policy would simply stipulate that the hospital does not wish to cooperate in any aspect of such arrangements. Obstetric services for surrogate mothers, who are by definition sponsored (i.e., paying) patients, surely would be available at other hospitals. Meanwhile, the witness value of not cooperating in a practice about which such serious and extensive reservations exist could be important.

Notes

1. Ethics Committee of the American Fertility Society, "Ethical Considerations of the New Reproductive Technologies," *Fertility and Sterility,* supp. 1, September 1986, pp. v, 58S–68S.

2. *Medical World News,* Jan. 9, 1984, p. 24.

3. Ibid., p. 24.

4. Sheila Cohen, "Surrogate Mothers: Whose Baby Is It?" *American Journal of Law and Medicine,* vol. 10, no. 3, 1984, pp. 243–285, footnotes 2 and 57.

5. When the situation is an emergency (e.g., serious threat to the woman's life or health) and no other provider is available, many commentators suggest that the conscientious objector (organization or individual) should reevaluate the refusal to cooperate in abortion.

6. The insight of Ralph Cushing, MD, a member of an institutional ethics committee deliberating hospital policy in this matter.

VIII

CASE STUDIES

This final part of the anthology presents a number of studies of actual cases illustrating problems that arise in the use of reproductive technology. These cases are just a small sampling of the troubling, often bizarre, disputes and conundrums that have arisen. Indeed, it has been said, with only slight hyperbole, that even the most fantastic scenarios that one might imagine have already in fact happened. The cases presented here, however, have not been chosen for their outlandishness, but rather to stimulate interest and to offer concrete situations in which to apply insights gained from the substantive articles and against which to test them for adequacy. It should be noted that though case studies can be fascinating, care must be taken in generalizing from unusual cases.

The first case presented is an extended study of the much-publicized case of Baby M, in which the parties to a contract for parenting all wanted the child and battled for over two years in and out of court for custody of the little girl. This case is described at length, including substantial excerpts from two court decisions, in order to provide a detailed record for analysis and to illustrate how emotional issues can, for better and for worse, be addressed though rational argument in public proceedings. Virtually all of the normative issues about parenting through contract raised and examined in the earlier articles arise here, including the splitting of genetic, gestational, and social parenting roles; commercialization; the oppression of women; and legal and constitutional issues. In considering the case of Baby M, particular attention should be given to the ways in which preconceived attitudes can color how "facts" are interpreted and distort inferences drawn from them.

Contrasting with the study of Baby M is the case "Parenting through Contract When No One Wants the Child," in which, as its title indicates, *neither* of the parties to a contract wanted the child. This case raises again, in a different context, many of the standard normative issues of parenting through contract. It also challenges preconceptions about parental attachment to children and reminds us of the wide range of exigencies that must be anticipated when innovation goes beyond established moral and legal norms.

The final selection, "Property or Persons?—The Status of Embryos in In

315

Vitro Fertilization," comprises four cases in which embryos created through IVF are at issue. In the Del Zio case, a hospital administrator deliberately destroyed embryos being used in an early attempt at IVF. In the Rios case, a couple died without having made arrangements for the disposition of embryos frozen during their attempts at IVF. The York case involves an IVF clinic's refusal to release an embryo to a couple who moved across the country. In *Davis v. Davis,* a divorcing couple sued for rights over embryos they created when their marriage was still intact. These cases, in different ways, raise questions about respect for human embryos and about how IVF practice should be regulated through professional guidelines, administrative regulations, and legal statutes.

Two further, very brief cases were offered earlier in this anthology as an appendix to Kenneth Alpern's "Genetic Puzzles and Stork Stories." There, instances of testicle and ovary transplantation were presented in order to focus questions about the meaning and significance of having children when natural genetic relations have been disrupted.

The Case of Baby M:
Parenting through Contract
When Everyone Wants the Child

In 1985, William Stern, Mary Beth Whitehead, and Richard Whitehead entered into an agreement for surrogate motherhood through the Infertility Center of New York (ICNY), headed by leading surrogacy broker Noel Keane. The agreement was arranged by ICNY, which had recruited Mrs. Whitehead, brought the parties together, provided all the contracts, and in general facilitated the arrangement, for which it received a fee of $7,500. By the terms of the agreement, Mrs. Whitehead would be artificially inseminated with Mr. Stern's sperm, carry a child to term, give up her parental rights to the child, thus allowing Mr. Stern's wife, Elizabeth, to adopt, and receive $10,000 in addition to all costs associated with her pregnancy. On March 27, 1986, Mrs. Whitehead gave birth to a healthy baby girl but decided not to give up the baby.

For nearly two years, the Sterns and the Whiteheads contended for the child, who became famous under her name in legal documents, "Baby M." Early on, the Sterns obtained a court order for temporary custody of the child, but the Whiteheads evaded police, at one point handing the baby out through their bedroom window with the Sterns and authorities in their living room. For three and a half months Mrs. Whitehead hid with the child in various locations in Florida. Finally discovered by detectives, she was forced to give over the child to Mr. Stern's temporary custody while the parties battled in the courts.

Four days after the baby's first birthday, Judge Harvey Sorkow of the New Jersey Superior Court for Bergen County held that the surrogacy contract was valid and enforceable, awarded Mr. Stern permanent custody, and completely terminated all Mrs. Whitehead's parental rights. Judge Sorkow, without giving notice to the Whiteheads, then called the Sterns into his chambers and immediately processed Mrs. Stern's adoption, making her the legal mother of the child.

The Whiteheads appealed these decisions, and finally, in February 1988, the New Jersey Supreme Court reversed the lower court's decision on the validity of the contract and, though concurring in the award of custody to Mr. Stern, refused to terminate completely Mary Beth Whitehead's[1] parental rights. She remains the child's legal mother, with weekly visitation rights.

The case of Baby M has commanded national attention, both because of the controversial nature of surrogacy—this being the first surrogacy case to be fully argued in court—and because of the sensational details of this particular case. Spectacular cases can distort underlying issues, but with care, the Baby M case can be used to examine, in concrete detail, many of the moral, legal, and policy issues raised by surrogacy. These issues include whether surrogacy is exploitive of the mother or child; whether surrogacy arrangements must be recognized under constitutional rights to privacy, reproductive freedom, and freedom of contract; and whether regulations should govern any surrogacy practices that are allowed. However, it must be remembered that any single case has its own peculiarities that complicate simple generalization, and that as a court case, the issues raised and the principles on which they are decided are (at least in theory) *legal,* and not directly principles of morality, theology, or public policy. Further, in evaluating the court's decision, it must be remembered that details and nuances of evidence and testimony cannot always be fully appreciated from a distance—which is one reason for trying cases in court rather than by public opinion. Still, we do have the court transcripts, the judges' long and detailed decisions in the cases, and extensive reports in the press. So with care, it may be possible to reach reasoned conclusions about what should have been decided in this case and, more important, about what policies should be in place to avoid or prepare for the problems of surrogacy generally.

Issues

In public discussion of the case, emotions tended to fix on one or another feature of the parties. The Sterns are well educated, reasonably well-to-do professionals: he is a biochemist, she a medical doctor with a Ph.D. in genetics. The Whiteheads are blue-collar: she dropped out of high school and has been a housewife with a number of menial part-time jobs; he served in Vietnam and drives a sanitation truck. The Whiteheads have suffered through financial problems, a bankruptcy, Richard Whitehead's drinking problem, and a short separation. On the other hand, the Whiteheads have two children, who by all accounts were reasonably well raised and cared for. The Sterns had put off starting a family until they had established their careers and then feared that Elizabeth Stern's recently self-diagnosed multiple sclerosis would make pregnancy too risky for her. Mr. Stern is the last in his family line, most of his relatives having died in the Nazi Holocaust. The Whiteheads had defied the law in absconding with the baby; Mrs. Whitehead was emotional, her appeals were appeals of love and, some claimed, of hysteria. The Sterns were controlled and rational. They had the contract[2] and the legal system on their side. They had used the police to force a mother to give up her child. Mrs. Whitehead had signed a contract and then reneged.

By the time the controversy came to court, two issues had emerged as the most basic legal concerns: the status of the contract and the custody of the child. As to the contract, many felt the simple principle was that when adults knowingly and freely sign a contract, they should do as they said they would. Furthermore, it was argued, constitutional recognition of freedom in matters of reproduction should be understood as extending to the freedom to make and have legal protection of surrogacy arrangements. According to this way of thinking, the terms of the contract settle all issues of custody and parental rights. Less recognized in public debates, however, was the fact that courts have discretion as to what remedy to impose in cases of breached contracts. In cases of contracts for personal services, it is more common for courts to demand payment of monetary damages than to demand specific performance (that is, that the parties do as they had contracted).

Opposed to the above line of thinking on the contract was the view that the contract was invalid and unenforceable because it violates public policy concerning adoption, baby-selling, and exploitation. If the contract were held to be invalid or unenforceable, then custody would have to be decided, presumably on the basis of the usual criterion of "the best interests of the child," though some felt that in this case the parents' interests should also be considered.

Though the discussion that follows is limited largely to court proceedings and legal issues, these legal matters are important for a number of reasons. First, one of the chief problems regarding surrogacy is what its status should be before the law. Second, the law, though technical, is a repository for concepts, distinctions, principles, and precedents developed in the attempt to bring principles of justice and equity to bear on the complexity of real life. Morality may not be simply read off of (or into) the law, but legal reasoning often can be a guide to moral truth. Finally, legal proceedings are fairly orderly and explicit, and so provide at least a starting point for reasoned consideration of controversial and emotional disputes such as surrogacy and the matter of Baby M. As in this case, disagreements between the trial court and the appeals court further highlight opposing lines of legal and moral argument.

The case of Baby M involved two primary court decisions, the initial trial[3] and its appeal,[4] as well as a number of motions and determinations concerning temporary custody and visitation rights. The initial trial was presented before Judge Harvey Sorkow, the judge who had awarded temporary custody to the Sterns at the beginning of legal wrangling over the child. Judge Sorkow's decision surprised virtually everyone by upholding the contract. He further ruled, with somewhat puzzling logic, that the proper enforcement of the contract was specific performance as long as that would be in the child's best interest. He then determined that the child's best interest required precisely what the contract had stipulated: that William Stern have custody and that Mary Beth Whitehead's parental rights, including any right to visitation, be completely terminated.

The Whiteheads appealed Judge Sorkow's decision directly to the New Jersey Supreme Court. In February 1988, this court unanimously ruled that the contract is *not* enforceable, indeed, that it may be illegal, that the best interest of the child required that Mr. Stern still be awarded custody, but that Mary Beth Whitehead be recognized as the child's legal mother (with visitation rights). This last judgment blocked adoption of the child by Elizabeth Stern. Mary Beth Whitehead pronounced herself satisfied with this decision and dedicated herself to the growing campaign against surrogacy. The Sterns took the child, Melissa Elizabeth Stern, back home and are trying to raise here in some semblance of stability and privacy.

Reasoning of the Trial Court

The following summarizes the reasoning on the key issues in the case, first as judged by the trial court and then as reviewed by the New Jersey Supreme Court on appeal. As much as practicable, quotations and paraphrase of the courts' decisions have been used.

Validity of the Contract

The Sterns sought specific performance of the contract. The Whiteheads argued that the contract should be declared invalid and unenforceable on a number of grounds, most importantly lack of informed consent and conflict with law and public policy. The Sterns countered that the surrogacy contract was protected by the constitutional right to privacy in procreative matters.

Informed Consent

The Whiteheads argued that Mary Beth could not have given informed consent to the contract, since she could not have anticipated her feelings for the child in advance of giving birth or of even becoming pregnant. Judge Sorkow held, however, that the concept of informed consent is irrelevant to the surrogacy situation, as no one in a superior position of knowledge withheld information from Mrs. Whitehead. But, as if to assuage lingering feelings of unfairness on this issue, he added that Mrs. Whitehead was under no time constraints and could obtain any legal, medical, or psychological advice she wished before entering the agreement.[5]

Surrogacy and Public Policy

Contracts of any sort will not be enforced by a court if the terms of the contract are against public policy, that is, if they are either illegal or against clear goals and values promoted by the state. The Whiteheads argued that the contract was against public policy for failing to protect the child, violating adoption laws, making the child an object of sale (commercialization), undermining the family, and contributing to economic elitism.

PROTECTION OF THE CHILD. Judge Sorkow reasoned that even given the absence of legislation designed with surrogacy in mind, children born through surrogacy will be protected because if the contract is complied with, the adoption will still have to be approved by the courts, and if the contract is not complied with, litigation will unavoidably turn on the best interests of the child.[6]

EXPLOITATION AND THE LAW OF ADOPTION. Adoption law, Judge Sorkow pointed out, is intended to protect mothers from having to make drastic and final decisions when they are under the stress and emotion of just having given birth, often in financial difficulty, and often without the support of a husband or other family members. In contrast, a surrogate mother "has an opportunity to consult, take advice and consider her act and is not forced into the relationship." Therefore, laws protecting mothers from exploitation in adoption are not applicable to surrogates.

COMMERCIALIZATION. Judge Sorkow rejected claims that "to produce or deal with a child for money denigrates human dignity" and that laws prohibiting payment in exchange for adoption are violated. "The biological father pays the surrogate for her willingness to be impregnated and carry his child to term. At birth, the father does not purchase the child. It is his own biological genetically related child. He cannot purchase what is already his."

UNDERMINES THE FAMILY. Judge Sorkow held that surrogacy does not undermine the family. The childless husband and wife desperately want a child and seek to make a family. The husband of the surrogate is a willing party to the agreement.

ECONOMIC ELITISM. Wrote Judge Sorkow: it is argued that "an elite upper economic group of people will use the lower economic group of woman to 'make their babies'. This argument is insensitive and offensive to the intense drive to procreate naturally and when that is impossible, to use what lawful means are possible to gain a child. This intense desire to propagate the species is fundamental. It is within the soul of all men and women regardless of economic status."

Constitutional Issues

The Sterns argued that the arrangements made in the contract are protected by the Constitution on the grounds of privacy and equal protection. The trial court took up these issues and, as well, the constitutionality of the clauses in the contract that sought to give William Stern the right to direct Mary Beth Whitehead to have an abortion.

PROCREATIVE AND PRIVACY RIGHTS. Judge Sorkow reviewed constitutional protection of the right to privacy in procreation as follows:[7]

"In 1923, the United States Supreme Court held that an individual in this country has a constitutional right to 'marry, establish a home and bring up children.' *Meyer v. Nebraska*, 262 U.S. 390. While one might read into *Meyer* a right to procreate so as to bring up children, the issue was faced squarely 19 years later, when in 1942, the United States Supreme Court struck down Oklahoma's statute permitting sterilization of certain criminals and held that the right to procreate was among the 'basic civil rights of man.' *Skinner v. Oklahoma*, 316 U.S. 535. These rights were later deemed by the Court to be 'rights far more precious . . . than property rights.' *Stanley v. Illinois*, 405 U.S. 645. In *Cleveland Board of Education v. LaFleur*, 414 U.S. 632, it was settled that 'freedom of personal choice in matters of marriage and family life is one of the liberties protected by the due process clause of the 14th Amendment.'

"At the same time these fundamental *family* rights were being secured in our constitutional matrix, the court held that individuals had a right of privacy entitled to constitutional protection. *Griswold v. Connecticut,* 381 U.S. 479. And finally in 1972, Justice William Brennan wrote in *Eisenstadt v. Baird,* 405 U.S. 438: 'If the right of privacy means anything it is the right of the *individual,* married or single, to be free from unwarranted governmental intrusion into matters so fundamentally affecting a person as the decision whether to bear or beget a child.'

"While it may appear from a reading of these cases that no mention of alternative reproductive methods means non-coital reproduction is excluded from the [C]onstitution's protections, this court does not so hold. Rather it must be reasoned that if one has a right to procreate coitally, then one has the right to reproduce non-coitally. If it is the reproduction that is protected, then the means of reproduction are also to be protected. The value and interests underlying the creation of family are the same by whatever means obtained. This court holds that the protected means extends to the use of surrogates. The contract cannot fall because of the use of a third party. It is reasoned that the donor or surrogate aids the childless couple by contributing a factor for conception and gestation that the couple lacks. The third party is essential if the couple is to rear a genetically related child. While a state could regulate, indeed, should and must regulate, the circumstances under which parties enter into reproductive contracts, it could not ban or refuse to enforce such transactions altogether without compelling reasons. It might even be argued that refusal to enforce these contracts and prohibition of money payments would constitute an unconstitutional interference with procreative liberty since it would prevent childless couples from obtaining the means with which to have families. Robertson, "Embryos, Families and Procreative Liberty: The Legal Structure of New Reproduction," 59 *S.Cal.L.Rev.* 501 (1986.)

"Continuing the analysis, the right of privacy was further expanded in *Roe v. Wade* [410 U.S. 113], where *inter alia* it was held to be solely the woman's decision in the first trimester whether to terminate pregnancy. If the law of our land sanctions a means to end life then that same law may be used to create and celebrate life. . . ."

Judge Sorkow then went on to point out that fundamental rights can be restricted only for *compelling,* not merely rational or worthy, state interests, that regulations must be *narrowly* drawn to have only those effects necessary to protect the compelling interests, and that classifications of persons by such categories as gender or legitimacy must bear "a fair and substantial relation to the object of the legislation." Applying these principles, Judge Sorkow continued: "Currently, males may sell their sperm. The 'surrogate father' sperm donor is legally recognized in all states. The surrogate mother is not. If a man may offer the means for procreation then a woman must equally be allowed to do so. The rule otherwise denies equal protection of the law to the childless couple, the surrogate, whether male or female, and the unborn child. . . ."

Judge Sorkow thus concluded that the surrogate-parenting agreement is a valid and enforceable contract constitutionally protected under the Fourteenth Amendment to the United States Constitution.

ABORTION. Though upholding the contract, Judge Sorkow held that the clauses regarding abortion (see note 2, paragraph b) are void and unenforceable on constitutional grounds. *Roe v. Wade* established that "only the woman had the constitutionally protected right to determine the manner in which her body and person shall be used." Thus, only the woman shall have a right to determine whether or not to abort.

Specific Performance

Having found the contract valid and enforceable, Judge Sorkow reasoned that specific performance was an equitable remedy: "If specific performance is ordered, the result will be just what the parties bargained for and the contract contemplated. Mr. Stern wanted progeny, a child. Mrs. Whitehead wanted to give the child she would bear to a childless couple. . . . The Whiteheads have two children. They did not want any more. . . . It is suggested that Mrs. Whitehead wanted a baby, now that she is older than when her first two children were born, to experience and fulfill herself again as a woman. She found the opportunity in the newspaper advertisement. She received her fulfillment. Mr. Stern did not."

Custody, Parental Rights, and the Best Interests of the Child

Though demanding specific performance, Judge Sorkow reasoned that no agreement between parents could be supported by the court unless it was also in the best interests of the child. The contract called for William Stern's custody and for complete severing of all of Mary Beth Whitehead's parental rights. But a number of other arrangements were possible, including awarding custody to Mary Beth Whitehead, or retention of some parental rights (such as visitation) by the noncustodial parent, or even joint custody.

The matter of custody was fiercely contested, both as to the qualities of the individuals and the criteria by which "best interests" should be determined. The Sterns called numerous expert witnesses to impugn Mary Beth Whitehead's character and the stability of the Whitehead household. The Whiteheads' lawyer chose not to attack the Sterns, and Judge Sorkow disallowed attempts to examine the Stern's motives for rejecting adoption. Their argument was thus reduced largely to an attempt to portray the Whiteheads as a warm and loving family. But most of the time they were on the defensive.

Judge Sorkow sided almost entirely with the Sterns. He accepted both the criteria and the judgments of character presented by Dr. Lee Salk,[8] expert witness for the Sterns. Dr. Salk asserted that the child would be best placed with parents who had planned for the child, are emotionally stable and able to make judgments rationally, can maintain a stable and peaceful home life, are able to respond to the physical and emotional needs of the child, can instill positive attitudes toward health, can encourage curiosity and learning and motivate the child toward education, and can help the child to understand and deal with the facts of her origin.

Accepting these criteria, Judge Sorkow concluded that on all counts the Sterns promised to be better parents for the child than the Whiteheads. The Sterns had planned for the child; the Whiteheads had not. The Sterns both hold graduate degrees, and Mrs. Stern is also a pediatrician; Richard Whitehead was an unenthusiastic high school graduate, Mary Beth Whitehead a high school dropout. The Sterns "have a strong and mutually supportive relationship" and make decisions rationally, with respect and cooperation; the Whiteheads "appear to have a stable marriage now" but have been plagued with separations, domestic violence, problems with alcohol, and severe financial difficulties requiring the family to move their home numerous times. The Whiteheads hardly showed cogent thought in their attempts to evade the law. Furthermore, "Mrs. Whitehead dominates the family . . . [and is] thoroughly enmeshed with Baby M, unable to separate out her own needs from the baby's. . . ." She has been shown to be impulsive (by, among other things, her flight to Florida in violation of a court order), manipulative (threatening, seriously or not, to harm herself and the child), and exploitive (e.g., in her attempts to use the media by exposing her older daughter to the media for sympathy and drawing her into a false charge of sexual abuse against William Stern). Finally, as for helping the child come to grips with her origins, Mrs. Whitehead "has shown little empathy for the Sterns and their role and even less ability to acknowledge the facts surrounding the original contract," and she has shown a propensity to mold facts to her own perceptions. "The Sterns, [on the other hand], have indicated a willingness to obtain professional advice on how and when to tell his daughter" the facts of her origin and have approached all matters rationally, whether routine or in crisis. Thus, Judge Sorkow concluded, "Melissa's best interests will be served by being placed in her father's sole custody."

Reasoning of the Supreme Court of New Jersey

The Whiteheads' appeal to the Supreme Court of New Jersey, the highest court in the state and a widely respected court throughout the nation, challenged virtually all parts of the lower court's decision.[9] The supreme court, consisting of seven members, ruled unanimously to reverse the lower court in key matters. It invalidated the contract and, though awarding primary custody to William Stern, reinstated Mary Beth Whitehead's parental rights, including visitation. Key parts of the supreme court's decision are as follows.

Validity of the Contract

"We invalidate the surrogacy contract because it conflicts with the law and public policy of this State. While we recognize the depth of the yearning of infertile couples to have their own children, we find the payment of money to a 'surrogate' mother illegal, perhaps criminal, and potentially degrading to women. . . .

"We find no offense to our present laws where a woman voluntarily and without payment agrees to act as a 'surrogate' mother, provided that she is not subject to a binding agreement to surrender her child. Moreover, our holding today does not preclude the Legislature from altering the current statutory scheme, within constitutional limits, so as to permit surrogacy contracts. Under current law, however, the surrogacy agreement before us is illegal and invalid. . . ."

Conflict with Legislation

BABY-SELLING. The contract stated and the Sterns contended that money was being paid for services and expenses, but the court had "no doubt whatsoever that the money is being paid to obtain an adoption" (baby-selling), which "is illegal and perhaps criminal." This use of the money is shown by the following: the money was not to be paid until the child had been surrendered, parental rights terminated, and adoption facilitated; no payment was to be made if the child was stillborn before five months, and only $1,000 if later, even though all supposed services would then have been rendered; Mr. Stern was to assume the Whiteheads' expenses in connection with the adoption. In addition, Mr. Stern's contract with ICNY stated that ICNY would coordinate the adoption, and that if Mr. Stern arranged a further pregnancy with Mrs. Whitehead, a further fee must be paid by Mr. Stern—clearly indicating that ICNY arranged not just services but adoptions.

The Supreme Court of New Jersey rejected the lower court's view that surrogacy avoids the evils of baby-selling: "The evils inherent in baby bartering are loathsome for a myriad of reasons. The child is sold without regard for whether the purchasers will be suitable parents. The natural mother does not receive the benefit of counseling and guidance to assist her in making a decision that may affect her for a lifetime. In fact, the monetary incentive to sell her child may, depending on her financial circumstances, make her decision less voluntary. Furthermore, the adoptive [or genetic] parents may not be fully informed of the natural parent's medical history.

"Baby-selling potentially results in the exploitation of all parties involved. Conversely, adoption statutes seek to further humanitarian goals, foremost among them the best interests of the child. The negative consequences of baby buying are potentially present in the surrogacy context, especially the potential for placing and adopting a child without regard to the interest of the child or the natural mother."

SURRENDER OF THE CHILD AND TERMINATION OF PARENTAL RIGHTS. The court noted that the legislature had carefully crafted the law to provide for voluntary surrender of custody of a child only to an approved agency, to make surrender irrevocable only after stringent conditions had been met, including thorough counseling for the natural mother, and to allow surrender only after the birth of the child. Contractual surrender of parental rights is not provided for and agreements to establish paternity are specifically invalidated. The court then judged that these statutory safeguards of the child's well-being are entirely ignored in the surrogate's "contractual concession, in aid of the adoption, that the child's best interests would be served by awarding custody to the natural father and his wife—all of this before she has even conceived, and, in some cases, before she has the slightest idea of what the natural father and adoptive mother are like." The surrogacy contract attempts to circumvent all these carefully crafted institutional protections of the child's well-being and of natural mothers against coercion.[10]

Conflict with Public Policy

Public policy is that children should remain with and be brought up by both natural parents, that deviations from this goal are to be decided on the basis of the best interests of the child, and that the mother and father have equal rights concerning their children. The surrogacy contract, however, guarantees the permanent separation of the child from one of its parents, replaces the child's best interests with an agreement signed in advance, and gives the father exclusive rights to the child. The impact of failure to follow public policy "is nowhere better shown than in the results of this surrogacy contract. A child, instead of starting off its life with as much peace and security as possible, finds itself immediately in a tug-of-war between contending mother and father."

New Jersey's policies call for extensive independent counseling and evaluation in termination and adoption proceedings. In this surrogacy arrangement, in contrast, Mary Beth Whitehead received one hour of legal counseling from a attorney retained for this purpose by ICNY. There is no indication that the psychological counseling she received was for her benefit at all. She was only told that "she had passed." The Sterns relied entirely on ICNY; they were not told that Mary Beth Whitehead had expressed misgivings, and they knew little about her psychological and medical history. The court concluded: "It is apparent that the profit motive got the better of the Infertility Center."[11]

"Worst of all, however, is the contract's total disregard of the best interests of the child." As the court observed, there is no indication of attempts to determine the fitness of the Sterns as parents, their superiority to the Whiteheads, or the effect on the child of not living with her natural mother. "Almost every evil that prompted the prohibition of the payment of money in connection with adoptions exists here." Indeed, continued the court, the payment of money causes *more* problems in surrogacy than in adoption. In adoption, unlike in surrogacy, money is not essential for the process to continue as a social institution; money does not initiate the creation of a child; nor does the child go to the highest bidder. Furthermore, in surrogacy, unlike adoption, "consent occurs so early that no amount of advice would satisfy the potential mother's need, yet the consent is irrevocable" according to the terms of the contract. "[A]ny decision prior to the baby's birth is, in the most important sense, uninformed, and any decision after that [is] compelled by a pre-existing contractual commitment, the threat of a lawsuit, and the inducement of a $10,000 payment. . . ." The surrogate, thus, does not, then, go into the arrangement "with her eyes open"; her need of money is used to take away her child, just as in the more common exchanges of money for adoption. "In the scheme contemplated by the surrogacy contract in this case, a middle man, propelled by profit, promotes the sale. Whatever idealism may have motivated any of the participants, the profit motive predominates, permeates, and ultimately governs the transaction."

Furthermore, the court continued, the surrogate's "consent is irrelevant. There are, in a civilized society, some things that money cannot buy. In America, we decided long ago that merely because conduct purchased by money was 'voluntary' did not mean that it was good or beyond regulation and prohibition [as exemplified in laws concerning child labor, the minimum wage, and equal pay for equal work]. There are, in short, values that society deems more important than granting to wealth whatever it can buy, be it labor, love, or life."[12]

"Beyond that is the potential degradation of some women that may result from this arrangement. In many cases, of course, surrogacy may bring satisfaction, not only to the infertile couple, but to the surrogate mother herself. The fact, however, that many women may not perceive surrogacy negatively but rather see it as an opporunity does not diminish its potential for devastation to other women.

"In sum, the harmful consequences of his surrogacy arrangement appear to us all too palpable. In New Jersey the surrogate mother's agreement to sell her child is void. Its irrevocability infects the entire contract, as does the money that purports to buy it."

Termination of Parental Rights

Though *custody* is to be determined by the best interests of the child, the only ground for *termination* of parental rights is "intentional abandonment or very substantial neglect of parental duties without a reasonable expectation of reversal of that conduct in the future." The court judged that nothing supports such a finding in the case of Mary Beth Whitehead; indeed, the trial court itself had "affirmatively stated that Mary Beth Whitehead had been a good mother to her children. . . . We therefore conclude that the natural mother is entitled to retain her rights as a mother."

Constitutional Issues

Though the court held constitutional claims to be moot in virtue of the invalidity of the contract, it offered certain brief observations contrary to the lower court's interpretation of the constitutional protection of procreation and privacy.

". . . The right to procreate very simply is the right to have natural children, whether through sexual intercourse or artificial insemination. It is no more than that. Mr. Stern has not been deprived of that right. Through artificial insemination of Mrs. Whitehead, Baby M is his child. The custody, care, companionship, and nurturing that follow birth are not parts of the right to procreation. To assert that Mr. Stern's right of procreation gives him the right to the custody of Baby M would be to assert the Mrs. Whitehead's right of procreation does not give her the right to the custody of Baby M; it would be to assert that the constitutional right of procreation includes within it a constitutionally protected contractual right to destroy someone else's right of procreation.

"We conclude that the right of procreation is best understood and protected if confined to its essentials, and that when dealing with rights concerning the resulting child, different interests come into play. There is nothing in our culture or society that even begins to suggest a fundamental right on the part of the father to the custody of the child as part of his right to procreate when opposed by the claim of the mother to the same child. We therefore disagree with the trial court: there is no constitutional basis whatsoever requiring that Mr. Stern's claim to the custody of Baby M be sustained. Our conclusion may thus be understood as illustrating that a person's rights of privacy and self-determination are qualified by the effect on innocent third persons of the exercise of those rights.

"In the present case, the parties' right to procreate by methods of their own choosing cannot be enforced without consideration of the state's interest in protecting the resulting child, just as the right to the companionship of one's child cannot be enforced without consideration of that crucial state interest. . . ."

Custody

"With the surrogacy contract disposed of, the legal framework becomes a dispute between two couples over the custody of a child produced by the artificial insemination of one couple's wife by the other's husband. . . . The applicable rule given these circumstances is . . . [that] the child's best interests determine custody. . . ."

The New Jersey Supreme Court recognized no serious contention that either party was unfit. "The issue here is which life would be better for Baby M, one with primary custody in the Whiteheads or one with primary custody in the Sterns." The court further admitted "considerable force" to the Whiteheads' argument that awarding temporary custody to the Sterns (in error) had precipitated the alleged failings in Mrs. Whitehead's character and had favored the Sterns by giving them custody during the whole period of litigation. But the court held that concern for the child requires that best interests be determined relative to the actual state of affairs—even if it resulted in part from judicial error.[13]

The New Jersey Supreme Court then agreed with the lower court that primary custody should be awarded to Mr. Stern. It did, however, go out of its way to comment on what it called the "harsh judgment" of Mrs. Whitehead by the lower court and by some of the experts who testified. Mary Beth Whitehead did break the agreement she had made, and she did wrongly violate a court order even if that order was erroneous,[14] but the court observed, "it is expecting something well beyond normal human capabilities to suggest that this mother should have parted with her newly born infant without a struggle. Other than survival, what stronger force is there? We do not know of, and cannot conceive of, any other case where a perfectly fit mother was expected to surrender her newly born infant, perhaps forever, and was then told she was a bad mother because she did not. We know of no authority suggesting that the moral quality of her act in those circumstances should be judged by referring to a contract made before she became pregnant. . . . We do not find it so clear that her efforts to keep her infant, when measured against the Sterns' effort to take her away, make one, rather than the other, the wrong-doer. The Sterns suffered, but so did she. . . . [H]ow much weight should be given to her nine months of pregnancy, the labor of childbirth, the risk to her life, compared to the payment of money, the anticipation of a child and the donation of sperm?"

The supreme court rejected the view that Mrs. Whitehead's actions during the legal battle showed her to be a selfish, grasping woman ready to sacrifice the interests of her children. It judged rather that the evidence suggested nothing other than a motive of love and that had she been allowed to keep the child, she would have acted unremarkably.

The supreme court did hold the child's educational prospects to be a legitimate concern, but added that "a best-interests test is designed to create not a new member of the intelligentsia but rather a well-integrated person who might reasonably be expected to be happy with life. . . . Stability, love, family happiness, tolerance, and ultimately, support of independence—all rank much higher in predicting future happiness than the likelihood of a college education."[15]

In its final decision to award primary custody to William Stern, the court cited the greater stability of the Stern household and noted that none of the expert witnesses called by the Whiteheads clearly asserted that the White-heads' custody would be in the child's best interests, while both of the experts called by the Sterns and, most persuasively, all three experts called by Baby M's court-appointed guardian *ad litem* "unanimously and persuasively recommended custody in the Sterns."

Visitation

The lower court had terminated Mary Beth Whitehead's parental rights and so did not consider the matter of visitation. The New Jersey Supreme Court ordered that this matter be considered but directed that a different trial judge be assigned to the case. The court did stipulate, though, that Mrs. Whitehead was entitled to some sort of visitation, which, given the established relationship between her and the child, would be in both their interests. The court added, finally, that Mrs. Whitehead "is not to be penalized one iota because of the surrogacy contract."

Mary Beth Whitehead's visitation rights were conclusively determined on April 6, 1988, when Judge Birger M. Sween, of the New Jersey Superior

Court, granted most of her requests. She was allowed to see the child unsuper-
vised at home, at first for one day a week for up to six hours; after five months
a second day would be added every two weeks, and after another seven
months an overnight stay would be allowed. In addition, she could be with the
child for an uninterrupted two weeks in the summer of 1989, and at certain
holidays as well. The Sterns were unhappy that their wish to bar visits until the
child was ten years old (unless she asked to see her mother) was not granted,
but they elected not to appeal. Judge Sween directed both Mary Beth Whitehead and the Sterns to undergo counseling to help them deal better with their
differences. He also prohibited the parties from public discussion of their
relationships with the child and urged Mary Beth Whitehead not to call the
child by the name "Sara," which she had chosen, but by the name "Melissa,"
given by the Sterns and recognized by the courts.

Conclusion

Advocates of surrogacy, including women who had been surrogates themselves, had hailed the trial court's initial decision. Broker Noel Keane noted
that in the period between the two trials his inquiries had quadrupled. Brokers in general pointed to a high rate of satisfaction among the parties to
surrogacy, citing a figure of only five or six disputes in over 600 cases. Even
after the New Jersey Supreme Court's reversal, brokers claimed that surrogacy would continue to flourish, especially in states that did not follow the
New Jersey Supreme Court's lead. Indeed, few brokers had *ever* thought that
surrogacy contracts were enforceable. The Sterns' lawyer, though, said he
would counsel his clients against surrogacy as too legally precarious.

Many opponents of surrogacy had rallied around Mary Beth Whitehead
during the first trial. Just before the first decision, a group of 135 prominent
American woman circulated an open letter under the title "By These Standards, We Are All Unfit," asserting that virtually no one's character could
withstand the hostile scrutiny Mary Beth Whitehead had received. The same
unsympathetic attitudes with which Judge Sorkow and the press[16] approached
the Whiteheads could also have painted an ugly portrait of the Sterns.[17] The
point here is not to claim that the Sterns are terrible people or that they will be
less than good parents. Rather, the point is that biases of class and gender
seriously prejudice judgments about this case and about surrogacy generally.
Mary Beth Whitehead breached a contract, absconded with her child, and
generally expressed her emotions openly. These actions occasioned outrage,
and her character was vilified in the press, in popular understanding, and by a
superior court judge. Yet disputes over contracts, even those involving children, rarely occasion *outrage*.[18] Defenders of Mary Beth Whitehead pointed
out that the odd behavior in these circumstances would be the ability to
sublimate one's emotions. Not until after the New Jersey Supreme Court
decision was there much of an attempt to imagine sympathetically what it
must be like to have the police appear without notice at one's door with a

court order to remove one's newborn child. It was a major breakthrough for the supreme court to finally recognize officially that Mary Beth Whitehead is *not* a surrogate mother or "surrogate uterus,"[19] but rather the natural, biological mother of the child.

In light of such observations, some commentators charged that appeals to violation of the contract and the court order were merely rationalizations for popular sentiment against Mary Beth Whitehead, and that the deeper motivation for such feelings was indignation that a blue-collar housewife got out of line and was so presumptuous as to fight by whatever means she could find against the structures of power and status—of money, lawyers, contracts, and courts—that were aligned against her.[20]

The decision by the New Jersey Supreme Court clearly calls out for legislation explicitly addressed to surrogacy. Though the court condemns commercial surrogacy, its decision leaves it open for the legislature to create new laws allowing surrogacy under various guises.[21] The court does, however, seek to instruct by showing that the rationale for close state regulation of adoption— to protect the interests of children, mothers, and the state—also applies to the surrogacy situation.[22]

As for this particular case, the outcome of the arrangement for the individuals directly involved is that none of the adults got what they wanted. The Sterns did not get a child to raise in privacy and in the illusion that the child is related to no one but themselves. Mary Beth Whitehead failed to find the fulfillment of providing a loving gift to others, and she refused the monetary compensation to which she was entitled. Noel Keane, the broker, received his fee and notoriety that may perversely have increased his business, but in the longer run the legal climate may have shifted significantly against surrogacy.[23] And Melissa Stern, who had no representative in the formulation of all the agreements, has lived through two years of disruption and instability. If we *hope* that she will now be able to grow up and live her life in peace and security, we must also *act* to create regulations and practices to ensure that children and parents in the future will not have to suffer as they have in this case.

Notes

1. By the time the appeal was decided, Mary Beth Whitehead had been divorced, remarried, and taken on the new surname of Whitehead-Gould. "Whitehead" continues to be her name in court records and will be used here.

2. There were in fact several contracts or agreements, involving William Stern, both Whiteheads, and ICNY. Elizabeth Stern was not a party to any of the agreements; her position was that she would seek to adopt the child once Mary Beth Whitehead relinquished her parental rights. The main provisions of the agreements were as follows:

a. ICNY will "use its best efforts to assist the Natural Father in the selection of a 'surrogate mother' " and receive a nonrefundable fee of $7,500 from Mr. Stern. ICNY will "coordinate arrangements for the adoption of the child by the wife." "ICNY does not guarantee or warrant that the 'surrogate mother' . . . will comply with the terms and provisions of [her agreements]. . . ."

b. Mary Beth Whitehead agrees to be artificially inseminated with Mr. Stern's sperm and carry any resulting pregnancy to term; "agrees that in the best interest of the child, she will not form or attempt to form a parent-child relationship . . . and shall freely surrender custody to William Stern . . . immediately upon birth of the child; and terminate all parental rights . . .;" agrees to follow doctors' instructions on prenatal care; and agrees "to assume all risks, including the risk of death, which are incidental to conception, pregnancy, [and] childbirth." Mary Beth Whitehead also agrees not to abort the child unless the inseminating physician deems abortion necessary for her physical health or the child has been determined to be physiologically abnormal. She agrees to undergo amniocentesis or similar tests and to abort if a genetic or congenital abnormality is found and Willian Stern demands abortion. In such a case, she is to receive her full payment.

c. Richard Whitehead agrees to execute all the documents necessary to establish that he is not the father of the child. William Stern is to be listed as the father on the child's birth certificate.

d. William Stern agrees to be responsible for the child once born, regardless of any abnormality; to deposit a check for $10,000 in an escrow account—payable to Mrs. Whitehead upon delivery of the child and after her "completion of the duties and obligations" under the agreement—and is to pay all legal and medical expenses. If the child is miscarried, dies, or is stillborn before the end of the fourth month, no part of the $10,000 fee is to be paid, if after that time, payment is to be $1,000.

3. New Jersey Superior Court for Bergen County, *In the matter of Baby M,* 525 A.2d 1128 (N.J.Super.Ch. 1987).

4. New Jersey Supreme Court, 537 A.2d 1227 (N.J. 1988).

5. The Whiteheads also argued against the contract on grounds of unconscionability—that its terms were unreasonable, unfair, and oppressive. The court rejected these claims: Mary Beth Whitehead "knew just what she was bargaining for." She agreed to the arguably small compensation of $10,000 and by virtue of her previous pregnancies had knowledge of the risks. Further, "Mrs. Whitehead says that Mr. Stern undertook no risks. To compare the risk of pregnancy in a woman to the donation of sperm by the man would be unconscionable. This, however, is the bargain Mrs. Whitehead sought and obtained. Mr. Stern did take a risk, however, whether the child would be normal or abnormal, whether accepted or rejected he would have a lifetime obligation and responsibility to the child as its natural and biological father."

6. Judge Sorkow did not consider whether it is good for the children and good policy to deliberately create children with different genetic and social parents.

7. Citations in the following quoted passages are shortened. [This constitutional status of procreative rights is further debated in this anthology in papers by Robertson and by Smith and Iraola in the part entitled "Constitutional Rights, Law, and Public Policy."]

8. Clinical professor of psychology, psychiatry, and pediatrics at New York Hospital-Cornell Medical Center. Dr. Salk had examined the records of other expert witnesses but had never examined or met Mary Beth Whitehead in person.

9. During the appeal, Mary Beth Whitehead was able to obtain limited visitation of two hours per week under a matron's supervision at a county-run institution.

10. The court did note that surrogacy differs from the usual case of adoption because in surrogacy the "adoptive couple" is the natural father and his wife. But it held that the relevant fact in both adoption and surrogacy is "the vulnerability of the natural mother who decides to surrender her child in the absence of institutional safeguards."

11. Though public attention focused on the Whitehead-Stern trial, Mary Beth

Whitehead was also suing Noel Keane's ICNY for fraud and negligence in brokering the arrangement. At the time, Keane was also being sued by three other women who had been surrogates in his program. Directors of several other commercial surrogacy programs claimed that they experienced few, if any, complaints, due to what they described as their more scrupulous screening and counseling procedures. See Malcolm Gladwell and Rochelle Sharpe, "Baby M Winner," *New Republic* 126 (Feb. 16, 1987), pp. 15ff.

12. The court added: "Whether this principle recommends prohibition of surrogacy, which presumably sometimes results in great satisfaction to all of the parties, is not for us to say. We note here only that, under existing law, the fact that Mrs. Whitehead 'agreed' to the arrangement is not dispositive."

13. Some commentators further pointed out that temporary custody orders are seldom overturned, especially by the judge who issued them. Thus, these commentators claimed, custody was for all practical purposes decided in April 1986, when Judge Sorkow issued the initial order without notice to or representation of the Whiteheads. See, for example, George Annas, "Baby M: Babies (and Justice) for Sale," *Hastings Center Report* 17(3) (1987), pp. 13–15.

14. The New Jersey Supreme Court stipulated that during future surrogacy disputes children should be removed from their natural mothers only on exceedingly strong proof "of unfitness, of danger to the child, or the like." The court judged that an erroneous transfer of custody presents greater risk to a child's well-being than does the child's being taken out of the court's jurisdiction. At most, courts should enjoin such flight, though if surrogate mothers know that their custody cannot be seriously challenged at this stage, they are less likely to even consider flight.

15. The court also noted Mary Beth Whitehead's separation from Richard Whitehead, her becoming pregnant by another man, and her marriage to him. Though stating that these developments did not affect their opinion, they added that in any case they do not necessarily show less fitness as a parent, only less stability in the Whiteheads' lives.

16. The Sterns received a three-minute standing ovation from the press at a news conference after the first trial; they remained seated and silent for Mary Beth Whitehead after the New Jersey Supreme Court's decision.

17. The Sterns could have been characterized as selfish and shortsighted in putting their careers before family and then contriving to avoid the consequences of their own free choice. They were arrogant in their self-diagnosis of Elizabeth Stern's medical condition and in rejecting adoption with hardly a thought. They sought a quick, no-risk (they thought) solution to their difficulties. Mr. Stern was obsessive and narcissistic in his desire to continue his bloodline, and he bullied his less than enthusiastic wife into the surrogacy arrangement. The Sterns were aggressive and authoritarian in engaging the police to tear a child literally from her mother's breast and in using the courts, a contract, and the penal law in an attempt to obliterate any vestige of relationship between a daughter and her mother. Finally, a couple so rigid, brittle, and unemotional would be in a poor position to participate in a young child's emotional life and nourish her emotional development.

Such a portrait, some commentators asserted, shows no greater distortion than most reporting and perceptions of the Whiteheads. See, for example, Phyllis Chesler, *Sacred Bond: The Legacy of Baby M* (New York: Times Books, 1988), especially pp. 26–30, and Michelle Harrison, "Social Construction of Mary Beth Whitehead," *Gender and Society* 1(3) (1988), pp. 300–311.

18. It is often held to be *fair* that sports figures be able to renegotiate their

contracts. Contested divorce and custody battles are often bitter, but neither party is commonly held *contemptible* for breaching the "marriage contract."

19. A term used by expert witness Lee Salk, upon whom Judge Sorkow relied.

20. For examples of such analysis, see Chesler, *Sacred Bond*, and Michelle Landsberg, "Judge in Baby M Case Spoke in Language of Feminists," *Globe and Mail* (Toronto) (February 6, 1988), p. A2.

21. A perhaps cynical reading is that the lesson of the New Jersey Supreme Court's decision to couples seeking a child is to hire a mother who is so poor and uninformed that she would not feel sufficiently empowered to contest the contract, and whom a judge would certainly determine to be unfit if she were to do so.

22. Nonetheless, the court allowed that a 10–15% rate of infertility (a figure often cited, but one for which the court found no reliable confirmation), and the corresponding demand for children by adoption *could* be enough to establish a compelling state interest in promoting (even commercial?) surrogacy, and that this compelling interest could override policy and constitutional concerns to the contrary.

23. Michigan, for example, after having proposed legislation on surrogacy buried for years in committee, passed a bill in the summer of 1988 outlawing commercial surrogacy under a penalty of up to $50,000 in fines and five years in prison for brokers. It has also been wondered whether lawyers/brokers are not guilty of legal malpractice and fraud for charging clients for contracts publicly admitted to be unenforceable. For this and other reflections on the New Jersey Supreme Court decision, see George Annas, "Death without Dignity for Commercial Surrogacy: The Case of Baby M," *Hastings Center Report* 18(2) (1988), pp. 21–24.

Parenting through Contract When No One Wants the Child

Alexander Malahoff, an accountant for the New York City school system, and his wife, Nadja, were childless, and they turned to a surrogate mothering arrangement through lawyer and surrogacy pioneer Noel Keane. The Malahoffs picked Judy Stiver of Lansing, Michigan, from Keane's album of potential surrogates. Judy Stiver was an inventory clerk, married to Ray Stiver, a part-time bus driver, with whom she had a young daughter. The Malahoffs liked the picture in the album, which presented Mrs. Stiver with her daughter.

By the terms of the arrangement, Mrs. Stiver was to be artificially inseminated with Mr. Malahoff's sperm, carry the child to term, and relinquish custody of the child to Mr. Malahoff at birth. In return, Mrs. Stiver was to receive $10,000 in addition to her medical costs. Noel Keane, for his part, was to be paid a nonrefundable fee of $5,000 by Mr. Malahoff, regardless of the outcome.

Under medical supervision, Judy Stiver was checked for pregnancy, with negative results, and artificially inseminated with Mr. Malahoff's sperm on April 15, 1982. Nothing unusual was reported during the pregnancy, and nine months after insemination, on January 10, 1983, Mrs. Stiver, following a long and difficult labor, gave birth to a baby boy, with both her husband and Mr. Malahoff present. In accordance with their agreement, Mr. Malahoff and Mrs. Stiver signed the birth certificate as legal parents.

The baby, however, had serious problems. Its umbilical cord had two knots; the baby himself was microcephalic, a condition which often indicates mental retardation; and he had a severe strep infection, which threatened to cause loss of hearing and eyesight and further mental retardation. The baby was taken from his mother for treatment and the pediatricians approached Mr. Malahoff for permission to begin medical treatment, without which the baby was likely to die.

At this point the facts of the case are disputed. According to the hospital, Mr. Malahoff sought to assert his right of custody under the surrogacy contract and instructed the hospital to "take no steps or measures to treat the strep infection or to otherwise care for" the baby.[1] In later public statements, Mr. Malahoff asserted that he only told the doctors not to perform a spinal tap, and that he never made a blanket request that the child not be treated at all.[2] Whatever Mr. Malahoff exactly said and meant, the hospital immediately filed a suit and obtained a temporary order allowing tests and treatment and barring Mr. Malahoff from interference.

During treatment, Mr. Malahoff had the baby baptized, naming him Alexander. Later he said that the baptism was in accordance with his Roman Catholic faith, as he believed that the child was going to die. He denied that having the child baptized signified his acceptance of the child as his own.

The Stivers, in the meantime, demanded and were paid the $10,000, but before they cashed the check, results of early blood tests suggested that Mr. Malahoff was in fact not the father of the child. They returned the check, and disputes began over who should have custody of and responsibility for the child.

Mr. Malahoff, now separated from his wife, contended that since he was not the child's father, he was in no way liable or responsible for it. The Stivers said that they felt that the child was not theirs and that they felt no maternal or paternal bond to it. "We feel sorry for it," they added, "but we don't want it."[3]

The case had been an item in the news from the time of Mr. Malahoff's apparent rejection of treatment for the child. But the incident escalated into a media spectacle when Mr. Malahoff and the Stivers appeared on the *Phil Donahue Show*. On the air, before a national television audience, it was announced to all parties for the first time that further tests of blood and tissue conclusively showed that Mr. Malahoff could not be the child's father.

When the facts finally emerged, it turned out that the Stivers had followed the instructions they had been given, or as they had understood them, and had refrained from sexual intercourse for 30 days following the artificial insemination. However, they had apparently not been told or had not understood that intercourse closely *before* the insemination could also result in a pregnancy through Ray Stiver's, and not Alexander Malahoff's, sperm. This is apparently what had happened. A pregnancy resulting from intercourse just before the preinsemination test would not necessarily have been detected by that test.[4]

When first confronted with the possibility that the child might be theirs, the Stivers considered placing him for adoption. But when it was proved that the child was certainly biologically theirs, they accepted the child, named him Christopher Ray, and sought help for him. Up to age three he lived at home, and in the spring of 1986 he entered the Beekman Center for Therapy. The Stivers were told that the child had the capabilities of a two- to four-month-old and probably would proceed little further.

Several suits and countersuits were filed against four of the physicians involved (in part for improper instructions before insemination); against two lawyers; and between the contracting parties for breach of contract, loss of privacy, and emotional damage. The Stivers had entered the arrangement, they said, to give others the gift of a child and to gain money to pay bills and take a vacation. In the end, they collected no payment and acquired responsibility for a severely handicapped child. Alexander Malahoff was reported to have thought that a child would help patch up his marriage. But summing up the incident from his perspective, he pointed out that he had no more of a child than he did when he began and was out of the brokering fee: "Instead of a baby," he concluded, "I end up with a lawyer."[5] Perhaps oddest of all, though, is that both parties indicated that under the right circumstances they would enter into a surrogacy agreement again.

Notes

1. *The Washington Post* (January 21, 1983), p. A11.
2. *The New York Times* (January 23, 1983), p. I19.
3. Ibid.
4. Also relevant were reports that Ray Stiver had some years earlier fathered another microcephalic child.
5. *Newsweek* (February 14, 1983), p. 76.

Property or Persons? The Status of Embryos in in Vitro Fertilization

Legal proceedings point up complicated problems that can arise from in vitro fertilization (IVF) and, in particular, illustrate conflicting judgments about the status of fertilized eggs and embryos.

Embryos Destroyed: The Del Zio Case

In an early court case,[1] fertilized ova were deliberately destroyed by the supervisor of a physician attempting IVF. The plaintiffs in the case, John E. Del Zio and Doris Del Zio, sought compensation for severe emotional distress and for destruction of their personal property. The jury awarded $50,000 for Mrs. Del Zio's emotional suffering but did not accept the Del Zios' claim for compensation for the destruction of their property. As the appeals court pointed out, however, this second part of the jury's decision need not have been a rejection of the claim that the embryos were the Del Zios' property. Rather, the jury may have merely been unable to fix an amount for an award of damages. Indeed, it might be claimed that the judge in the case in fact regarded the embryos as personal property, since he instructed the jury that any award for damages to the plaintiffs would have to be based on market or replacement value.

Orphaned Embryos: The Rios Case

In June 1981, Mario Rios, 54, and Elsa Rios, 37, of Los Angeles traveled to Australia to enter the IVF program at the Queen Victoria Medical Center in Melbourne in the state of Victoria. Both Rioses had had children during previous marriages: Mr. Rios, a grown son, Michael, and Mrs. Rios, a daughter, whom the Rioses had been raising until her accidental death in 1978, at the age of 10.

After the daughter's death, the Rioses very much wanted to have another child, but Mr. Rios was infertile, reportedly due to an earlier vasectomy, and Mrs. Rios was unable to conceive naturally. Because of her age, Mrs. Rios was not eligible to participate in an IVF program in the United States.

338

In the IVF program in Australia, Mrs. Rios was stimulated by hormones to superovulate, and three eggs were obtained. Sperm was provided by an anonymous sperm donor from Melbourne with the Rioses' consent. All three eggs were fertilized in vitro. One was implanted in Mrs. Rios's uterus, and two were frozen (at the two- to eight-cell stage) for possible future use.

Approximately 10 days after implantation of the embryo, Mrs. Rios miscarried. Because at that time she did not feel emotionally ready for a second attempt, the Rioses left Australia. They said that they might return, but they made no definite arrangements and indicated no special wishes as to the disposition of the frozen embryos. According to documents, the Rioses subsequently adopted a child in South America, but in April, 1983, the parents and their adopted child died in a plane crash.

After the Rioses' deaths, questions were raised about what should be done with the frozen embryos and about how they should be regarded. The problems were further complicated by the discovery that the Rioses had left a considerable estate (estimated at over $1 million) and had died without a will. These facts made more pressing the issue of whether the embryos, if implanted and brought to term, would have a right of inheritance.

Legal issues were potentially governed by the laws of California (the Rioses' home) and the laws of Australia and the state of Victoria, where the frozen embryos were stored. California had no laws specifically dealing with embryos created by IVF. Furthermore, though California law does recognize posthumous children as heirs and recognizes children conceived through artificial insemination by donor (AID) as legitimate children of a husband who has given consent to the insemination, California law does not address a further complication in this case, namely, that the embryos, if thawed and implanted, would have to be gestated by a woman other than Mrs. Rios. Under Australian law at that time, when both parents are dead and have not left specific instructions for the disposition of frozen embryos, the hospital assumes responsibility. Professor Russell Scott, a member of the medical research committee that formulated Australia's guidelines for IVF in August 1982, offered the opinion that children resulting from a successful implantation and gestation would be the legal offspring of the woman who gestated them, not of the woman from whom the ova were taken.[2]

Among the many positions put forth on the status and treatment of the embryos were the following: (1) Regard the embryos as objects or personal property having economic value, and so as subject to being inherited. In that case, the heirs, presumably Michael Rios and/or Mrs. Rios's mother, as owners, would have the right to decide what to do with the embryos. (2) The courts should appoint a guardian *ad litem* (i.e., a guardian for the purposes of the suit) to decide in the best interests of the embryos. (3) Treat the embryos as having a right to life, a right to be thawed, implanted, born, and adopted.[3] (4) Consider Queen Victoria Hospital to be the Rioses' constructive trustee, appointed by the court to ensure that any actions taken not be inconsistent with what the Rioses would have wished. (5) Solicit the ad hoc recommendations of professional groups (e.g., lawyers, doctors). (6) Pass special legislation to deal with the case.[4]

What in fact did happen?

The Australian and Victoria governments stepped in. Premier John Cain of the state of Victoria created the Waller Committee (named for its chairman, Louis Waller, professor of law at Monash University in Melbourne) to study the case and make recommendations. While the committee deliberated over the summer of 1984, scores of women volunteered to gestate the embryos, including Loca Genrich, mother of the first IVF twins born through the Queen Victoria program.

At the end of the summer of 1984, the Waller Committee recommended that the embryos be destroyed. The committee reasoned that attempts to gestate the embryos and bring them to term would require the Rioses' consent, which was not given. Further, the fact that the Rioses left no instructions as to the disposition of the embryos was held to indicate that they did not recognize the fertilized ova as persons. One member of the committee argued that since the Rioses had agreed in writing to experimentation on their embryos, the couple must have regarded the two- to eight-cell embryos as having no rights. In any event, the Waller Committee concluded that the disposition of stored embryos should not be determined by the hospital; that the embryos should not be regarded as possessing legal rights or as having any right of inheritance; and that where an "embryo is stored which cannot be transferred as planned, and no agreed provision has been made at the time of storage . . . the embryos shall be removed from storage."[5]

Upon receiving the Report of the Waller Committee, Premier Cain announced that a three-month period of inaction would be instituted to allow an opportunity for public reaction. However, soon thereafter, the Upper House of the Victoria Parliament passed a measure directing that the attempt be made to thaw and implant the embryos in surrogates and to place them for adoption if they came to term alive. The legislature stipulated that any child resulting from the attempt would be a child only of its adoptive parents and thus would have no claim of inheritance from the Rioses as far as the law of Victoria was concerned.[6]

In the wake of the Rios case, Australian authorities have banned the use of IVF facilities to overseas couples, and throughout the world, professional organizations and hospitals have formulated guidelines suggesting ways to avoid or prepare for such cases in the future. The American Fertility Society, for example, now urges that cryopreservation not be sustained beyond the reproductive life of the mother and that the disposition of any frozen eggs should be decided prior to freezing: they may be discarded, used for research up to 14 days into embryonic development, or offered for adoption, in which case anonymity should be required and the rights of biological parents waived.[7] These guidelines, however, have not been sanctioned by law or accepted by society at large.

Debate, reports, directives, legislation, and guidelines notwithstanding, as of this writing, the embryos remain in their frozen state at the Queen Victoria Medical Center in Melbourne.

Clinic Refuses to Release Clients' Embryos: *York v. Jones*

A more recent case raises further issues about the status of embryos. In this case, Risa and Steven York are battling the Howard and Georgeanne Jones Institute for Reproductive Medicine in Norfolk, Virginia, for possession of a frozen embryo.[8] The Yorks had gone through three failed attempts at IVF at the Jones Institute. After moving from New Jersey to California, they requested that the one remaining frozen embryo be sent to another program they wished to enter in Los Angeles. But the Jones Institute refused, claiming that the agreement the Yorks had signed gave the Yorks no right to the embryo outside the institute. The Yorks' options, then, were (all at the Jones Institute) to try again, to donate the embryo to another couple, to offer it for experimentation, or to have it destroyed. While the case goes through the courts, the embryo becomes less likely to be viable and Risa York risks a greater likelihood of miscarriage during any attempted pregnancy.

Embryos and Divorce: The Davis Case

In a further case, a Tennessee trial court rejected the argument that fertilized ova or embryos should be treated as property, and went so far as to declare that four- to eight-cell embryos should be treated as children are in custody disputes.[9] This case evolved out of the attempts of Mary Sue Davis and her husband, Junior Lewis Davis, to have a child through IVF. Mrs. Davis had undergone five tubal pregnancies, a ruptured fallopian tube, several operations including, for reasons of health, ligation of her remaining fallopian tube, and six failed attempts at IVF during her marriage to Mr. Davis. The six attempts at IVF, at the Fertility Center of Eastern Tennessee under the direction of Dr. Ray King, involved considerable stress for Mrs. Davis. Each attempt included lengthy preparation, hormonal injections, and surgery to obtain eggs, as well as substantial expenses for the Davises—$4,000 to $6,000 per attempt, for a couple of modest means (he was earning approximately $17,500 per year and she about $18,000).

After being disappointed in an attempt to adopt (the mother decided to keep the child), the Davises returned to the Fertility Center to enter Dr. King's new cryopreservation program, which allowed multiple attempts at implantation without continual surgery. In December 1988, nine ova were surgically removed, fertilized, and allowed to develop to the four- to eight-cell stage. Two were introduced into Mrs. Davis's womb without success, and the remaining seven were frozen for possible future use.

The Davises were aware that the practical storage life of the frozen embryos was probably about two years. Testimony conflicted on the extent to which they had discussed the disposition of any embryos that they did not use, but in any event, they made no decision and their contract with the Fertility Center did not specify what should be done with the frozen embryos in case of death or divorce.

In February 1989, Junior Davis filed for divorce. The disposition of the embryos then became a matter of contention. Mary Sue Davis wanted the opportunity to use the embryos in further attempts to have a child. But Junior Davis did not want to become a father and asked in court that joint custody be awarded, with the stipulation that the embryos remain in storage until he and his wife could reach a mutual decision. He indicated that he did not want the embryos destroyed—in case he changed his mind later and because he was strongly against abortion—but he would rather that they be destroyed than implanted in an anonymous recipient. Junior Davis further testified that he would feel "raped of my reproductive rights" if Mary Sue Davis were allowed to implant the embryos without his consent[10] and that because of the pain of his own parents' divorce, he strongly objected to bringing a child into the world to share the same fate.

Mary Sue Davis, in contrast, contended that the embryos should be treated as "pre-born children," and that the best interests of the embryos consisted in her having the opportunity to bring them to term. She added that the embryos represented her best chance for becoming a mother, now aged 28 and divorced. Dr. King testified that Mary Sue Davis could still undergo further aspirations of ova and attempts at IVF, though there was no guarantee that she could produce further usable ova. He did say that if the court awarded the embryos to Mary Sue Davis, he would suspend his clinic's policy against accepting single persons into his IVF program.

Commentators and expert witnesses offered a number of further solutions and approaches. One argument was that if the embryos were property, then they should be treated as property normally is in contested divorce proceedings, that is, they should be divided equally among the litigants or awarded to one, with monetary or other compensation being given to the other. Alternatively, it was asserted that the embryos should be awarded to Mary Sue Davis, since she had contributed the most to their creation. Other opinions included holding that the clinic should be allowed to make the decision or that the embryos should be destroyed or allowed to "die a passive death" by being left in the frozen state until they were no longer viable. An expert witness, law professor John A. Robertson, argued that though the embryos are not property, it is still proper to regard them in terms of "ownership" and to award the right to make decisions concerning them. It was also pointed out that Mary Sue Davis's difficulties in initiating and carrying a pregnancy to term should be considered in judging the best interests of the embryos.

In October 1989, Judge W. Dale Young of the Tennessee State Circuit Court decided the case at the trial level, ruling, among other things, (1) that the embryos were "human beings, *in vitro*," that "life begins at the moment of conception," (2) that existing public policy did not specify the legal status of children in vitro, and so, in the absence of a guiding public policy, (3) the doctrine of *parens patriae*—"the best interests of the child"—should determine the disposition of the embryos. Thus, since Junior Davis strongly objected to the implantation of the embryos, in Mary Sue Davis or in any other recipient, and since Mary Sue Davis wanted to bring the children to term, the court awarded temporary custody of the embryos to Mary Sue Davis for the purpose of implantation.

The ruling that the embryos are "human beings, *in vitro*" was based on the unique genetic makeup of the cells of the embryo from the earliest point of the union of sperm and egg, so that "[f]rom fertilization, the cells of a human embryo are differentiated, unique and specialized to the highest degree of distinction."[11] As the embryos were "children, *in vitro,*" the court applied the standard doctrine of *parens patriae,* as in cases of disputed custody of children in divorce.[12] In applying the doctrine of *parens patriae,* the Court stressed:

> The thrust of the equitable nature of this doctrine is that it turns its full focus on the best interests of the child; its concern is not for those who claim "rights" to the child, nor for those who claim custody of the child, nor for those who may suffer perceived or real inequities resulting from scrupulously guarding the child's best interest.[13]

Judge Young withheld any judgment concerning visitation, child support, and final custody pending the actual birth of a child. At one point in his decision, Judge Young observed that Mr. Davis had participated in the IVF program in order to have a child, and that in that aim he had already succeeded. In closing, Judge Young recalled the wisdom of Solomon, which was to give a disputed child to the person who would preserve its life. He added that in the present case, wisdom and justice might correspond.

As might be expected, not all parties agreed: Junior Davis appealed the trial court's decision. While the appeal was pending, Mary Sue (Davis) Stowe, now remarried, sought, but did not receive, release from the court to donate the embryos to other infertile couples for implantation.

In September 1990, the Tennessee Court of Appeals rendered its decision, reversing the trial court's decision.[14] The Appeals Court ruled that Mary Sue and Junior should have "joint control of the ova and with equal voice over their disposition," adding:

> it would be repugnant and offensive to constitutional principles to order Mary Sue to implant these fertilized ova against her will. It would be equally repugnant to order Junior to bear the psychological, if not the legal, consequences of paternity against his will.[15]

The court based its decision on its construal of the legal status of the embryos and on its construal of Junior Davis's procreative rights. As to the legal status of the embryos, the Appeals Court reasoned that state and federal court rulings and legislative acts (most notably, the U.S. Supreme Court in *Roe v. Wade* and the Tennessee legislature and Supreme Court concerning claims of wrongful death in the case of the death of fetuses) accord greater respect to embryos only as they develop. The conclusion clearly intended, if not explicitly stated in its entirety by the Appeals Court, is that the undifferentiated, unimplanted preembryos[16] at issue in this case cannot be said to have a legal right to implantation.

As to Junior Davis's procreative rights, the Appeals Court cited U.S. Supreme Court cases commonly held to establish certain procreative rights and drew from them the conclusion that awarding the fertilized ova to Mary Sue for implantation would be "in violation of Junior's constitutionally protected right not to beget a child where no pregnancy has taken place."[17]

Though Judge Young's decision was decisively overturned in the Davis case, we might still hope that in all these cases, the sound and humane judgment that he called wisdom, and the fairness and equity in the eyes of the law that he called justice, might correspond. But we should also recognize that for justice in the widest sense, that is, for true fairness and equity, to prevail, wisdom may have to be exercised not just by courts called in after the fact to resolve disputes, but by all parties involved at all stages of their activities—by the people who seek help through reproductive technology, by lawyers and others who facilitate transactions, by health care personnel who carry out the sophisticated techniques, and also by society at large, which may to a great extent form and direct our attitudes and aspirations.

Notes

1. *Del Zio v. The Presbyterian Hospital,* United States District Court, Southern District of New York, Nov. 14. 1978. 74 Civ. 3588 (memorandum decision).

2. *The New York Times* (June 23, 1984), p. A30.

3. Practically speaking, Dr. Carl Wood, head of Queen Victoria's IVF unit, said that it was extremely unlikely that the embryos would survive thawing and implantation. Though the Rios story broke just as the clinic was achieving its first live birth from a frozen embryo, the techniques used for the Rioses in 1981 were less sophisticated and much less likely to succeed.

4. For comments on several of these alternatives, and on the case in general, see George P. Smith III, "Australia's Frozen 'Orphan' Embryos: A Medical, Legal, and Ethical Dilemma," *Journal of Family Law* 24 (1985), pp. 27–41.

5. Australia: *Committee to Consider the Social, Ethical, and Legal Issues Arising from In Vitro Fertilization: Report on the Disposition of Embryos Produced by In Vitro Fertilization,* Louis Waller, chairman (Victoria, 1984).

6. In fact, the estates were distributed under California's law of succession, with no regard to the embryos.

7. See American Fertility Society, Ethics Committee, "Ethical Considerations of the New Reproductive Technologies," *Fertility and Sterility* 46, suppl. 1 (1986), p. 55S.

8. See *York v. Jones,* 717 F.Supp. 421 (E.D. Va 1989).

9. *Davis v. Davis,* No. E-14466, Circuit Court for Blount County, Tennessee, at Maryville, Equity Division (Division I), 9/21/89, reported in 15 FLR 2108.

10. *Davis* (Circuit Court), p. 2108.

11. *Davis* (Circuit Court), p. 2097; see also p. 2103.

12. Judge Young argued that statutes concerning the status of the unborn in cases of wrongful death (according status only to a child viable outside the uterus) and abortion (according no status during the first three months) do not establish a public policy for IVF. In this policy vacuum, he claimed not to be forming public policy, but to be developing the common law to deal with a new situation confronting the court. He did note (p. 2103), however, that the Supreme Court in the recent *Webster* case on abortion "saw no reason why the state's interest in protecting potential human life should come into existence only at the point of viability" [*Webster v. Reproductive Health Services,* et al., 109 *Supreme Court Reporter* 3040 (1989)].

13. *Davis* (Circuit Court), p. 2104.

14. *Davis v. Davis,* Tennessee Court of Appeals, No. 180, 9/13/90, 16 FLR 1535 (1990).

15. *Davis* (Appeal), p. 1536.

16. The court uses this term apparently to refer to the product of conception from the time of fertilization until implantation. See *Davis* (Appeal), p. 1536, note 2.

17. The Appeals Court's decision provides no details on how this particular conclusion was reached. The full relevant text of the court's presentation of this issue is as follows (with legal citations shortened):

> The United States Supreme Court in *Skinner v. Oklahoma* recognized [that] the right to procreate is one of a citizen's "basic civil rights." Conversely, the court has clearly held that an individual has a right to prevent procreation. "The decision whether to bear or beget a child is a constitutionally protected choice. *Cary v. Population Serv. Int'l, Eisenstadt v. Baird;* see *Griswold v. Connecticut.*" *Matter of Romero,* (Colo. 1990). (*Davis* (Appeal), p. 1535).

Glossary

For more detailed explanations of the terminology of natural and aided reproduction, see Lawrence Kaplan and Carolyn Kaplan, "Natural Reproduction and Reproduction-Aiding Technologies" in this anthology.

Amniocentesis. A procedure in which, under local anesthesia, a needle is inserted into the womb of a pregnant woman and a sample of the amniotic fluid surrounding the fetus is removed. Various tests can then be performed, including identification of the sex of the fetus. Usually performed at around the fifteenth or sixteenth week of pregnancy.

Artificial insemination (AI). The introduction of semen into a woman's reproductive tract by mechanical means for the purpose of conception. *AID:* artificial insemination using the sperm of a man other than the woman's husband. *AIH:* artificial insemination using the sperm of the woman's husband.

Blastocyst. See "Embryo."

Breach of contract. Failure to live up to the terms of a contract.

Cervix. The passage from a woman's uterus to her vagina.

Chromosomes. Strands of DNA in the nuclei of cells on which genes are located.

Commercialization. To regard or treat something as appropriate to own, price, buy and sell, and in general subject to other market activities such as advertising, production management, and so on.

Commodification. To turn something into a commodity; to commercialize it. See "Commercialization."

Conception. Fertilization, the point at which sperm and egg unite.

Conceptus. See "Embryo."

Cryopreservation. Storage of reproductive materials—sperm, eggs, embryos—at very low temperatures ($-200°$F), for later thawing and use.

Damages. One of two actions a court of law may take to remedy a breach of contract. An award of damages, usually in the form of money, compensates for actual losses suffered as a result of the breach of contract. Contrast "Specific performance."

DNA. Deoxyribonucleic acid. The chemical compound that, arranged in various patterns (called "genes"), encodes an organism's genetic formation.

Donor. A person who provides, whether for a fee or gratis, reproductive materials (sperm, eggs, embryos, etc.) for use by a person who is not the spouse of the donor.

Ectogenesis. Development of an embryo or embryonic tissue outside the body. Often used to refer to generation of an organism entirely outside the body.

Egg. See "Ovum."

Egg follicle. A small, fluid-filled pocket at the surface of an ovary in which an egg matures prior to ovulation.

Embryo. One of a number of terms used to designate different stages of development from conception until birth. The most inclusive single term is:

> *Conceptus.* The product of conception at any time or stage of development from conception until birth, usually including extraembryonic membranes as well as the developing organism itself.

Commonly used terms include:

> *Zygote.* The fertilized one-celled egg before it divides. Sometimes used more loosely to include later stages of development.
> *Blastocyst.* The stage at about five days after fertilization and just before implantation in the uterine wall, when the developing organism takes the form of a fluid-filled ball of cells in which a cavity has developed.
> *Pre-embryo.* A popular term for the developing organism from fertilization until the appearance of the embryonic axis at about 14 days after fertilization.
> *Embryo.* The developing organism from about day 14, when the embryonic axis appears, until all major structures are represented in the seventh or eighth week after fertilization. Often used more loosely to include other stages of development as well.
> *Fetus.* The developing organism from the time when all major structures are present until birth.

Embryo transfer (ET). The transfer to a woman's womb of an embryo (actually a pre-embryo) to which she did not contribute the egg. The pre-embryo may have been retrieved from another woman or may have been developed in vitro.

Fallopian tubes. Thin tubes leading from each of a woman's two ovaries to her uterus, through which eggs travel and in which they are fertilized.

Fertilization. Conception, the point at which sperm and egg unite.

Fetus. See "Embryo."

Gamete (germ cell, sex cell). A reproductive cell—a man's sperm or a woman's egg, the union of which is necessary in sexual reproduction for the development of a new individual.

Genes. Portions of chromosomes, the biological units of heredity.

Gestation. The period of development from conception until birth.

GIFT (gamete intrafallopian transfer). A variation on in vitro fertilization in which eggs are retrieved and mixed with sperm, and the mixture is reintroduced into the fallopian tube for fertilization there rather than outside the body, as in in vitro fertilization.

Guardian ad litem. A person appointed by a court of law to look after the interests of an infant in legal proceedings.

Implantation. The embedding of a fertilized egg in the lining of the uterus, occurring about seven days after fertilization.

Infertility. Failure of reproductive function. Clinically defined as failure to have contributed to the live birth of a child after one year of regular intercourse. Infertility, in contrast to sterility, is not necessarily a permanent condition.

Informed consent. In medicine and law, the agreement of the recipient to a particular medical treatment with information that a reasonable patient would consider adequate. (In England the standard is more commonly information that a reasonable doctor would consider adequate.)

In vitro fertilization (IVF). Fertilization of eggs outside the woman's body, generally for subsequent implantation in the uterus. The Latin term "in vitro" literally means "in glass," referring to the fact that in IVF sperm and egg are usually brought together in a glass petri dish.

In vivo. From Latin, literally "in body," referring to processes going on inside the body.

Laparoscopy. A surgical procedure carried out under general anesthesia to examine the pelvic region and commonly used in connection with in vitro fertilization to retrieve eggs from a woman's ovaries. Two incisions are made in the abdomen, one for a tube through which carbon dioxide is pumped to distend the abdomen, the other for a laparoscope (a fiberoptic telescope) and other instruments, which allow examination and the aspiration of eggs.

Normative. Concerning values, good and bad, better and worse, in contrast to being purely factual or descriptive, as in "a normative issue."

Objectification. A term that has many uses but that is commonly used in connection with reproductive technology in the sense of regarding or treating something, such as a person or a human embryo, as if it were a mere thing, a mere object.

Oligospermia. Scarcity of sperm in a man's semen.

Oocyte.   Female reproductive cell before full maturation.

Oogenesis.   The process through which ova (eggs) mature.

Oviducts.   Another term for the fallopian tubes.

Ovaries.   The two female sex glands located on either side of a woman's lower abdomen in which eggs develop and the hormones estrogen and progesterone are produced.

Ovulation.   The discharge of an ovum (egg) from an ovary.

Ovum, (plural, ova).   Egg; a general term for a female reproductive cell, which when united with a male reproductive cell (sperm) has the potential to grow into a fully developed organism. Ova carry the woman's contribution to the genetic makeup of any offspring, and the ovum provides the initial substance of and sustenance for the developing organism.

Parens patriae.   The legal doctrine of the state as protector of persons unable to protect themselves, as when a court decides a case in the best interests of a child.

Parenting through contract.   An arrangement in which a woman (commonly, though misleadingly, called "the surrogate mother") agrees to bear a child and then turn over the child to others to be raised by them. In the most common form of parenting through contract, the contract stipulates that the "surrogate mother" is to be artificially inseminated with the contacting man's sperm and, upon birth of the child, relinquish her legal rights to the child. The child is then adopted by the man's wife, and they raise the child as their own.

Parthenogenesis.   Development of an egg without fertilization from the sperm.

Parturition.   The process of giving birth.

Pre-embryo.   See "Embryo."

Pregnancy.   In medical practice often dated from the first day of the last menstrual cycle, pregnancy is a 40-week period during which a woman gestates a child to birth or until the pregnancy is otherwise terminated.

Semen.   Seminal fluid and sperm together, as in a normal male ejaculate.

Seminal fluid.   The fluid added to sperm by various glands in the male reproductive system.

Sex preselection.   Procedures by which the sex of an offspring may be selected. To date no generally reliable procedures have been developed.

Slippery slope argument (thin edge of the wedge, camel's nose argument).   Metaphorical labels for the argument that a certain course of action should be curtailed not because it is itself bad, but because it will lead by degrees to practices that are without a doubt unacceptable.

Specific performance. One of two actions a court of law may take to remedy a breach of contract. An order of specific performance requires the party that breached the contract to do as the contract stipulated. Contrast "Damages."

Sperm. Mature male germ cells, which carry a male's contribution to the genes of an offspring. When united with a female reproductive cell (ovum), the resulting cell has the potential to grow into a fully developed organism.

Sperm donor. See "Donor."

Sterility. Inability to perform the reproductive function successfully, often due to absence of or severe damage to a part of the reproductive system. Sterility, in contrast to infertility, is generally a permanent condition.

Surrogate mother. See "Parenting through contract."

Surrogate motherhood, surrogate parenthood, surrogacy. Popular terms for parenting through contract.

*Testis (*plural, *testes).* Two glandular organs in a man's scrotal sac that produce sperm and the male hormone testosterone.

Test-tube baby. A popular term for a child conceived through in vitro fertilization. Not to be confused with complete gestation of a child outside the womb, which has not yet been achieved.

Ultrasound. A painless, noninvasive procedure that uses high-frequency sound waves to form an image of the contents of a woman's uterus.

Unenforceable contract. A contract that a court of law will not recognize as binding in deciding the outcome of disputes, for example, a contract for actions that are illegal or against public policy.

Uterus. The womb, where the conceptus implants and develops until birth.

Vagina, vaginal canal. A canal extending from a woman's cervix to outside her body.

Womb. See "Uterus."

Zygote. See "Embryo."

Suggestions for Further Reading

In addition to the works cited below, see works cited in the Introduction and the introductions to each of the eight parts of the anthology. See also the full texts of works excerpted in this anthology.

Andrews, Lori B. *New Conceptions*. New York: St. Martin's Press, 1984.

> Review of techniques, criteria of selection, and state of the law, with many bibliographical references to cases, laws, and discussions.

Bartels, Dianne M., ed. *Beyond Baby M: Ethical Issues in New Reproductive Techniques*. Clifton, NJ: Humana Press, 1990.

> Anthology reviewing the nature of the techniques and reflecting on normative issues from a variety of perspectives, including philosophy, religion, and public policy.

Biolaw.

> A looseleaf journal with up-to-the-minute reports on all legal-medical issues, with frequent analytical and review articles.

"Developments in the Law: The Constitution and the Family," 93 *Harvard Law Review* 1156 (1980).

> Comprehensive review of constitutional law on the family.

Feinberg, Joel. *Social Philosophy,* Englewood Cliffs, N.J.: Prentice-Hall, 1973.

> Includes an examination of justifications for laws limiting individual liberty.

Hastings Center Report. Bimonthly journal published by the Institute of Society, Ethics and the Life Sciences, Hudson, New York.

> Review of the latest controversies, with commentary and short analyses.

Holmes, Helen B. "Sex Preselection: Eugenics for Everyone." In James M. Humber and Robert F. Almeder, eds., *Biomedical Ethics Reviews—1985*. Clifton, NJ: Humana Press, 1985, pp. 38–71.

> Review of techniques of sex preselection and arguments against the morality and desirability of the practice.

Hull, Richard T., ed. *Ethical Issues in the New Reproductive Technologies*. Belmont, CA: Wadsworth, 1990.

> Philosophical anthology focusing on normative issues raised by specific techniques.

King, Patricia. "Reproductive Technologies." *BioLaw* 1 (1986), pp. 113–148; updated in *BioLaw* 4 (July 1989), pp. R:165–182.

> Review of the state of the law relating to reproductive technology, both in the United States and abroad.

MacIntyre, Sally. " 'Who Wants Babies?' The Social Construction of 'Instincts'." In Diana Leonard Barker and Sheila Allen, eds., *Sexual Divisions and Society: Process and Change*. London: Tavistock, 1976, pp. 150–173.

Examination of women's supposed drive to have children.

Menning, Barbara Eck. *Infertility: A Guide for the Childless Couple*. Englewood Cliffs, NJ: Prentice-Hall, 1977.

Describes the condition of infertility, its causes, and psychological responses to this condition.

O'Neill, Onora, and William Ruddick, eds. *Having Children: Philosophical and Legal Reflections on Parenthood*. New York: Oxford University Press, 1979.

Wide-ranging anthology on the nature, value, and regulation of having children.

Overall, Christine. *Ethics and Human Reproduction: A Feminist Analysis*. Boston: Unwin Hyman, 1987.

Considers a wide range of issues related to reproduction, with an extensive bibliography.

Page, Edgar. "Parental Rights." *Journal of Applied Philosophy* 1 (1984), pp. 187–203.

Examination of parental rights, including the relative importance of natural and adoptive relations. Addresses issues of children as property and as valued for their qualities, in contrast to being valued for their mere existence.

"Reproductive Technology and the Procreative Rights of the Unmarried." 98 *Harvard Law Review* 3 (January 1985).

Review of Supreme Court cases on procreative rights, finding support for the rights of unmarried individuals.

Schoeman, Ferdinand D. *Philosophical Dimensions of Privacy: An Anthology*. Cambridge: Cambridge University Press, 1984.

Basic perspectives on the meaning, value, and scope of privacy.

Singer, Peter, and Deane Wells. *Making Babies: The New Science and Ethics of Conception*. New York: Charles Scribner's Sons, 1985.

Examination of reproductive technology from the point of view of utilitarian ethics by individuals involved in clinical decisions about reproductive technology.

Stanworth, Michelle, ed. *Reproductive Technologies: Gender, Motherhood and Medicine*. Minneapolis: University of Minnesota Press, 1987.

Anthology addressing a wide range of normative issues raised by the reproduction-aiding techniques and services, with an extensive bibliography.

Trebilcot, Joyce, ed. *Mothering: Essays in Feminist Theory*. Totowa, NJ: Rowman & Allanheld, 1983, pp. 199–212.

Anthology of many excellent essays examining the nature of motherhood.

Warnock, Mary. *A Question of Life: The Warnock Report on Human Fertilisation and Embryology*. Oxford: Blackwell, 1985.

Report of the British Committee of Inquiry, headed by philosopher Mary Warnock. Contains brief, inclusive overviews of the problem of infertility, the practices in question, the pros and cons of each practice, and recommendations for public policy.

Wood, Carl, and Alan Trounson, eds. *Clinical In Vitro Fertilization*. Berlin: Springer-Verlag, 1984.

Detailed descriptions of the clinical procedures of IVF, including criteria for selecting patients, edited by leading practitioners.

Zelizer, Viviana A. *Pricing the Priceless Child*. New York: Basic Books, 1985.

Sociological account of the changing terms in which children have been valued.